Color Atlas of Neuroscience

Neuroanatomy and Neurophysiology

Ben Greenstein, Ph.D.
Director of Endocrine Research
Lupus Research Unit
Rayne Institute
St. Thomas' Hospital
London, UK

Visiting Research Professor,
Arizona Arthritis Center,
University of Arizona,
Tucson, Arizona, USA

Adam Greenstein,
BSc (Hons) Mb, ChB
Hope Hospital
Manchester, UK

194 Illustrations

Thieme
Stuttgart · New York 2000

Library of Congress Cataloging-in-Publication Data

Greenstein, Ben, 1941 –
    Color atlas of neuroscience : neuroanatomy and neurophysiology / Ben Greenstein, Adam Greenstein.
        p. cm.
    Includes bibliographical references and index.
    ISBN 0-86577-710-1 (TNY). –
    ISBN 3-13-108171-6 (GTV)
    1. Neuroanatomy Atlases.
    2. Neurophysiology Atlases.
    I. Greenstein, Adam. II. Title.
    [DNLM: 1. Nervous System—anatomy & histology Atlases. 2. Nervous System Physiology Atlases. WL 17 G815c 1999]
QM451.G74   1999
611'.8'0222—dc21
DNLM/DLC
for Library of Congress   99-37655
                                                      CIP

© 2000 Georg Thieme Verlag,
Rüdigerstrasse 14,
D-70469 Stuttgart, Germany
Thieme New York, 333 Seventh Avenue,
New York, NY 10001, USA

Cover drawing by Cyclus, Stuttgart

Typesetting by primustype R. Hurler GmbH,
D-73274 Notzingen, Germany
typeset on Textline/HerculesPro
Printed in Germany by Staudigl-Druck,
Donauwörth

ISBN 3-13-108171-6 (GTV)
ISBN 0-86577-710-1 (TNY)   1 2 3 4 5 6

To the very many wonderful,
critical students and to our patient
and forgiving family,
Lorraine and Saul.

Preface

A book like this could not have been possible without the work of a great many people, some of whom have long since passed on. We refer to the enormous body of knowledge that has been built up over the years, upon which all our efforts are based. We were given excellent advice when we started out with this book, and in particular, we want to thank Dr Roger Carpenter of Cambridge University for his enthusiasm and encouragement. Dr Phil Aaronson of Kings College, London was most helpful in the early stages.

For those who are interested in computer-generated artwork, this book was not only written by us but also illustrated by us to camera-ready material. We therefore needed plenty of help with the hardware through sundry crashes, electrical surges and the other hair-tearing glitches that bedevil the computer artist. We could not have been better served than we were by the entire staff of PC Microfix Ltd, which is a wonderful firm of dedicated enthusiasts in North London. Thanks, you were always there when we needed you.

We also want to thank Dr Clifford Bergman of Georg Thieme Verlag, who originally signed us up, and who has been constantly encouraging and supportive. Virtually the entire book has been scrutinised by Dr Markus Numberger, whose critical comments, suggestions and timely netting of author's errors has improved the final product immeasurably. We are grateful to the many students who took the time to read sample spreads. If the book is user-friendly, clear and concise, it is thanks largely to those constructive comments. A big thank you also to the production team at Georg Thieme Verlag who so professionally have turned the material we sent to them into the book you are holding now. It goes without saying that any errors remaining are the responsibility of the authors, who would be grateful to be alerted about any. This book was designed to be a cohesive, fairly comprehensive undergraduate syllabus in Neuroscience, and we hope that it makes the life of the student an easier and more interesting one.

Adam Greenstein
Ben Greenstein

Contents

Acknowledgements

The authors are grateful for permission to use the images on pages 3, 7, 9, 31, 79, 93, 281, 339, 361, reproduced from the following publications:

Carpenter MB. *Core text of Neuroanatomy*. 1st ed. Philadelphia PA: Lippincott Williams and Wilkins; 1975

Carpenter RHS. *Neurophysiology*. 3rd ed. London: Arnold Publishing, Hodder Headline Group; 1996

Kuffler SW, Nicholls JG, Martin AR. *From Neuron to Brain*. 2nd ed. Sunderland MA: Sinauer Associates Inc.; 1984

Snell RS. *Clinical Neuroanatomy for Medical Students*. 2nd ed. Philadelphia PA: Lippincott Williams and Wilkins; 1987

In addition, the authors acknowledge the contribution of the **Corel Corporation**, 1600 Carling Avenue, Ottawa, Ontario, Canada for the use of clip art supplied with CorelDraw8, licensed to Ben Greenstein; serial number: DR8XR.OP948839

Atlas

Meninges and Tracts

The nervous system consists of two main divisions: the **central nervous system** (CNS), consisting of **brain** and **spinal cord**, and the **peripheral nervous system**, consisting of **cranial** and **spinal nerves**, and their associated **ganglia**.

Three membranes surround both spinal cord and brain: **dura mater**, **arachnoid mater**, and **pia mater**. The dura mater is a tough, fibrous coat that encloses the spinal column and cauda equina, which is a bundle of nerve roots from the lumbar, sacral and coccygeal spinal nerves. The dura mater runs rostrally and is continuous beyond the foramen magnum with the dural meninges, which cover the brain. Caudally, the dura ends on the filum terminale at the level of the lower end of the second sacral vertebra. The dura is separated from the walls of the vertebral canal by the extradural space, which contains the internal vertebral venous plexus. The dura extends along the nerve roots and is continuous with the connective tissue that surrounds the spinal nerves. The inner surface of the dura is in direct contact with the arachnoid mater.

The arachnoid mater is a relatively fragile, impermeable layer that covers the spinal cord, the brain and spinal nerve roots, and is separated from the pia by the wide subarachnoid space, which is filled with cerebrospinal fluid. The pia mater is a highly vascularized membrane closely apposed to the spinal cord. It thickens on each side between the nerve roots to form lateral supports, anchored to the arachnoid, which suspend the spinal cord securely in the center of the dural sheath.

The **spinal cord** is an approximately cylindrical column, continuous with the medulla oblongata, that extends in adults from the foramen magnum to the lower border of the first lumbar vertebra. Structurally, the cord contains central gray matter, roughly H-shaped, consisting of the **anterior** and **posterior horns** and joined by a thin commissure containing the **central canal**, which is connected to the fourth ventricle. The gray matter is surrounded by white matter, which consists mainly of ascending and descending tracts, and has been divided arbitrarily into **anterior**, **lateral**, and **posterior columns**. The individual tracts will be dealt with in more detail later.

In the peripheral nervous system, there 12 pairs of **cranial nerves**, which leave the brain through foramina (apertures) in the skull, and 31 pairs of **spinal nerves**, which leave the spinal cord through vertebral foramina. There are eight cervical, 12 thoracic, five lumbar, five sacral, and one coccygeal pair of spinal nerves. The spinal nerves are linked to the cord by **dorsal** (**posterior**) nerve roots, which carry afferent nerves into the CNS, and **ventral** (**anterior**) nerve roots, which carry efferent nerves away from the CNS. Afferent fibers are also called sensory fibers, and their cell bodies are situated in the swellings or **ganglia** on the dorsal roots.

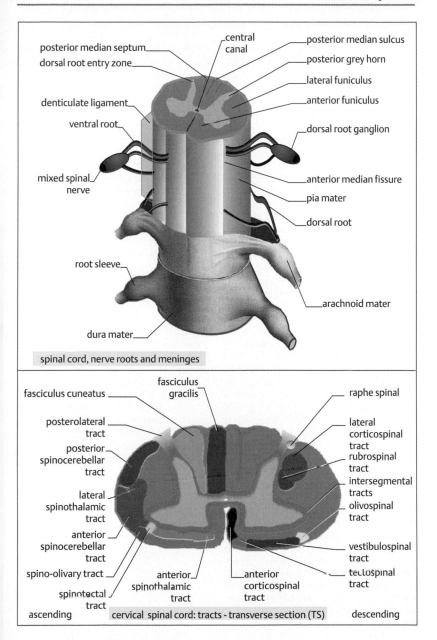

posterior median septum

dorsal root entry zone

denticulate ligament

ventral root

mixed spinal nerve

central canal

posterior median sulcus

posterior grey horn

lateral funiculus

anterior funiculus

dorsal root ganglion

anterior median fissure

pia mater

dorsal root

root sleeve

arachnoid mater

dura mater

spinal cord, nerve roots and meninges

fasciculus cuneatus

fasciculus gracilis

raphe spinal

posterolateral tract

posterior spinocerebellar tract

lateral spinothalamic tract

anterior spinocerebellar tract

spino-olivary tract

spinotectal tract

lateral corticospinal tract

rubrospinal tract

intersegmental tracts

olivospinal tract

vestibulospinal tract

tectospinal tract

anterior spinothalamic tract

anterior corticospinal tract

ascending

cervical spinal cord: tracts - transverse section (TS)

descending

Laminae and Nuclei of the Spinal Cord Gray Matter

The gray matter of the cord is butterfly-shaped, with the so-called **dorsal (posterior) horns** forming the upper wings of the butterfly shape. These are linked by a thin gray commissure in which lies the **central canal**. In the thoracic and upper lumbar segments the gray matter extends on both sides to form **lateral horns**. The lower wings of the butterfly shape are formed by the **ventral (anterior) horns** of the gray matter. (The size of the gray matter is greatest at segments that innervate the most skeletal muscle. These are the cervical and lumbosacral, which innervate upper and lower limb muscles, respectively.)

Structurally, the gray matter is composed of neuronal cell nuclei, their processes, neuroglia (see p. 76) and blood vessels. The overall arrangement of the gray matter of the cord was systematized by Rexed, who proposed the generally accepted laminar arrangement, commonly referred to as the **cytoarchitectonic** organization of the spinal cord. The gray matter is divided arbitrarily into nine visually distinct laminae, labeled I through IX, and an area X, which surrounds the central canal. Most laminae are present throughout the cord, but VI, for example, is apparently absent from T4 to L2.

Lamina I is at the apex of the dorsal horn, and contains the **posterior marginal nucleus**. These cells respond to thermal and other noxious stimuli, and receive axosomatic connections from lamina II. Near the apex, in lamina II, is the **substantia gelatinosa**, which is found throughout the length of the cord, and which receives touch, temperature and pain afferents, as well as inputs from descending fibers. Both I and II are rich in substance P, considered to be an excitatory neurotransmitter of pain impulses, in opioid receptors and the enkephalin.

Ventral to the substantia gelatinosa, extending through III and IV, is the largest dorsal horn nucleus, the **nucleus proprius**, which also exists at all cord levels. This receives inputs concerning movement, position, vibration and two-point discrimination from the dorsal white column. The **nucleus reticularis** is present in the broad lamina V, which is divided into medial and lateral zones, except in thoracic segments. Lamina VI, seen only at cord enlargements, receives group I muscle afferents in its medial zone, and descending spinal terminations in its lateral zone. Lamina VII contains the **nucleus dorsalis of Clark (Clark's column)**, a group of relatively large multipolar or oval nerve cells that extends from C8 through L3 or L4. Most of the cells respond to stimulation of muscle and tendon spindles. Layer VIII is a zone of heterogeneous cells most prominent from T1 through L2 or L3, associated with autonomic function.

Lamina IX is situated in the anterior or ventral horn of the gray matter, and contains clusters of large, motor nerve cells. The larger cells send out a efferent motoneuron axons, which innervate the extrafusal skeletal muscle fibers, while smaller cells send out g motoneuron axons, which innervate the intrafusal spindle fibers.

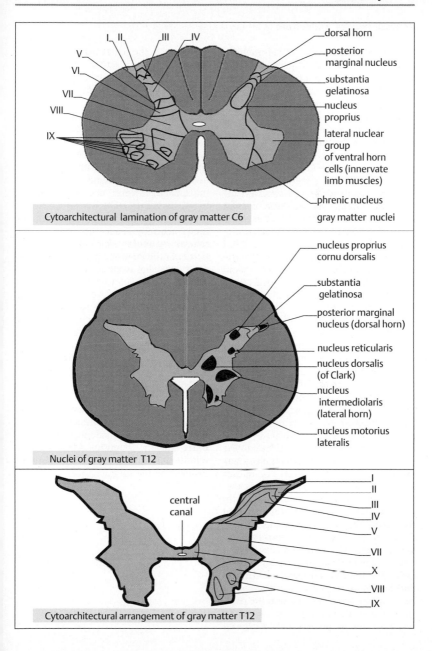

Cytoarchitectural lamination of gray matter C6

- dorsal horn
- posterior marginal nucleus
- substantia gelatinosa
- nucleus proprius
- lateral nuclear group of ventral horn cells (innervate limb muscles)
- phrenic nucleus

gray matter nuclei

I II III IV
V
VI
VII
VIII
IX

Nuclei of gray matter T12

- nucleus proprius cornu dorsalis
- substantia gelatinosa
- posterior marginal nucleus (dorsal horn)
- nucleus reticularis
- nucleus dorsalis (of Clark)
- nucleus intermediolaris (lateral horn)
- nucleus motorius lateralis

Cytoarchitectural arrangement of gray matter T12

central canal

I
II
III
IV
V
VII
X
VIII
IX

Ventral View of Brain Stem

The **brain stem** consists of the **medulla oblongata** (or **medulla**), the **pons** and the **midbrain**. The three brain areas each contain cranial nerve nuclei, and the fourth ventricle lies partly in the pons and partly in the medulla. The brain stem may occasionally be referred to as the 'bulb' in such terms as the 'corticobulbar' tract.

The medulla is around 3 cm long in adult humans and widens rostrally. It is continuous with the spinal cord from just below the foramen magnum, at the level of the upper rootlet of the **first cranial nerve**, and extends through to the lower (caudal) border of the pons. The medulla lies on the basilar part of the occipital bone, and is obscured from view by the cerebellum. Externally, the spinal cord and medulla appear to merge imperceptibly, but internal examination reveals extensive reorganization of white and gray matter at the junction. In the medulla the central canal widens into the fourth ventricle.

From the **ventral aspect**, the **central median fissure** appears as a central groove, which is a continuation of that of the spinal cord. The progress of the fissure is interrupted by the **decussation** (crossing over) of the fiber tracts of the corticospinal tract, where they cross over at the **pyramid** of the medulla to form the lateral corticospinal tract (see p. 2). Lateral to the pyramids on each side is the **olive**, made up of a convoluted mass of gray matter called the inferior olivary nucleus (see p. 2). The olive is separated from the pyramids by the rootlets of the **hypoglossal nerve** (**XII**). Rootlets of the **vagus** (**X**) and the cranial accessory (XI) nerves arise lateral to the olive, the latter two being united with the **spinal accessory nerve** (**XI**). The facial (VII) and **vestibulocochlear** (**VIII**) nerves arise at the border between the lateral medulla and the pons.

The pons is about 2.5 cm in length. Its name is Latin for 'bridge', since it appears to connect the cerebellar hemispheres though this is not actually the case. Ventrally, the pons is a sort of relay station, where cerebral cortex fibers terminate ipsilaterally on pontine nuclei, whose axons become the contralateral middle cerebellar peduncles. Thus the ventral (or basal) pons is a sort of massive synaptic junction that connects each cerebral hemisphere with the contralateral cerebellar hemisphere. Functionally, this system maximizes efficiency of voluntary movement.

The ventral surface of the midbrain extends rostrally from the pons to the **mamillary bodies**, which mark the caudal border of the diencephalon. On either side are prominent swellings called the **crus cerebri** (basis pedunculi). These are made up of the fiber tracts of the descending pyramidal motor system, and fibers from the cortex to the pons (corticopontine fibers). Although not shown here, the midbrain is penetrated by several small blood vessels in the floor of the interpeduncular fossa, and the area has been named the posterior **perforated substance** because of these blood vessels. The **oculomotor nerve** (**III**) to the eye leaves the brain through the cavernous venous sinus from each side of the interpeduncular fossa. The **optic chiasm** and **optic nerves**, together with the diencephalic **tuber cinereum** are exposed on the ventral surface.

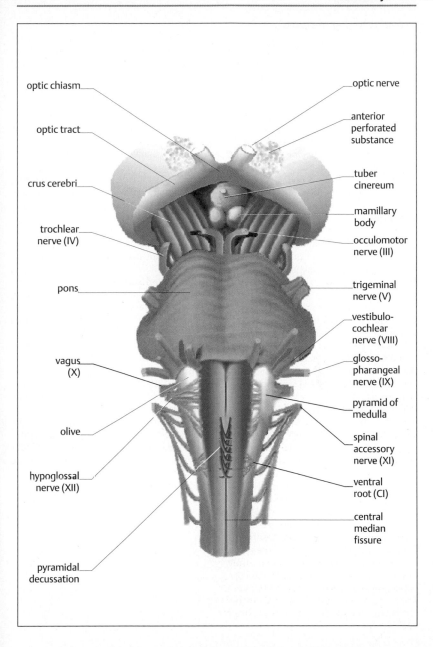

optic chiasm

optic nerve

anterior perforated substance

optic tract

crus cerebri

tuber cinereum

mamillary body

trochlear nerve (IV)

occulomotor nerve (III)

pons

trigeminal nerve (V)

vestibulo-cochlear nerve (VIII)

glosso-pharangeal nerve (IX)

vagus (X)

pyramid of medulla

olive

spinal accessory nerve (XI)

hypoglossal nerve (XII)

ventral root (CI)

central median fissure

pyramidal decussation

Dorsal View of Brain Stem

The **dorsal surface** of the brain stem, and particularly that of the medulla and pons, is obscured by the cerebellum. When this is removed, the bilateral swellings caused by the ascending **cuneate** and **gracile fasciculi** can be seen, as well as the corresponding tubercles, which are the swellings caused by their nuclei. Dorsal to the olives are the **inferior cerebellar peduncles**, which climb to the lateral aspect of the **fourth ventricle** and then swing into the cerebellum between the **middle and superior cerebellar peduncles**. The inferior cerebellar peduncle receives fibers in the **stria medullaris**, a tract from the hypothalamic arcuate nucleus. The stria medullaris fibers pass dorsally through the midline of the medulla and cross the floor of the fourth ventricle.

The floor of the fourth ventricle (also called the rhomboid fossa) is in part the dorsal surface of the pons; the dorsal surface of the pons (also called the tegmentum of the pons) forms the rostral half of the floor of the ventricle, and is divided longitudinally by a **medial sulcus** into two symmetrical halves. The ventricle is broad in the middle and narrows caudally to the **obex**, the most caudal end of the fourth ventricle, and rostrally towards the aqueduct of the midbrain. Caudally, the ventricle narrows into two triangles or trigones. Beneath the medial area of the ventricle are several motor nuclei; the rostral ends of both the **vagal** and **hypoglossal** nuclei lie beneath these **trigones**. There is a swelling at the lower end of the **medial eminence**, the **facial colliculus**, which is formed by fibers from the motor nucleus of the facial nerve. The roof of the fourth ventricle is tent-shaped and extends upwards towards the cerebellum. The roof is formed rostrally by the superior cerebellar peduncles and by a sheath called the superior medullary velum. The rest of the roof consists of another sheath, the inferior medullary velum, which is often found adhering to the underside of the cerebellum. The sheath may be incomplete, creating a gap called the median aperture of the fourth ventricle or the foramen of Magendie, which constitutes the main communication between the ventricular system and the subarachnoid space. The lateral walls of the fourth ventricles are provided mainly by the inferior cerebellar peduncles. There are recesses in the lateral walls, which extend around the medulla, and these open ventrally as the foramina of Luschka, through which cerebrospinal fluid can enter the subarachnoid space.

The dorsal surface of the midbrain is defined by four rounded swellings: the **superior** and **inferior colliculi** (the corpora quadrigemina). The colliculi make up the roof or tectum, and define the length of the dorsal surface, around 1.5 cm. The inferior colliculus is mainly a relay nucleus in the transmission of auditory impulses *en route* to the thalamus and cerebral cortex. The superior colliculus mediates control of voluntary eye movements and the head in response to visual and other forms of stimuli. The lateral surface of the midbrain is formed principally by the cerebral peduncle. Parts of the epithalamus (see p. 68), the **habenular** nuclei and the **stria medullaris** are seen rostral to the midbrain. The **third ventricle** of the diencephalon and the **pineal body** are also shown.

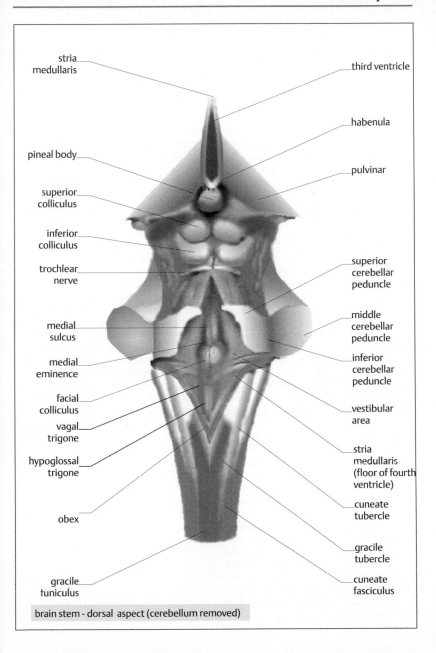

stria medullaris

third ventricle

habenula

pineal body

pulvinar

superior colliculus

inferior colliculus

trochlear nerve

superior cerebellar peduncle

middle cerebellar peduncle

medial sulcus

inferior cerebellar peduncle

medial eminence

facial colliculus

vestibular area

vagal trigone

hypoglossal trigone

stria medullaris (floor of fourth ventricle)

cuneate tubercle

obex

gracile tubercle

cuneate fasciculus

gracile tuniculus

brain stem - dorsal aspect (cerebellum removed)

Transverse Section of Medulla Oblongata

The spinal cord becomes the **medulla oblongata**, which also contains white and gray matter, but the arrangement changes, due to the embryonic expansion of the **central canal** to form the hindbrain vesicle, which will become the fourth ventricle. Development of the ventricle pushes dorsally situated structures more dorsolaterally. The transition is clearly seen in transverse section. The spinal cord becomes the medulla, which initially resembles the upper cervical segments. The substantia gelatinosa is now much larger in size and has become the **spinal nucleus of the trigeminal nerve**. In transverse section, descending fibers of the **spinal trigeminal tract** can be seen immediately dorsolateral to the nucleus. There is an increase in the amount of gray matter surrounding the central canal.

At low medullary level (A; see Figure opposite), the most prominent sign of transition to medulla is the appearance of the **decussation at the pyramids**. This is where the descending corticospinal motor tracts cross over. These fibers cross ventral (anterior) to the central gray matter and project dorsolaterally across the base of the ventral horn of the medulla. The pyramidal decussation almost eliminates the spinal anterior median fissure. (In the human, approximately 90% of the descending corticospinal fibers decussate and descend the cord in the lateral corticospinal tract, while about 10% do *not* cross, and descend in the uncrossed lateral and ventral corticospinal tracts.) The decussation explains the contralateral control of body movements by the motor cortex. At this level can also be seen the tracts of the **gracile** and **cuneate fasciculi**, which are the CNS projections of the cells of the spinal ganglia, and the lower ends of the **gracile** and **cuneate nuclei** where they terminate. At this level are also the cut fibers of the ascending ventral (ante-

rior) and lateral **spinocerebellar tracts**, which carry information from the sense organs in tendons and muscle spindles, the **inferior olivary nucleus**, and the **spinal root of the accessory nerve**.

Transaction at a higher level of the medulla (B) reveals another prominent decussation, that of the **medial lemniscus**. This is where fiber tracts from the ascending gracile and cuneate nuclei cross the midline of the medulla on their way up to higher centers. The nuclei are complex and arranged to correspond topographically with the body areas from which the ascending fibers come. Ascending fibers from the nuclei curve round the central gray matter and decussate to form the **medial lemniscus**. At this level, the **spinal nucleus of the trigeminal nerve**, which innervates the head region, is prominent, and immediately dorsolateral to it are the fibers of the descending **trigeminal nerve**. At both levels, the **ascending spinocerebellar** and **spinothalamic tracts** are both visible, and in B the **medial accessory olivary nucleus** lies medial to these tracts.

In summary, the transition from spinal cord to medulla is marked by (i) the expansion of the central canal; (ii) decussation at the pyramids; (iii) formation of the medial lemniscus through the decussation of ascending fibers arising from the cuneate and gracile nuclei; (iv) dorsolateral displacement of the dorsal horn of gray matter; (v) appearance of cranial nerve nuclei and various relay nuclei projecting to the cerebellum.

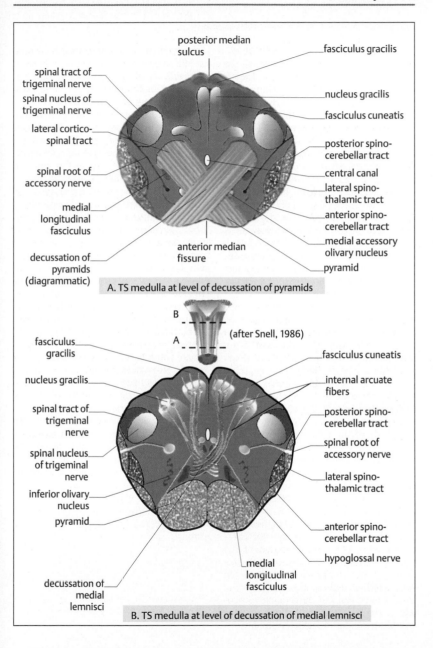

A. TS medulla at level of decussation of pyramids

- posterior median sulcus
- fasciculus gracilis
- spinal tract of trigeminal nerve
- spinal nucleus of trigeminal nerve
- lateral cortico-spinal tract
- spinal root of accessory nerve
- medial longitudinal fasciculus
- decussation of pyramids (diagrammatic)
- nucleus gracilis
- fasciculus cuneatis
- posterior spino-cerebellar tract
- central canal
- lateral spino-thalamic tract
- anterior spino-cerebellar tract
- medial accessory olivary nucleus
- anterior median fissure
- pyramid

(after Snell, 1986)

B. TS medulla at level of decussation of medial lemnisci

- fasciculus gracilis
- nucleus gracilis
- spinal tract of trigeminal nerve
- spinal nucleus of trigeminal nerve
- inferior olivary nucleus
- pyramid
- decussation of medial lemnisci
- fasciculus cuneatis
- internal arcuate fibers
- posterior spino-cerebellar tract
- spinal root of accessory nerve
- lateral spino-thalamic tract
- anterior spino-cerebellar tract
- hypoglossal nerve
- medial longitudinal fasciculus

Transverse Section of Medulla Oblongata II

Higher transection of the medulla oblongata at the level of the middle of the **olivary nuclei** clearly shows the **fourth ventricle**, the roof of which is formed by the choroid plexus in the **inferior medullary velum** at the base of the cerebellum. The floor of the ventricles is pushed up by the **hypoglossal** and **dorsal vagal nuclei**. The **reticular formation**, a network of nerve cells in the brain stem, is now clearly visible, as are the major fiber tracts.

The **pyramids**, **medial lemnisci,** and **tectospinal tract** lie medially in section. The tectospinal tract carries descending fibers from the tectum, which is the roof of the midbrain, consisting of superior and inferior colliculi. Also prominent is the **inferior vestibular nucleus**, which lies just medial to the **inferior cerebellar peduncle**.

The most prominent feature of the transverse section at this level is the convoluted **inferior olivary nucleus**, which has a massive input to the cerebellum through the **olivocerebellar tract** which constitutes most of the inferior cerebellar peduncle. If it could be dissected entirely, the inferior olive would resemble a collapsed purse or bag. Axons of olivary cells leave the nucleus and decussate to the other side of the medulla and sweep up into the peduncle. The fibers radiate to virtually all parts of the cerebellum and many have an excitable effect on cerebellar Purkinje cells. The inferior olivary complex has been divided into the **principal, medial accessory** and **dorsal accessory olivary nuclei**, based mainly on their cerebellar connections. For example, the fibers arising from the medial portion of the principal nucleus and those from the accessory nuclei terminate mainly in the vermis of the cerebellum.

The olive receives descending cortico-olivary fibers from the occipital, parietal, and temporal cortex, which terminate bi-laterally mainly in the principal olivary nucleus. The principal olive also receives rubro-olivary fibers from the red nucleus, and fibers in the central tegmental tract from the periaqueductal gray matter in the midbrain, some of which also terminate in the medial accessory nuclei. The dorsal and medial accessory olives receive ascending fibers in the spino-olivary tract, which runs up the cord in the anterior (ventral) funiculus of the white matter.

There are other nuclei at this level. The **nucleus ambiguus** is a longitudinal column of nerve cells within the reticular formation, extending through the medulla from the medial lemniscus to the mid-rostral portion of the inferior olive. The cells are multipolar motoneurons, and the efferents from this nucleus arch upward to join efferents from the dorsal vagal nucleus and from the **nucleus of the tractus solitarius**. Efferents from the rostral part of the nucleus ambiguus become visceral efferents of the glossopharyngeal nerve, which innervate the stylopharyngeus muscle. The more caudal portion of the nucleus gives rise to fibers of the spinal accessory nerve. The nucleus of the tractus solitarius gives rise to fibers, which, among other destinations, target the hypothalamic nuclei which release the peptide vasopressin. The reticular formation contains several important raphe nuclei which extend in the pons, and which project 5-HT neuronal processes to the midbrain, diencephalon and cerebral cortex. These central gray projections appear to mediate rhythmic processes such as arousal.

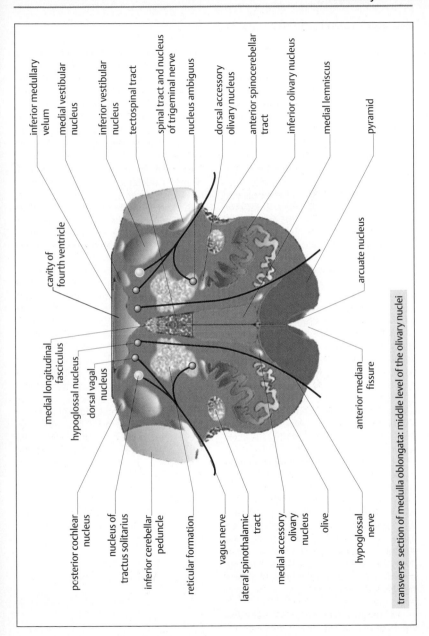

transverse section of medulla oblongata: middle level of the olivary nuclei

inferior medullary velum

medial vestibular nucleus

inferior vestibular nucleus

tectospinal tract

spinal tract and nucleus of trigeminal nerve

nucleus ambiguus

dorsal accessory olivary nucleus

anterior spinocerebellar tract

inferior olivary nucleus

medial lemniscus

pyramid

cavity of fourth ventricle

medial longitudinal fasciculus

hypoglossal nucleus

dorsal vagal nucleus

arcuate nucleus

anterior median fissure

posterior cochlear nucleus

nucleus of tractus solitarius

inferior cerebellar peduncle

reticular formation

vagus nerve

lateral spinothalamic tract

medial accessory olivary nucleus

olive

hypoglossal nerve

Transverse Section of Pons

The **pons** (metencephalon) lies beneath (anterior to) the cerebellum and is around 2.6 cm in length. The pons has been arbitrarily divided into the dorsal or posterior tegmentum, and a basal or anterior part, sometimes referred to as the pons proper.

Transection of the caudal pons at the level of the **facial colliculi** shows the **fourth ventricle** prominently, as well as the **middle cerebellar peduncles**. (The term **colliculus** refers to the visible swellings caused by the mass of the nucleus.) The **superior** and **inferior cerebellar peduncles** and the nuclei and spinal tracts of several cranial nerves are also visible. The **medial lemniscus** runs at the base of the tegmentum, and above it the area occupied by the **reticular formation** is now much larger than that of the medulla. The **trapezoid body** consists of fibers from the cochlear nuclei and the nuclei of the trapezoid nucleus in the pons; these convey, for example, auditory information arriving in the pons. Ascending and descending fiber tracts, such as the **corticospinal tract,** course through the pons.

The basal (anterior or ventral) portion of the pons consists of transverse and longitudinal bundles of fibers. The fibers constitute, mainly, a massive relay system from the cerebral cortex to the contralateral cerebellar cortex.

Dorsolateral to the reticular formation, lying in the floor of the fourth ventricle are the **vestibular nuclei**, which receive afferent inputs concerning equilibrium and balance and which are then well placed to be relayed to the cerebellum. The cerebellum in turn sends afferents from Purkinje cells to the vestibular nucleus; these are inhibitory, and release the neurotransmitter γ-aminobutyric acid (GABA). The vestibular nuclei project efferent fibers to the middle ear.

The **motor nucleus of the facial nerve** innervates facial muscles, and its function is clearly manifested when the facial nerve is damaged. This results in partial paralysis of the facial muscles (Bell's palsy), and possibly autonomic disturbances. Transverse section through the pons higher up (rostrally) reveals similar structural features, except that the **motor** and **sensory nuclei** of the **trigeminal nerve** are now clearly visible. The principal sensory nucleus of the trigeminal nerve lies lateral to the **motor nucleus**, and its sensory incoming fibers lie laterally to the efferent fibers of the trigeminal nerve, which leave the trigeminal motor nucleus. The **superior cerebellar peduncle** is now more prominent, as is the **lateral lemniscus,** which runs dorsolateral to the medial lemniscus.

Damage to the pons results, typically, in muscle paralysis or weakness of structures innervated by cranial nerves. For example, a childhood tumor of the pons called astrocytoma of the pons, is the most prevalent brainstem tumor, and causes a number of symptoms that reflect the paralysis of the ipsilateral cranial nerve; thus there may be weakness (hemiparesis) of facial muscles due to damage to the facial nucleus. The pons may be damaged by hemorrhage of the cerebellar arteries or of the basilar artery, and, depending on whether the damage is unilateral or bilateral, will result in facial paralysis and contralateral paralysis of lower limbs, through damage to corticospinal fibers which traverse the ventral pons.

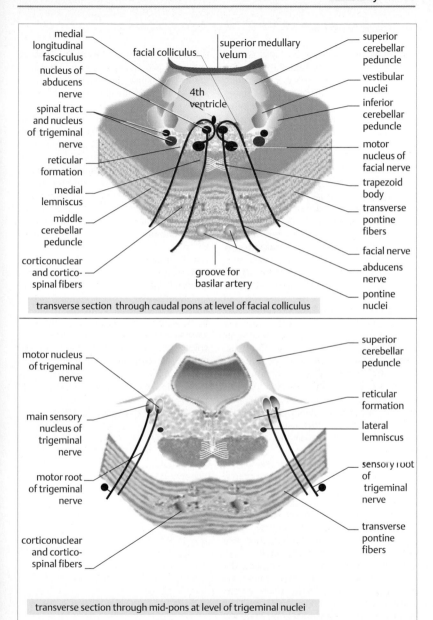

transverse section through caudal pons at level of facial colliculus

transverse section through mid-pons at level of trigeminal nuclei

The Fourth Ventricle

The **fourth ventricle** is an expansion of the central canal of the medulla oblongata. It is a roughly tent-shaped cavity filled with cerebrospinal fluid (CSF), situated beneath the cerebellum, above the **pons** and above the rostral half of the medulla. Laterally, the ventricle is bounded by the superior and inferior **cerebellar peduncles**.

The **roof** or dorsal surface of the fourth ventricle consists of a sheet of white non-nervous tissue called the **inferior medullary velum**. A layer of pia mater covers the inner lining or ependyma. Situated at the caudal part of the roof is an opening, the median eminence or **foramen of Magendie**, which connects the subarachnoid space and the interior of the ventricle. The ventricle communicates with the subarachnoid space also through two lateral openings called the foramen of Luschka (see also p. 8). Situated caudally above the ventricular roof is a double layer of pia mater, called the tela choroidea, which lies between the cerebellum and the ventricular roof. The tela choroidea is highly vascularized, and its blood vessels project through the roof of the caudal part of the ventricle to form the **choroid plexus**. The choroid plexus together with others situated in the lateral and third ventricles produce the CSF.

The floor or rhomboid fossa of the fourth ventricle is formed by the rostral half of the medulla and the dorsal surface of the pons, and is divided longitudinally into symmetrical halves by the **median sulcus**. The floor is raised because of the nucleus and the fiber tracts that run beneath it in the pons and medulla. Thus, there is a slight swelling in the floor, the **facial colliculus**, caused by the fibers leaving the motor nucleus of the facial nerve as they arch over the abducens nucleus (see p. 15). Although not shown here, there are other nuclei situated immediately below the floor of the fourth ventricle. These include the vagal and hypoglossal nuclei, together with their fiber connections.

The ventricle is filled with fluid, and if it is overfilled, as can occur through abnormal production of CSF, hydrocephalus may result. This is a clinically significant increase in the volume of CSF, due to the obstruction of the foramina of the roof of the fourth ventricle, or to displacement of the medulla by a tumor, or adhesions of tissues through meningitis, or through the presence of a congenital septum. The increase in fluid increases pressure on the nuclei and fiber tracts immediately below the floor of the fourth ventricle, and can result in autonomic and motor disturbances such as cardiac, respiratory, and vasomotor problems.

Tumors may arise in the ependymal lining of the fourth ventricle, or in the pons, or the vermis of the cerebellum and may spread to the fourth ventricle. Alternatively tumors of ependymal origin may invade the cerebellum, causing locomotor disturbances.

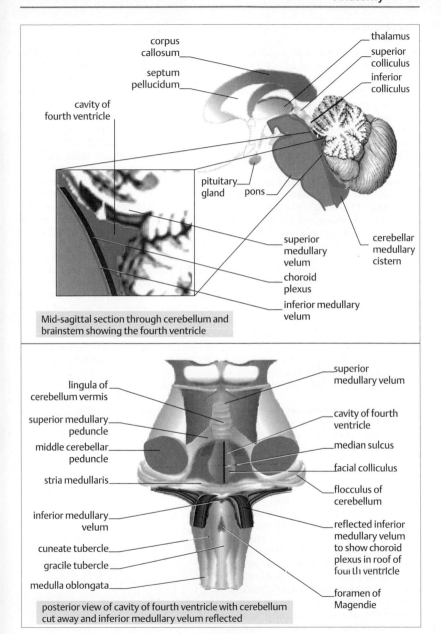

corpus callosum

septum pellucidum

cavity of fourth ventricle

thalamus

superior colliculus

inferior colliculus

pituitary gland

pons

superior medullary velum

choroid plexus

inferior medullary velum

cerebellar medullary cistern

Mid-sagittal section through cerebellum and brainstem showing the fourth ventricle

lingula of cerebellum vermis

superior medullary peduncle

middle cerebellar peduncle

stria medullaris

inferior medullary velum

cuneate tubercle

gracile tubercle

medulla oblongata

superior medullary velum

cavity of fourth ventricle

median sulcus

facial colliculus

flocculus of cerebellum

reflected inferior medullary velum to show choroid plexus in roof of fourth ventricle

foramen of Magendie

posterior view of cavity of fourth ventricle with cerebellum cut away and inferior medullary velum reflected

The Cerebellum I

The hindbrain or rhombencephalon consists of the medulla (myelencephalon), **pons** (metencephalon), and the **cerebellum** as its largest structure. The cerebellum consists of two hemispheres joined medially by a relatively narrow **vermis**, sits in the posterior cranial fossa of the skull beneath the tentorium cerebelli, and is separated from the medulla and pons by the fourth ventricle. The cerebellar cortex has many curved transverse fissures in the form of narrow infoldings called **folia**. Structurally, the cerebellum is covered by a cortex of gray matter with a medulla of white matter, which holds four intrinsic pairs of nuclei (see below). Observation of the superior surface shows two deep transverse fissures, the primary and the posterior superior **fissures**. Viewed from the ventral surface, the cerebellum is divided approximately into superior and inferior halves by the **horizontal fissure**. Three pairs of cerebellar peduncles connect the cerebellum to the three lower brain segments. The inferior, middle, and superior cerebellar peduncles connect it to the medulla, pons, and midbrain, respectively.

The **superior vermis** lies between the hemispheres as a longitudinal ridge; it is more clearly differentiated visually from the hemispheres on the ventral surface, where it is divided by fissures into the **nodule**, **uvula,** and **pyramid**. A stalk extends from the nodule on each side to the **flocculus**, which forms the flocculonodular lobe. The **tonsil** is a lobule that lies over the inferior vermis. The inferior medullary velum is exposed if the tonsil is removed.

From an embryological and functional viewpoint, the cerebellum can be divided into three main parts. (i) The archicerebellum, or flocculonodular node, is made of the pairs of flocculi and their peduncular connections. The flocculonodular node is the most ancient part of the cerebellum, present in fish as well as humans, and is connected with the vestibular nuclei and system. It is connected particularly with the dentate nucleus, one of the intrinsic medullary cerebellar nuclei. (ii) The paleocerebellum, or **anterior lobe** of the cerebellum, lies dorsal to the **primary fissure**. The lobe also includes the pyramid and uvula of the inferior vermis. The anterior lobe receives inputs via the spinocerebellar tract, originating in stretch receptors, and is the lobe most involved in the control of involuntary muscle tone. This lobe is connected principally to the globose and emboliform nuclei, which project to the red nucleus (see also p. 22), and thence to the central tegmental, rubroreticular, rubsospinal, and rubrobulbar efferent pathways (see p. 185). The paleocerebellum evolved in terrestrial vertebrates, which need to use limbs to support the body against the pull of gravity; therefore its connections are mainly spinal, and its functions are concerned with such stereotyped movements such as posture, locomotion, and muscle tone. (iii) The neocerebellum, which, as its name implies, is the phylogenetically newest part of the cerebellum, communicates with the thalamus and motor cortex. This lobe is made up of virtually all the posterior lobe, except for the pyramid and uvula of the vermis. The neocerebellum modulates non-stereotyped, learned behavior such as the learning of manual skills.

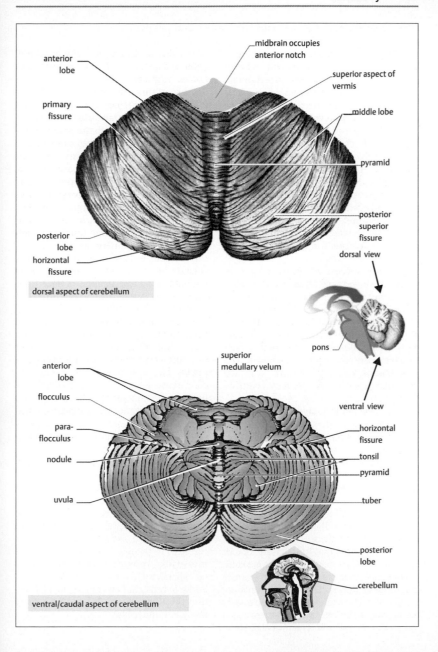

midbrain occupies anterior notch

anterior lobe

superior aspect of vermis

primary fissure

middle lobe

pyramid

posterior superior fissure

posterior lobe

horizontal fissure

dorsal aspect of cerebellum

dorsal view

pons

ventral view

anterior lobe

superior medullary velum

flocculus

para-flocculus

horizontal fissure

nodule

tonsil

pyramid

uvula

tuber

posterior lobe

cerebellum

ventral/caudal aspect of cerebellum

The Cerebellum II: Cellular and Lobular Arrangement

The lobules and fissures of the cerebellum are more easily understood if it is imagined that the surface of the cerebellum has been flattened as shown opposite. Using this representation, many of the areas of the cerebellum can be quickly and easily drawn schematically, and their relationship to other cerebellar structures understood.

The medial vermal cerebellum has been subdivided into **lobes** running down the middle. These are, from dorsal to ventral, the **lingula**, **culmen**, **declive**, **folium**, **tuber**, **pyramid**, **uvula**, and **nodule**. The various lobular subdivisions and the main lobes and **fissures** are also distinguished using this view.

Most of the cerebellar cortex is buried in the folia, and only about 15% is visible. In section, the cerebellar cortex is seen to be uniformly structured throughout, with three clearly defined layers that contain five different types of neurons. The **cerebellar cortical layers** are, from the surface inwards, the **molecular**, **Purkinje cell** (sometimes called piriform), and the **granular layers**. The medullary layer lies beneath the granular layer.

The **molecular layer** is relatively sparsely populated with two types of nerve cells: **basket cells** and outer **stellate cells**. The axons and dendrites of the outer stellate cells do not leave the molecular layer, and neither do the dendrites of basket cells. These processes run roughly horizontally in the layer, transverse to the long axis of the depth of the folia or infolding. The basket cell bodies are close to those of the Purkinje cells in the next layer, and project fibers that form basket shapes around the cell bodies of the Purkinje cells. Below this layer is the relatively narrow **Purkinje cell layer**. The Purkinje cells are large Golgi type I neurons; their cell bodies lie in rows along the folia, and their axons project to the intracerebellar nuclei. Some of these Purkinje axons in the archicerebellum project to the brainstem vestibular nuclei. Purkinje dendrites proliferate densely, transverse to the plane of the folia. Immediately below is the relatively wide **granular layer**, whose cells are very tightly packed and send axons up into the molecular layer, where they branch in T-shapes and run as parallel fibers along the horizontal axis of the folia. Each Purkinje dendritic tree may form synapses with up to half a million parallel fibers that have projected up from the granular layer. Also in the granular layer is a relatively small population of inhibitory **Golgi neurons**, which project their dendritic trees up into the molecular layer. One Golgi cell may synapse with a row of ten to twelve Purkinje cells, and it appears that Golgi cells do not overlap with respect to the innervation of the Purkinje cells.

There are two main types of **afferent input** to the cerebellum, and both are excitatory. Each Purkinje cell is supplied by one **climbing fiber** from the contralateral inferior olive (see p. 13). The phylogenetically more ancient archicerebellum and paleocerebellum are served by the correspondingly older accessory olivary nuclear cells. The neocerebellum is supplied with fibers by the newer inferior olive. The second afferent input is through the mossy fibers from many different sources, including the pontine nuclei. These fibers diverge extensively, and one mossy fiber may serve several folia. The mossy fiber axons form multiple **rosettes**, which synapse with several granular cell dendrites. Inhibitory Golgi axons synapse in these rosettes. It follows, therefore, that since mossy fiber rosettes synapse with granular fibers, which in turn synapse with Purkinje cells, that one mossy fiber can indirectly affect electrical activity in very many Purkinje cells.

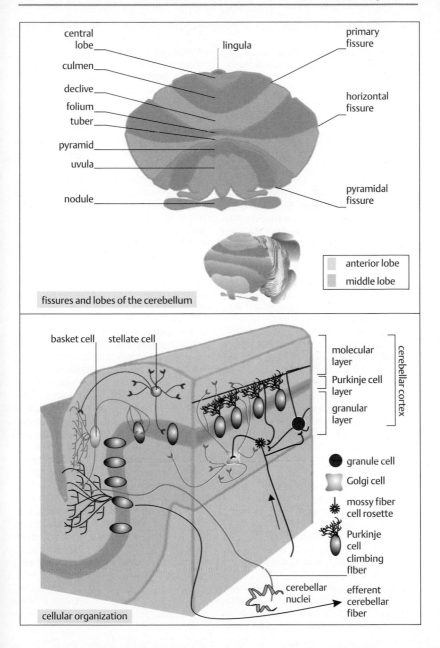

central
lobe

culmen

declive

folium

tuber

pyramid

uvula

nodule

lingula

primary
fissure

horizontal
fissure

pyramidal
fissure

anterior lobe

middle lobe

fissures and lobes of the cerebellum

basket cell   stellate cell

molecular
layer

Purkinje cell
layer

granular
layer

cerebellar cortex

granule cell

Golgi cell

mossy fiber
cell rosette

Purkinje
cell
climbing
fiber

cerebellar
nuclei

efferent
cerebellar
fiber

cellular organization

The Midbrain

The **midbrain** can be divided into three main parts: the **tectum** (quadrigeminal plate); the **tegmentum**, which is a continuation of the pons tegmentum; and the very large **crus cerebri**, which contains the corticofugal fibers. The midbrain contains two **cranial nerve nuclei**, the **oculomotor** and **trochlear** nuclei. The most prominent nuclear mass in the midbrain is the **substantia nigra**, a huge area darkly pigmented with melanin, a metabolic by-product of dopamine breakdown. The substantia nigra, which sends dopaminergic projections to the basal ganglia, is very important clinically since its degeneration produces a loss of dopamine terminations in the basal ganglia, resulting in the extra-pyramidal disorder Parkinson's disease. The structure of the midbrain is most usually demonstrated using transverse sections at the level of the **inferior** and **superior colliculi**.

Transection at the level of the **inferior colliculus** reveals that the pontine tectum or covering, i.e., the superior medullary velum, is now replaced by the inferior and superior colliculi, swellings caused by the masses of nuclei serving as relay stations for transmission of auditory and other signals to the brain. At this level the **cerebral aqueduct** replaces the fourth ventricle and **decussation** of the fibers of the **superior cerebellar peduncles** is visible.

Several tegmental nuclear groups surround the cerebral aqueduct in the periaqueductal gray matter. These include the **locus ceruleus**, a pigmented cell mass which sends many norepinephrine-containing projections to the cerebellum and cerebral cortex. The locus ceruleus appears to be involved in modulation of cortical sensory and association areas, and in sleep activation. (Parts of several nuclei, including the nucleus ceruleus, are also seen in rostral sections of pontine areas; it is wrong to compartmentalize brain stem nuclei as strictly pontine or midbrain etc.) Also in this region is the **mesencephalic nucleus of the trigeminal nerve**, a collection of unipolar sensory neurons, and the **dorsal nucleus of the raphe**. The trochlear nucleus lies ventrally in the periaqueductal gray matter and sends efferents to the superior oblique muscle of the eye.

Several tracts can be seen in transverse section. The most prominent is the **decussation of the cerebellar peduncles**. The **lateral lemniscus** is seen where it enters the inferior colliculus and the **medial lemniscus** *en route* to the thalamus. Just medial is the **ventral trigeminothalamic tract**. Clustered medially are the **dorsal trigeminothalamic tract**, **central tegmental tract**, **the medial longitudinal fasciculus**, and the **tectospinal tract**. The ventrally placed crus cerebri contains the massive descending **corticospinal** and **corticobulbar tracts**, and **temperopontine** fibers.

Transection at the level of the **superior colliculi** shows the prominent bilateral **red nucleus**, so called because it appears pinkish red in freshly cut sections. The red nucleus runs continuous with the crossed superior cerebellar peduncle, and it is the origin of descending motor tracts, which decussate in the ventral tegmentum to become the **rubrospinal tract**.

The superior colliculi communicate through the posterior commissure and integrate auditory, cortical, spinal, and retinal afferents in the control of eye movements and reflex reflexes. The **superior brachium** carries the retinal inputs. The **oculomotor nucleus** lies ventrally in the periaqueductal gray matter, and its efferent projections cross the red nucleus, emerge in the interpeduncular fossa and run to optic and extra-optic muscle.

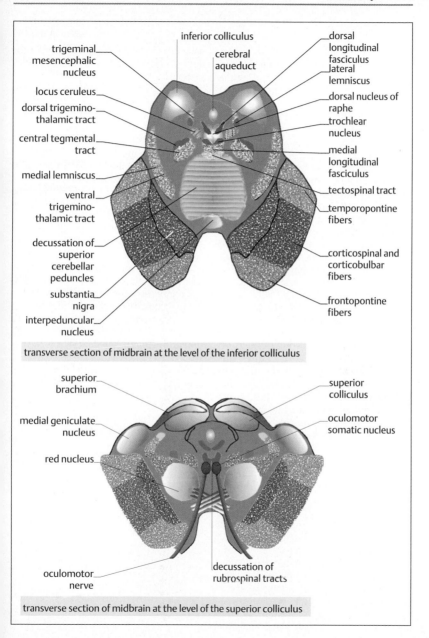

trigeminal mesencephalic nucleus

locus ceruleus

dorsal trigemino-thalamic tract

central tegmental tract

medial lemniscus

ventral trigemino-thalamic tract

decussation of superior cerebellar peduncles

substantia nigra

interpeduncular nucleus

inferior colliculus

cerebral aqueduct

dorsal longitudinal fasciculus

lateral lemniscus

dorsal nucleus of raphe

trochlear nucleus

medial longitudinal fasciculus

tectospinal tract

temporopontine fibers

corticospinal and corticobulbar fibers

frontopontine fibers

transverse section of midbrain at the level of the inferior colliculus

superior brachium

medial geniculate nucleus

red nucleus

superior colliculus

oculomotor somatic nucleus

oculomotor nerve

decussation of rubrospinal tracts

transverse section of midbrain at the level of the superior colliculus

The Cerebrum

The **cerebrum** or forebrain is the largest part of the human brain and is housed in the concavity produced by the vault of the skull. It consists of the **diencephalon** and **telencephalon**.

The **diencephalon** consists of the **third ventricle** and the structures that define its rostral, caudal, superior, and inferior boundaries. It is situated in the midline of the brain, and most of its components are bilateral and symmetrically arranged, with free communication between the two sides of a given diencephalic structure.

The **telencephalon** consists of the **cerebral hemispheres**. These are two bilaterally and symmetrically arranged structures separated by a sagittal midline fissure, and are connected across their midline by the commissural fibers of the **corpus callosum**.

The structures of the diencephalon are dealt with in more detail in later sections; the components of the diencephalon can be summarized as consisting of the **third ventricle**, and the major structures surrounding it, namely the **thalamus**, **subthalamus**, **epithalamus**, and the **hypothalamus**. Within each of these structures are nuclei, pathways and subsidiary structures which are considered in more detail later. The **thalamus** is a complex, highly organized and compartmentalized relay station for ascending tracts, situated centrally in the cerebrum, and plays an important part in the integration of somatic and visceral function. The **hypothalamus** forms the floor and part of the lateral walls of the third ventricle, and plays a critical role in endocrine, metabolic, autonomic, and emotional function. The **subthalamus**, which lies immediately below the thalamus, is concerned with the modulation of involuntary movement, and is considered to be one of the extrapyramidal motor nuclei. The **epithalamus** consists of the pineal gland and the habenular nuclei, which play a part in the integration of somatic and olfactory information.

Each **cerebral hemisphere** of the telencephalon has a highly convoluted and folded surface covering of **gray matter**, the **cerebral cortex**, and inner core of **white matter** consisting of fiber tracts. Deep with the hemispheres are masses of gray matter, the **basal nuclei** (also called **basal ganglia**) and the **lateral ventricles**. The infoldings of the surface greatly increase the surface area of the cortex; these folds are termed **gyri** (singular, gyrus), separated from each other by fissures called **sulci**.

The basal nuclei occur bilaterally and symmetrically in the hemispheres, and consist of the **amygdaloid nucleus**, situated in the temporal lobe, the **claustrum** and **corpus striatum**, which lies lateral to the thalamus. The corpus striatum is split by the **internal capsule**, a band of nerve fibers, into the **caudate nucleus** and **lentiform nucleus**. These nuclei are further subdivided by nerve fiber sheets into other nuclei, which are dealt with in more detail later (see, for example, p. 322).

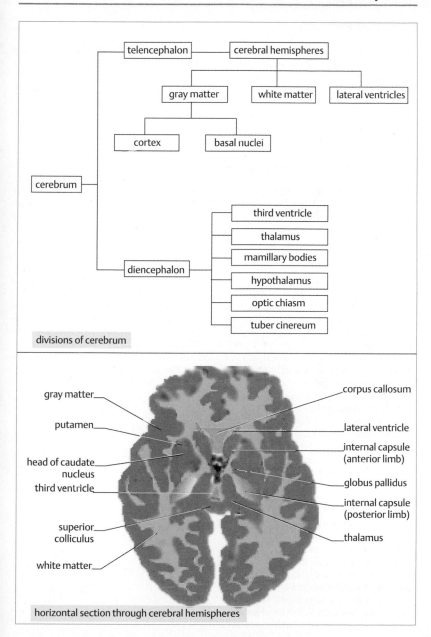

divisions of cerebrum

horizontal section through cerebral hemispheres

The Diencephalon

The **diencephalon** extends from the region of the **mamillary bodies** and the **posterior commissure** at its caudal end to the interventricular foramen at its most rostral end. It forms the lateral wall of the third ventricle and is made up principally of the hypothalamus, epithalamus, **thalamus**, and subthalamus (also termed ventral thalamus). The thalamus lies above the hypothalamic sulcus, and the hypothalamus below it. The thalamus makes up the dorsal wall and the hypothalamus the ventral wall of the ventricle. Little can be seen of the diencephalon, since most of it is surrounded by the cerebral hemispheres, and it is best seen in sagittal section. The only part that is visible on the brain surface is in the ventral view, when the **infundibulum**, bilateral **mamillary bodies** and **the tuber cinereum** can be seen, as well as a surface rostral boundary, the **optic chiasm**. The mamillary body holds the mamillary nuclei of the hypothalamus.

In sagittal section, the hypothalamus is seen from the mamillary body at its caudal end to the interventricular foramen rostrally. Functionally, the hypothalamus is critical for normal life, since it controls body temperature, fluid and water balance, and neuroendocrine function, and has an important role in the control of the autonomic nervous system and emotional and sexual behavior. At the base of the hypothalamus is the **infundibulum** or pituitary stalk, which connects the hypothalamus to the pituitary gland through blood portal and nervous links (see also p. 291). Several small but important nuclei have been identified in the hypothalamus.

The thalamus is the largest member of the diencephalon, and if it were dissected free might resemble a hen's egg in shape (see also p. 29). It is separated from the hypothalamus by a groove, the hypothalamic sulcus. There are two thalami, joined by a massa intermedia or interthalamic adhesion. The thalamus is a huge relay station, and has massive reciprocal connections with the cerebral cortex. The thalamus extends forward to the interventricular foramen, and is bounded laterally by the posterior limb of the internal capsule (see p. 35), and the head of the caudate nucleus. Internally, the thalamus consists of several nuclei, which project to the ipsilateral cerebral cortex, and the cortex in turn sends reciprocal fibers back to the areas from which it received them. Functionally, this relationship serves to control the organism's response to inputs from the special and the general senses, and to ensure a proper motor response to them.

Immediately below the thalamus lies the subthalamus, which is situated dorsolaterally to the hypothalamus. The epithalamus consists of the habenular nucleus and the **pineal gland** (see p. 9). The pineal gland synthesizes the hormone melatonin, which may modulate sleep-waking rhythms, and in recent years melatonin has been advocated to alleviate the condition known as jet lag.

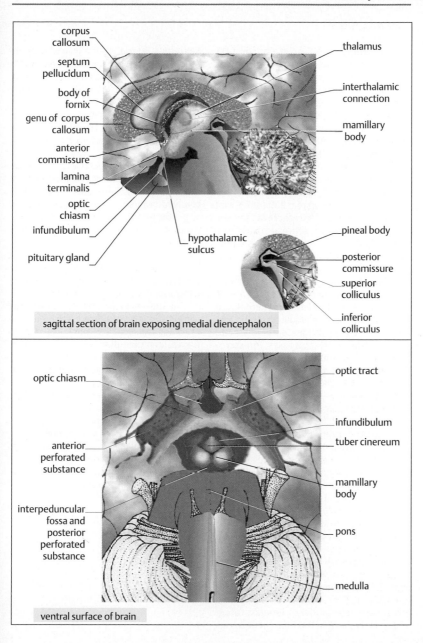

corpus callosum

septum pellucidum

body of fornix

genu of corpus callosum

anterior commissure

lamina terminalis

optic chiasm

infundibulum

pituitary gland

thalamus

interthalamic connection

mamillary body

hypothalamic sulcus

pineal body

posterior commissure

superior colliculus

inferior colliculus

sagittal section of brain exposing medial diencephalon

optic chiasm

anterior perforated substance

interpeduncular fossa and posterior perforated substance

optic tract

infundibulum

tuber cinereum

mamillary body

pons

medulla

ventral surface of brain

Thalamic Nuclei

The **thalamus** is the largest mass of CNS nuclei and lies at the center of the brain. It consists of two bilateral egg-shaped lobes on opposite sides of the third ventricle. Their upper surfaces comprise the floor of each lateral ventricle, and their lateral surfaces are contiguous with the posterior limb of the internal capsule. The thalamus contains within it several **nuclei** with very diverse and often independent functions. The thalamic nuclei may be somatosensory, receiving inputs from sensors of the somatosensory system and the special senses. From these nuclei there are projections to the primary sensory cortex (see next spread). Motor nuclei receive inputs from the **cerebellum** and the basal ganglia.

Each thalamus has a Y-shaped internal **medullary lamina** consisting of nerve fibers which are some of the afferent and efferent connections of the thalamic nuclei. The lamina divides each lobe into three main nuclear masses: **posteromedial** (or **mediodorsal**), **anterior** and **lateral**. Lateral to these nuclear masses is a thin, shield-like layer of neurons called the **reticular nucleus**. The reticular nucleus is the only thalamic nucleus that does not correspond with the cortex. Lying posteriorly (at the back) of the thalamus are the **lateral** and **medial geniculate bodies**. For convenience, the thalamic nuclei may be grouped as **relay** or **specific**, **association** and **non-specific**.

Specific nuclei are those which correspond reciprocally with the sensory and motor areas of the cerebral cortex. The **ventral posterior nucleus** is the termination site for fibers of the lemniscal system. A **somatosensory homunculus** has been mapped in the **lateral** and **medial** divisions of this nucleus. The head is mapped medially, and the trunk laterally. In both divisions, nociceptive inputs occur towards the back of the homunculus, tactile inputs lie in the middle, and proprioception lies at the front. In other words, there is **modality segregation**. The **ventral anterior nucleus** receives inputs from the globus pallidus

The **lateral geniculate nucleus** receives afferents from the retina, and the **medial geniculate nucleus** receives afferents from the ear.

The **association nuclei** are (i) the **anterior nucleus**, which receives inputs from the mammillothalamic tract and may be involved in memory, (ii) the **mediodorsal** or **posteromedial nucleus**, which receives afferents from the limbic and olfactory systems and seems to mediate mood and judgment, and (iii) the **pulvinar** and **lateral posterior nuclei**, which are grouped as a single nucleus and receive afferents from the superior colliculus.

The **non-specific nuclei** include the **intralaminar medullary nuclei** and the **reticular nucleus**. The **nuclei of the intralaminar medulla** (see above) seem to be a rostral projection of the brain stem reticular formation involved in arousal. The **reticular nucleus** is separated from the other nuclei by the **external medullary lamina**; it receives collaterals from the thalamocortical fibers as they pass through on their way to the cerebral cortex. The reticular nucleus in turn projects efferent GABAergic inhibitory fibers to the corresponding thalamic nuclei from which it received the collaterals.

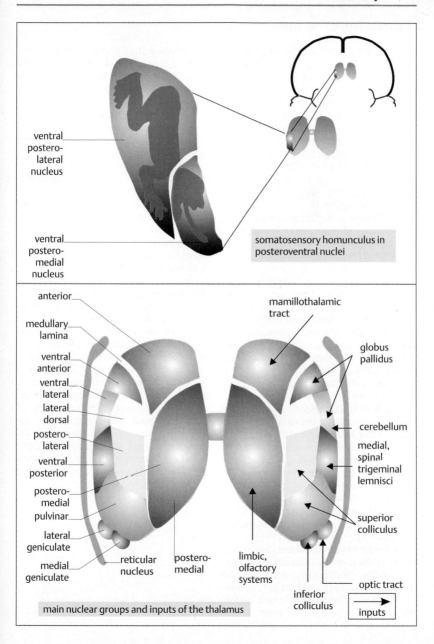

ventral
postero-
lateral
nucleus

ventral
postero-
medial
nucleus

somatosensory homunculus in
posteroventral nuclei

anterior

medullary
lamina

ventral
anterior

ventral
lateral

lateral
dorsal

postero-
lateral

ventral
posterior

postero-
medial

pulvinar

lateral
geniculate

medial
geniculate

reticular
nucleus

postero-
medial

limbic,
olfactory
systems

mamillothalamic
tract

globus
pallidus

cerebellum

medial,
spinal
trigeminal
lemnisci

superior
colliculus

inferior
colliculus

optic tract

inputs

main nuclear groups and inputs of the thalamus

Thalamic Nuclei: Projections to Cerebral Cortex

There are highly precise point-to-point **reciprocal connections** between **thalamic nuclei** and the **cerebral cortex**. All thalamic nuclei except the **reticular nucleus** send ipsilateral projections to the cerebral cortex, and all cortical areas receive inputs from the thalamus. Thalamic nuclei that communicate with cortical regions are termed **specific nuclei**. All the specific nuclei lie in the ventral tier of the lateral nuclear group. The thalamus projects efferents to the cortex in the **thalamic peduncles**.

The **ventral posterior nucleus** projects **efferents** via thalamocortical projections through the posterior limb of the internal capsule and the corona radiata (see p. 178), which terminate in the primary somatosensory cerebral cortex in the postcentral gyrus. There is a lesser projection to the secondary somatosensory area at the inferior end of the postcentral gyrus. The **ventral anterior nucleus** projects widely to the frontal cortex, including the supplementary motor area. The **ventral lateral nucleus** projects mainly to the motor and premotor areas of the cerebral cortex.

The **anterior nuclear group** is the most anterior part of the thalamus and is actually part of the limbic system. It receives inputs from the mamillary bodies of the hypothalamus via the mamillothalamic tract, and projects principally to the **cingulate gyrus**, which is seen on the medial surface of the cerebral hemisphere. This nuclear group appears to be associated with emotional status and recent memory.

The **ventral lateral nucleus** lies caudal to the anterior nucleus. This nucleus projects to the frontal lobe, including the areas of the primary and premotor cortex.

The bilateral **lateral geniculate nuclei** (also called the lateral geniculate bodies) form small but noticeable swellings or eminences near the posterior pole of the thalamus, just ventral to the pulvinar. These nuclei are the termination site of fibers of the optic tract from the retina, and are thus part of the visual system. Each nucleus projects efferents to the primary visual cortex in the occipital lobe via the retrolenticular portion of the internal capsule, and through the optic radiation.

The **medial geniculate nucleus** receives fibers carrying auditory information from the **inferior colliculus**. The medial geniculate nucleus projects this information to the primary auditory cortex in the temporal lobe via the retrolenticular portion of the internal capsule and the auditory radiation.

The **medial** (**mediodorsal**) **nuclear group** receives inputs from the amygdala, hypothalamus, and from other thalamic nuclei. This nuclear group projects extensively and reciprocally to the prefrontal cortex and mediates emotion and mood.

The **intralaminar nuclei** lie in the **internal medullary lamina** of the thalamus. These nuclei include the centromedian nucleus and parafascicular nucleus. These nuclei receive afferents from the spinothalamic and trigeminothalamic tracts, and also from the brain stem reticular formation. They send efferents to the basal ganglia, namely the caudate nucleus and the putamen. They also project very extensively to the cerebral cortex. Lesions to these nuclei result in a reduction of the level of consciousness and the perception of pain.

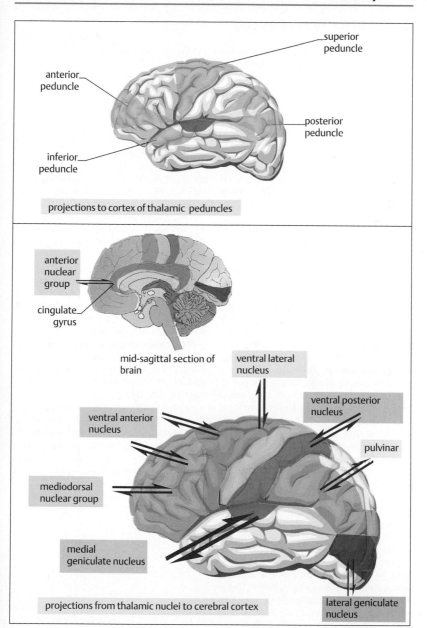

superior peduncle

anterior peduncle

posterior peduncle

inferior peduncle

projections to cortex of thalamic peduncles

anterior nuclear group

cingulate gyrus

mid-sagittal section of brain

ventral lateral nucleus

ventral posterior nucleus

ventral anterior nucleus

pulvinar

mediodorsal nuclear group

medial geniculate nucleus

lateral geniculate nucleus

projections from thalamic nuclei to cerebral cortex

Cerebral Cortex: Surface Features

The **cerebral cortex** is phylogenetically the youngest part of the brain, and carries out a huge range of discriminative and cognitive processes relating to affective behavior, motor function, somatosensory perception, integration, and mnemonic function. It is structurally highly organized in layers of nerve cells and processes.

In external appearance, the cerebral cortex has a convoluted, corrugated appearance both *in situ* and after removal from the cranial vault. The surface of the cortex is deeply folded, which greatly increases its surface area. The visible crest of a fold is called a **gyrus**, and the invisible depression between folds is called a **sulcus**. One of the main landmark sulci of the brain is the **central sulcus** (or sulcus of Rolando). Some sulci are relatively deep, and are termed **fissures**. The main fissures include the very large one separating the two hemispheres, the interhemispheric fissure. Another is the fissure that runs approximately horizontally along the lateral surface of the brain, called, appropriately, the **lateral fissure** or fissure of Sylvius. Viewed laterally, the surface is composed of four lobes: the frontal lobe, the parietal lobe, the temporal lobe, and the occipital lobe.

The frontal lobe is the largest of the cortex and extends from the **central sulcus** to the front or rostral end of the cortex. Several gyri can be distinguished on the frontal lobe surface. These are the **precentral gyrus**, which is defined by the **central** and **precentral sulci**, and which holds within itself the motor cortex (see p. 176); rostral to the precentral sulcus are the **superior**, **middle**, and **inferior frontal gyri**.

The parietal lobe is the area immediately behind or caudal to the central sulcus and it runs caudally, approximately to the **parieto-occipital sulcus**. It is bounded ventrally by the lateral fissure. The somatosensory cortex (see p. 174) is con-tained within the postcentral gyrus in the parietal lobe, just caudal to the central sulcus. Caudal to the postcentral gyrus is the **superior parietal lobule**, and ventral to that is the inferior parietal lobule.

The temporal lobe lies ventral to the lateral fissure, and includes the **inferior**, **middle**, and **superior temporal gyri**. These run approximately parallel to the lateral fissure. The superior temporal gyrus holds the area of the primary auditory cortex.

The occipital cortex occupies the most caudal end of the brain and may be considered to lie caudal to a line drawn through the parieto-occipital sulcus and the occipital notch. The visual cortex (see p. 286) is located in this lobe, around the **calcarine sulcus**.

Although not shown here, there is an area of cerebral cortex called the **insula**, which is buried, deep in the lateral fissure. Its borders are defined by the frontal, parietal and temporal cortex. The rostral end of the insula is a poorly understood part of the limbic system and the caudal end of the insula is involved in somatosensory processing.

There is also a limbic lobe, defined by Broca. The limbic lobe is made up of the **cingulate**, hippocampal and parahippocampal gyri. The cingulate gyrus is a primitive form of the cerebral cortex, having fewer layers of cells and is involved in the mediation of behavioral components of endocrine, olfactory, skeletal, and visceral function, and in aspects of memory.

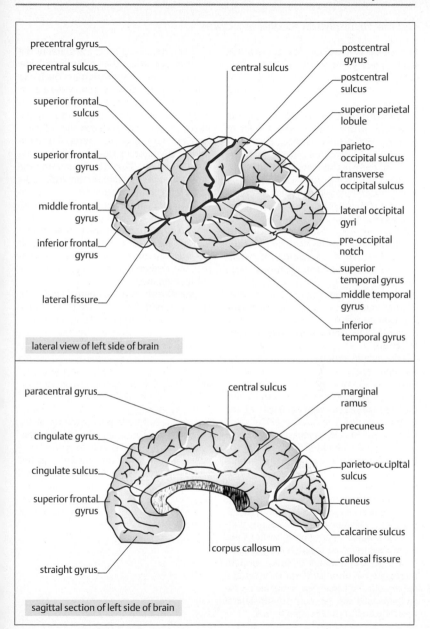

precentral gyrus
precentral sulcus
superior frontal sulcus
superior frontal gyrus
middle frontal gyrus
inferior frontal gyrus
lateral fissure
central sulcus
postcentral gyrus
postcentral sulcus
superior parietal lobule
parieto-occipital sulcus
transverse occipital sulcus
lateral occipital gyri
pre-occipital notch
superior temporal gyrus
middle temporal gyrus
inferior temporal gyrus

lateral view of left side of brain

paracentral gyrus
cingulate gyrus
cingulate sulcus
superior frontal gyrus
straight gyrus
central sulcus
corpus callosum
marginal ramus
precuneus
parieto-occipltal sulcus
cuneus
calcarine sulcus
callosal fissure

sagittal section of left side of brain

Cerebral Hemispheres: Internal Structures

The **cerebral hemispheres** contain the **lateral ventricles, white matter**, which consists of nerve fibers embedded in the neuroglia, and the **basal nuclei** (**basal ganglia**).

Each hemisphere possesses a **lateral ventricle**, which is lined with a layer of ependyma and filled with cerebrospinal fluid (CSF). The ventricle has a **body** located in the parietal lobe, and **horns**, the anterior, posterior and inferior horns, which extend into the frontal, occipital and temporal lobes respectively. The body of the ventricle has a floor, roof, and a medial wall. The body of the **caudate nucleus** forms the floor of the ventricle, and the lateral margin of the **thalamus** and the inferior surface of the **corpus callosum** form the roof.

The **basal nuclei or ganglia** are masses of gray matter lying inside each cerebral hemisphere. These masses are the amygdaloid nucleus, **claustrum,** and the **corpus striatum**.

The **corpus striatum** lies lateral to the thalamus and is divided phylogenetically into the neostriatum, which consists of the **caudate nucleus** and the **putamen,** and the paleostriatum, which consists of the **globus pallidus**. The caudate nucleus and the putamen are separated almost completely by a band of fibers called the **internal capsule**. The caudate nucleus has a large head and a tail, rather like a tadpole, and the tail ends in the amygdaloid nucleus in the temporal lobe. The globus pallidus lies medial to the putamen, and consists of medial and lateral segments.

The putamen and globus pallidus are sometimes referred together as the lentiform nucleus, although in more modern textbooks the term *lentiform* is being disregarded as archaic terminology. The caudate nucleus lies laterally to the lateral ventricle and to the thalamus.

The corpus striatum has important connections with the substantia nigra, thalamus and the subthalamus. The major afferent inputs to the corpus striatum are from the substantia nigra, the thalamus and the cerebral cortex. Nigrostriatal fibers are dopaminergic, and have both excitatory and inhibitory effects. Degeneration of this system results in Parkinson's disease (see p. 370). The thalamostriatal projections arise in the intralaminar nuclei of the ipsilateral thalamus. The corticostriatal afferents are extensive; there are afferents from motor areas of the frontal lobe to the putamen. Fibers from cortical association areas project to the caudate nucleus. The most prominent white matter (see also next spread) consists of the association and the commissural fibers connecting the corresponding regions of the hemispheres.

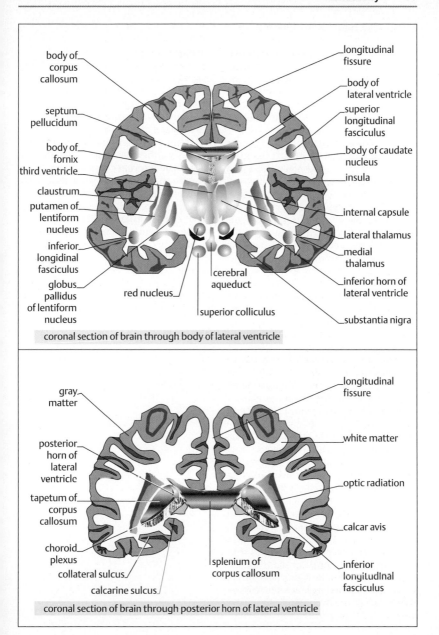

coronal section of brain through body of lateral ventricle

coronal section of brain through posterior horn of lateral ventricle

Tracts of Cerebral Hemispheres

Cerebral tracts are **association, commissural,** or **projection** in nature. In the brain, commissures run from one part to the corresponding part on the opposite side of the brain. Projection fibers carry information to and from the cortex. Association fibers connect different cortical areas.

The **corpus callosum** is the major **commissure** of the cerebrum. It is a massive band of myelinated nerve fibers and most of them interconnect symmetrical regions of the cerebral cortex. The different regions of the corpus callosum are termed the **splenium,** at the posterior end, the **body,** which is the main part, and the **genu,** which is the Latin word meaning 'knee' and is the bend at the anterior part of the corpus callosum. From the corpus callosum, fibers radiate out to the **cerebral cortex.** The corpus callosum forms part of the roof of the lateral ventricle and also the floor of the longitudinal fissure. The corpus callosum carries the interhemispheric transfer of memory, sensory experience, and learned discrimination. Damage to the corpus callosum does not appear to affect performance, except that destruction of the splenium causes **alexia,** or the inability to understand written words. This may be due to disconnection of the verbal processing in the left hemisphere from visual processing in the right hemisphere.

The **anterior commissure** is a compact fiber bundle that crosses the midline in front of the columns of the fornix and connects the olfactory bulbs and regions of the temporal gyri. The hippocampal commissure is a transverse commissure linking the posterior columns of the fornix.

Projection fibers are afferents carrying information to the cerebral cortex, and efferents carrying information away from it. The most prominent are the **corona radiata,** which radiate out from the cortex and then come together in the brain stem. These fibers become highly condensed in the **internal capsule,** which runs medially between the caudate nucleus and the thalamus and laterally between the thalamus and the lentiform nucleus. The **anterior limb of the internal capsule** carries connections between the frontal lobe and the basal part of the pons and between the prefrontal cortex and the mediodorsal nucleus of the thalamus. The **posterior limb of the internal capsule** carries fibers between the ventral posterior nucleus of the thalamus and the primary somatosensory cortex and also carries corticospinal and corticobulbar fibers.

The **association fibers** connect different areas of the cerebral cortex. Some are relatively large, such as the superior longitudinal fasciculus, which connects the occipital and frontal lobes. Part of the fasciculus, the arcuate fasciculus (see also p. 265) connects temporal and frontal lobes, and is important for language. The inferior longitudinal fasciculus connects the temporal and occipital lobes, and is involved in visual recognition function.

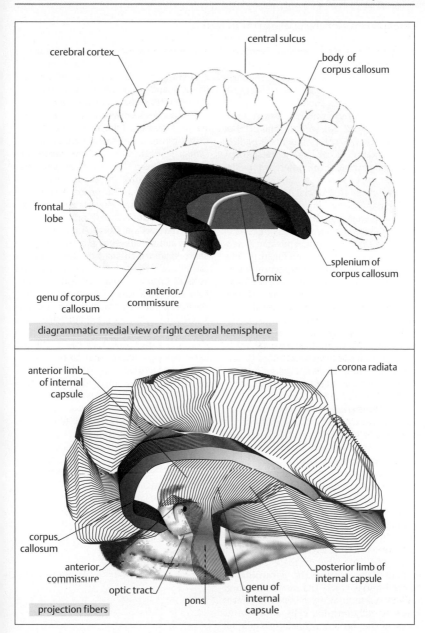

diagrammatic medial view of right cerebral hemisphere

projection fibers

Cerebral Hemispheres: Cellular Architecture

The gray matter of the cerebral cortex contains about 10 billion neurons. It varies in thickness from about 4.5 mm at the crest of a gyrus, to about 1.5 mm in the recess of a sulcus. The cortex contains five different types of cells: **pyramidal, fusiform, horizontal cells of Cajal, stellate,** and **cells of Martinotti.** The cortex has been divided into **six layers** according to the density and arrangement of the different types of cells.

The most superficial layer is the **molecular** (plexiform) **layer.** It has a dense network of tangentially oriented fibers and cells, made of axons of cells of Martinotti, stellate cells, and apical dendrites of pyramidal cells and fusiform cells. Afferent fibers from the thalamus terminate here, as do many commissural fibers. This is a layer of intense synapsing. The **external granular layer** has several small stellate and pyramidal cells, and the **external pyramidal layer** has larger pyramidal cell bodies than in more superficial layers. Their apical dendrites reach into the molecular layer, and their axons descend into the white matter as projection, commissural or association fibers.

The **internal granular layer** is densely packed with stellate cells, and there is a horizontal band of fibers called the **external band of Baillarger.** The **internal pyramidal** (**ganglionic**) **layer** contains medium-sized and large pyramidal cells. In between these cells are cells of Martinotti and stellate cells. There is also another band of fibers called the **inner band of Baillarger.** The internal pyramidal layer in the precentral gyrus of the motor cortex contains very large pyramidal cells, called **Betz cells.** The axons of these cells contribute about 3-4% of the **pyramidal** or **corticospinal tract.** The innermost layer of the cerebral cortex is the **multiform layer of polymorphic cells.** Most of the cells in this layer are fusiform cells but pyramidal cells and cells of Martinotti are also present.

Pyramidal cells are so called because of the shape of the cell body. The apex is oriented towards the outer layers and from it a thick apical dendrite projects upwards, giving out several collaterals. Dendrites possess many dendritic spines for synapsing with other cells. An axon projects down from the base of the cell body and may terminate in deeper cortical layers, but more usually descends into the white matter as a projection, commissural, or association fiber.

Stellate cells have small polygonal cell bodies and radiate several dendrites and a short axon which may terminate in the same or a neighboring layer. **Horizontal cells of Cajal** are small cells horizontally oriented in the superficial layers. **Fusiform cells** (*fusiform* means spindle shaped or tapering at both ends) are oriented perpendicular to the layers, have dendritic projections from each pole, and occur principally in deeper cortical layers. **Cells of Martinotti** are small multipolar cells, with an axon projecting upwards to the surface, and short dendrites.

The **bands of Baillarger** are made up principally of collateral nerve fibers given out by incoming afferents, and of stellate cells and horizontal cells of Cajal. They include some pyramidal and fusiform collaterals as well. They are prominent in sensory cortical areas because of high densities of thalamocortical fiber terminations. The outer band of Baillarger is especially prominent in the visual cortex, where it is sometimes called the stria of Gennari.

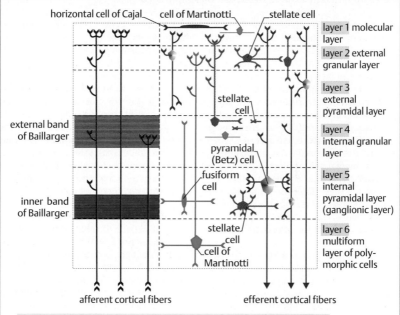

horizontal cell of Cajal — cell of Martinotti — stellate cell

layer 1 molecular layer

layer 2 external granular layer

layer 3 external pyramidal layer

stellate cell

external band of Baillarger

layer 4 internal granular layer

pyramidal (Betz) cell

inner band of Baillarger

fusiform cell

layer 5 internal pyramidal layer (ganglionic layer)

stellate cell

cell of Martinotti

layer 6 multiform layer of polymorphic cells

afferent cortical fibers   efferent cortical fibers

layers of cerebral cortex showing nerve fibers (left) and neurons (right)

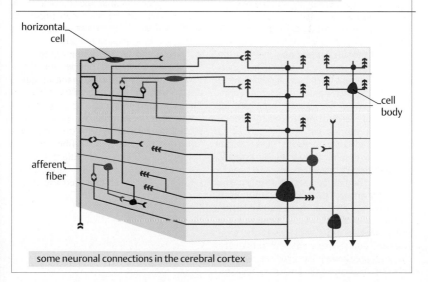

horizontal cell

cell body

afferent fiber

some neuronal connections in the cerebral cortex

Blood Supply and Venous Drainage of Spinal Cord

The **spinal cord** is supplied with arterial blood by descending arteries that run the length of the spinal cord, and by **radicular** arteries that arise at the segmental level. The descending arteries comprise the paired **posterior spinal arteries**, and the unpaired **anterior spinal artery**. The **posterior spinal arteries** arise either from the posterior inferior cerebellar arteries (see p. 43), or from the vertebral arteries. They descend the cord on the dorsal (posterior) surface, medial to the dorsal roots. The posterior spinal arteries are of variable diameter as they descend, and at some points become so fine that they seem to be discontinuous. These arteries supply the dorsal horns and the posterior (dorsal) columns (see p. 2).

The **anterior spinal artery** is formed by a confluence of the anterior spinal arteries at medullary level. The vessel descends the cord in the midline, and supplies the midline rami to the lower medulla oblongata. It also gives off **sulcal** branches, which enter the spinal cord via the anterior median fissure. Some of the sulcal branches are given off from the anterior spinal artery alternately to right or left, or the sulcal artery may itself divide to form right and left branches. These sulcal branches supply the spinal cord central gray matter, the lateral and anterior (ventral) columns, the lateral and ventral horns, and the basal portion of the dorsal (posterior) horn.

The **radicular arteries** arise from segmental vessels, including the ascending and deep cervical arteries, and the intercostal, lumbar, and sacral arteries. The radicular arteries gain access to the cord via the intervertebral foramina, and then divide into anterior and posterior radicular arteries which run together with the ventral and dorsal nerve roots, respectively. They supply the main arterial input to the thoracic, lumbar, sacral, and coccygeal spinal segments. In the cervical region, blood is supplied equally by left and right radicular arteries, while in thoracic and lumbar regions of the cord the radicular arteries occur more commonly on the left side.

There may be from two to ten **anterior radicular arteries**. One anterior radicular artery is larger than the others; this is the artery of the **lumbar enlargement**, or the **artery of Adamkiewicz**, which may arise from an intercostal artery or a lumbar artery anywhere from segments T8–L3. This artery commonly runs on the left side of the cord together with lower thoracic or upper lumbar spinal roots. The **posterior radicular arteries** divide on the dorsolateral surface of the cord and join the paired posterior spinal arteries. Their distribution with respect to left or right of the cord is not as marked as that seen with the anterior radicular arteries.

The distribution of the **spinal veins** is similar in general to that of the spinal arteries. There are two major longitudinal venous trunks running along the cord in the midline, the **anterior** and **posterior spinal veins**. These receive cord venous drainage via the sulcal veins. The posterolateral and posteromedial veins drain the dorsal horns and posterior funiculi. Ventral areas of the cord are drained by **anteromedian** and **anterolateral** veins. The internal vertebral venous plexus drains into the external vertebral venous plexus and from there into the ascending lumbar, azygos, and hemiazygos veins.

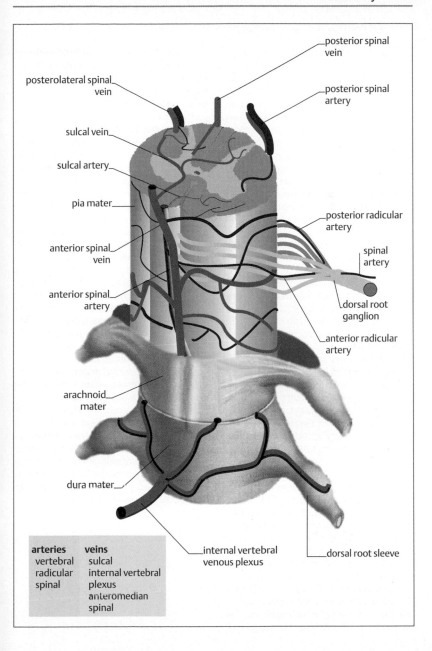

posterior spinal vein

posterolateral spinal vein

posterior spinal artery

sulcal vein

sulcal artery

pia mater

posterior radicular artery

spinal artery

anterior spinal vein

anterior spinal artery

dorsal root ganglion

anterior radicular artery

arachnoid mater

dura mater

internal vertebral venous plexus

dorsal root sleeve

arteries	**veins**
vertebral	sulcal
radicular	internal vertebral
spinal	plexus
	anteromedian
	spinal

Brain Vascularization: Arterial Supply

The brain receives its blood supply via two pairs of arteries, the **internal carotid** and **vertebral arteries**. The internal carotid arises from the common carotid and courses upward to the surface of the brain, giving off numerous preterminal branches, until it appears just laterally to the **optic chiasm**. The vertebral arteries run upwards and unite to form the **basilar artery**, which extends along the pons. As it runs up the pons, the basilar artery gives off small **pontine** tributaries, and the larger **anterior inferior cerebellar artery**, which feeds the inferior and anterior parts of the cerebellum. The basilar also gives rise to the **labyrinthine artery**, which travels to the internal acoustic meatus to supply the inner ear. The main terminal branches of the basilar artery, where the pons runs into the midbrain, are the **posterior cerebral arteries**, which run to the occipital lobe of the cerebral hemisphere, including the visual cortex, and the **superior cerebellar arteries**, which feed the superior part of the cerebellum.

The internal carotid gives rise to the **anterior** and **middle cerebral** arteries. The **anterior cerebral artery** runs medially above the optic chiasm, and then between the frontal lobes in the longitudinal fissure. This artery supplies the medial surface of the parietal and frontal lobes, and feeds both the sensory and motor cortex. It is linked to the opposite anterior cerebral artery by the **anterior communicating artery**. The **middle cerebral artery**, which is the largest of the cerebral arteries, divides and branches to supply most of the lateral surfaces of the frontal, parietal and temporal lobes, including the sensory and motor cortex, the insula and the auditory cortex.

The **vertebral arteries** arise from the subclavian artery and enter the cranium cavity via the foramen magnum. As they rise rostrally, the vertebral arteries give off, among others, the **posterior** and **anterior spinal arteries**, which feed the spinal cord and the medulla. The largest of these branches is the **posterior inferior cerebellar artery**, which supplies the inferior part of the cerebellum.

The two main arterial supply systems are termed the **internal carotid** and **vertebrobasilar** systems, and the posterior communicating arteries links these two systems. This anastomosis creates a vascular near circle at the base of the brain, called the **circle of Willis**, or circulus arteriosus. The circle of Willis covers the base of the hypothalamus and the optic chiasm. The arteries of the circle of Willis give off the **perforating arteries**.

Occlusion of the **anterior spinal artery** causes damage to the thoracic cord, and produces incontinence and paraplegia. The spinothalamic tracts, which carry pain and temperature information to the brain, are especially vulnerable, while the dorsal columns, which carry proprioceptive information, are more resistant to occlusion. Occlusion of a major brain artery may cause **rupture**, **hemorrhage**, and **stroke**. An **aneurism** is a ballooning of an artery, which may rupture allowing blood to penetrate the brain and subarachnoid space. Rupture of vessels, cerebral hemorrhage, causes a focal neurological problem. When cerebral vessels are involved this may present as a psychological problem such as aphasia (see p. 346), focal epilepsy, or contralateral motor deficits.

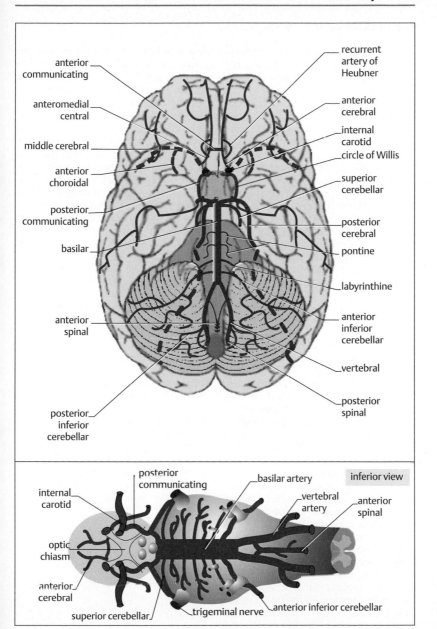

Venous Drainage of the Brain

Venous blood is drained from the brain through fine veins, which form themselves in pial venous plexuses. These drain into larger **cerebral veins** that traverse the subarachnoid space and drain into the **sinuses** of the dura mater, which lie between the meningeal and periosteal layers of the dura. The dural sinuses drain posteriorly and superiorly and meet at the **confluence of the sinuses**, which is situated near the internal occipital protuberance. Two transverse sinuses arise from the confluence and carry the venous blood to the **internal jugular vein** on each side.

The fine **superficial cerebral veins** arise from the subcortical white matter and the gray matter of the cerebral cortex and anastomose in the pia to form the veins, which drain into the sinuses. Examples of these superficial veins are the **superior** and **inferior cerebral veins**. The superior cerebral veins drain into the **superior sagittal sinus**. The inferior cerebral veins arise from ventral areas of the lateral surface and from the basal surface of the hemispheres and drain into the basal sinuses. In addition, a large number of fine veins arise on the medial and inferior surfaces of the cortex, and these drain into the **internal cerebral veins**, or into the great cerebral vein.

The main deep cerebral veins are the **great cerebral vein**, the **basal vein**, and the **internal cerebral vein**. The paired **internal cerebral** veins run rostrally in the midline in the tela choroidea (see p. 46) of the third ventricle from the interventricular foramina to the medial, superior surface of the thalamus. A number of veins drain into each internal cerebral vein; these are the **choroidal vein**, epithalamic vein, lateral ventricular vein, the septal vein and the thalamostriate vein. These veins in turn receive several smaller veins. The epithalamic vein drains the dorsal diencephalic structures. The thalamostriate vein runs rostrally from the junction of the caudate nucleus and the thalamus and a number of smaller veins drain into it. The choroidal vein runs into the inferior horn of the lateral ventricle and the **septal vein** receives venous blood from the septum pellucidum and part of the corpus callosum. The two internal cerebral veins eventually become confluent to form the great cerebral vein. The great cerebral vein is the drainage vessel for a number of lesser paired veins, these being the internal cerebral veins, the basal internal cerebral veins, occipital veins and the posterior callosal veins.

The **basal vein** is the drainage vessel for a number of other veins, these being the anterior cerebral vein, the deep middle cerebral vein and the inferior striate veins. The anterior cerebral vein runs alongside the anterior cerebral artery and drains venous blood from the rostral parts of the cingulate gyrus, the corpus callosum, and from the orbital surface of the frontal lobe. The deep middle cerebral vein is found in the lateral sulcus and drains the insula. The inferior striate vein drains part of the ventral striatum.

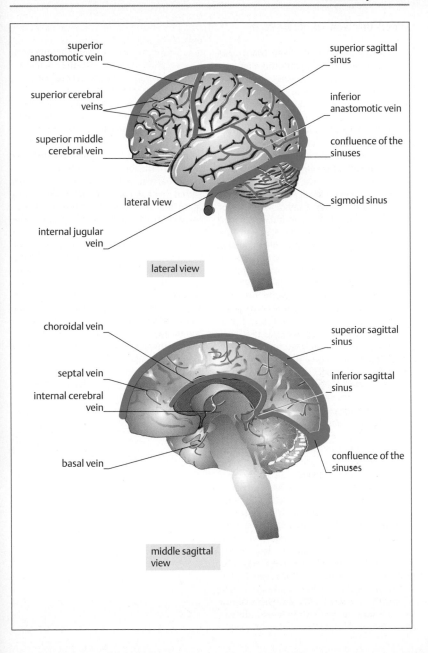

superior anastomotic vein

superior cerebral veins

superior middle cerebral vein

lateral view

internal jugular vein

superior sagittal sinus

inferior anastomotic vein

confluence of the sinuses

sigmoid sinus

lateral view

choroidal vein

septal vein

internal cerebral vein

basal vein

superior sagittal sinus

inferior sagittal sinus

confluence of the sinuses

middle sagittal view

Ventricular System of the Brain

The ventricular system of the brain consists of a continuous communicating system of five fluid-filled cavities whose inner walls are lined with ependymal cells. Each ventricle possesses a choroid plexus (see p. 17). The cavities are numbered and comprise the **cerebral aqueduct**, the unpaired **third** and **fourth ventricles**, and the paired **lateral ventricles**.

The **fourth ventricle** is a roughly pyramid-shaped cavity that is bounded ventrally by the medulla and pons and its floor is called the rhomboid fossa. The roof of the ventricle is incomplete and is formed from the anterior medullary velum and the posterior medullary velum (see also p. 17). The apex passes upward into the cerebellum at a point called the apex or fastigium. Cerebrospinal fluid (CSF) can flow from the fourth ventricle into the subarachnoid space through two apertures. The foramen of Luschka is an opening of the lateral recess into the subarachnoid space in the region of the cerebellar flocculus. There is a more important aperture, the foramen of Magendie, which lies caudally in the ventricular roof. Most of the CSF outflow from the ventricle occurs via this aperture.

From the fourth ventricle a narrow channel called the **cerebral aqueduct** runs into the **third ventricle**. This is a relatively narrow channel that runs between the two medial walls of the diencephalon. The roof of the ventricle consists of a tela choroidea and a lining of ependyma and pial cells, from which a choroid plexus protrudes into the cavity of the ventricle. The medial walls of the paired thalami form most of the walls of the third ventricle, and the hypothalamus supplies the floor and the basal part of the lateral walls. Rostrally, the boundary of the third ventricle is defined by the lamina terminalis and the anterior commissure. At the rostral end there is a small extension of the ventricle called the optic recess, and there is a small downward extension called the infundibular recess where the infundibulum extends downwards towards the pituitary gland.

The third ventricle communicates with the **lateral ventricles** though two **interventricular foramina**, or **foramina of Monro**. These are apertures between the anterior end of the thalamus and the column of the fornix. The lateral ventricles are the largest of the ventricles, and have a paired, irregular appearance. On each side there are **anterior** and **posterior horns** and a central **body**. The roof of the anterior horns is formed by the corpus callosum and its medial wall by the septum pellucidum. Each lateral wall and the floor is supplied by the head of the caudate nucleus. The body extends rostrally from the interventricular foramina to the splenium of the corpus callosum. The corpus callosum forms the roof of the body portion, and the floor is contributed to by a number of structures, these being from lateral to medial the caudate nucleus, vena terminalis, stria terminalis, thalamus, choroid plexus, and fornix. The posterior horn extends caudally into the occipital lobe; its roof is formed by part of the corpus callosum.

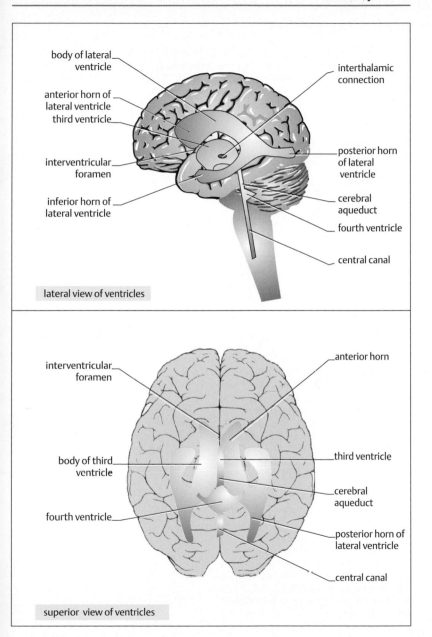

body of lateral ventricle

anterior horn of lateral ventricle

third ventricle

interventricular foramen

inferior horn of lateral ventricle

interthalamic connection

posterior horn of lateral ventricle

cerebral aqueduct

fourth ventricle

central canal

lateral view of ventricles

interventricular foramen

body of third ventricle

fourth ventricle

anterior horn

third ventricle

cerebral aqueduct

posterior horn of lateral ventricle

central canal

superior view of ventricles

Flow of Cerebrospinal Fluid

The **cerebrospinal fluid** (**CSF**) is an ultra-filtrate of plasma actively secreted into the cerebral **ventricles** by the **choroid plexus**, a highly vascularized and perfused lining of the ventricles. Average blood flow through the cerebral circulation is about 0.5 ml/min/g of brain tissue, and flow to the choroid plexus is about ten times higher. The choroid plexus supplies at least 75% of the CSF, which is also derived from the **interstitial fluid** (**ISF**), which is produced by the endothelial cells of the blood-brain barrier in the choroid plexus. The transformed ISF is pumped into the subarachnoid space as CSF across the pial-glial membranes. CSF passes through the ventricles and into the **subarachnoid space** through the foramina of **Magendie** and Luschka (see also p. 16). A third source of water for CSF is provided by the complete oxidation of glucose by brain parenchymal cells. The subarachnoid space is a cavity between the arachnoid membrane and pia mater surrounding the brain and spinal cord. CSF flows through the **cisternae** and **trabeculae** of the subarachnoid space, which, when filled with CSF, provides buoyancy for the brain, effectively reducing its weight from around 1400 g to about 45 g when it is suspended in CSF. The trabeculae are delicate columns of tissue bridges tethered to the arachnoid mater, which strengthen the subarachnoid space and they provide stable support for the brain within its fluid cushion of CSF.

CSF flows into the ventricles and through the subarachnoid space, driven by two forces. There is (i) the gradient set up between the point of secretion of CSF into the ventricles from the choroid plexus to the point where CSF drains through the **arachnoid villi** into the **venous sinuses**, and (ii) the mechanical propulsion provided by the pulsing of the cerebral arteries in the subarachnoid space and the movement of the trabecular tethers. CSF is propelled through the choroid plexus into the ventricles with a driving pressure of about 15 cm of water. CSF exits the subarachnoid space back into the venous system through the arachnoid villi by means of a hydrostatic pressure-dependent mechanism.

The flow of CSF must be regulated to prevent the build-up of excess pressure on brain tissue. This is achieved through the regulation of water flow across the blood–brain barrier, both at the level of the ISF and the level of glial and neuronal and intracellular fluid. ISF constitutes about 15–20% of the total tissue weight, and is the principal source of extracellular fluid in the brain. Cerebral capillary walls are less permeable than those of peripheral capillaries, and the flow across into the CSF is balanced by the return of CSF to the plasma compartment. CSF flows through the ventricles and the subarachnoid space at the rate of about 0.3 ml per minute. Neurons and glia contribute to the maintenance of normal hydrostatic pressures through the activity of their membrane ion transporters (see next spread). CSF flow is turned over about three times in 24 hours. CSF provides not only a buffering and cushioning system for brain, but also carries many substances such as trophic factors and nutrients.

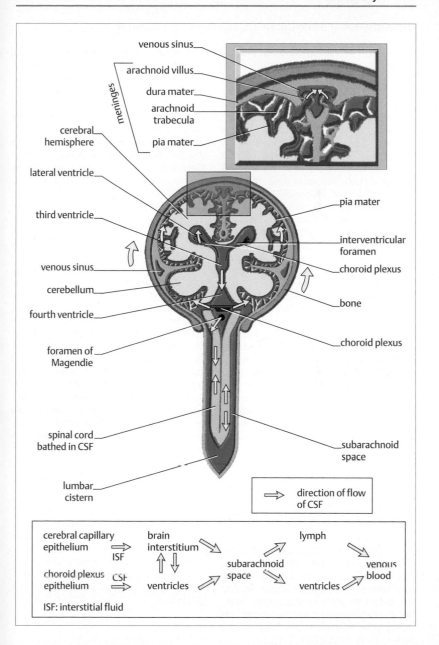

Cerebrospinal Fluid Composition, Secretion, and Pathology

CSF is derived from **extracellular** sources (see p. 48), and has been subclassified, depending on its whereabouts in the ventricles. Newly formed CSF is called **nascent CSF**. In the ventricles it is called **ventricular CSF**, and in the subarachnoid spaces, **subarachnoid CSF**. This classification is relevant because the composition of CSF changes as it passes from the choroid plexus to its exit sites and back into the venous system. The main ionic constituents of CSF are **Na^+, Cl^-**, and **HCO_3^-**. The concentration of Cl^- in nascent CSF is initially very similar to that in plasma (about 134 mEq/kg H_2O), but by the time it reaches the cisterna magna it is about 145 mEq/kg H_2O. Concentrations of Ca^{2+} and Mg^{2+} are held more constant by tighter exchange controls, since relatively small fluctuations in Ca^{2+} and Mg^{2+} could cause changes in membrane and hence CNS excitability. Changes in CSF ionic composition occur because of the more permeable membranes of the pial-glial and ependymal cell linings, which allow exchange of interstitial fluid and CSF in the subarachnoid and ventricular spaces.

The ionic composition of CSF is determined by the activity of ion transport mechanisms in the choroidal epithelial cell membrane. **Ion transporters** and **channels** work together to distribute ions and water between the **apical membrane**, which separates the choroidal cell from the ventricles, and the **basolateral membrane**, which separates the choroidal cell from plasma. The most important transporter is the apical Na^+/K^+-ATPase pump, which keeps intracellular Na^+ concentrations low by pumping the ion into the CSF. This creates an inwardly directed gradient that drives Na^+ into the cell from the blood in exchange for **H^+**, which is generated in the cell by the action of **carbonic anhydrase**. In addition, Na^+ and Cl^- are pumped in through the basolateral membrane by a co-transport mechanism.

Protein concentrations in CSF are very much lower than in blood, and urea and **glucose** concentrations are between 60-70% of those measured in plasma. The pH of CSF (7.35) is slightly lower than in plasma (7.4) because of a slighter higher pCO_2. Protein concentrations do, however, increase with travel through the ventricles and subarachnoid space due to regional differences in re-absorptive and secretory patterns along the length of the blood–CSF barrier.

CSF is sampled from patients by **lumbar puncture** (spinal tap), and is of diagnostic value. Normally, CSF is very **clear** and **colorless**. There are very few cells although a few monocytes, B and T lymphocytes may be observed. The presence of erythrocytes suggests either contamination of CSF during sampling or brain trauma, in which case CSF may be red in color. Cloudiness especially with yellow discoloration indicates disease, possibly of viral or bacterial origin, for example acute purulent meningitis. Poliomyelitis may yield a clear, yellow-tinged CSF, and virological examination is indicated.

CSF pressure reflects intracranial pressure (**ICP**), and increased CSF pressure is indicative of disease. Pulsation of flow of CSF creates a **waveform,** which is useful to measure. Obstruction to flow of CSF through occlusion produced, for example, by a brain tumor, or hemorrhage, can be life threatening. CSF pressure can be measured by invasive techniques, for example in the **lateral ventricle**, or through the less invasive **epidural space**. Tumors in the cerebellum, for example, may put pressure on the roof of the fourth ventricle. Increased CSF volume in the cranial cavity is called **hydrocephalus**. Measurement of ICP is therefore an important diagnostic tool.

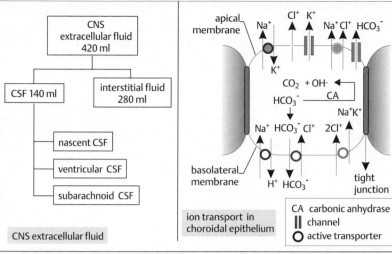

CNS extracellular fluid

ion transport in choroidal epithelium

CA carbonic anhydrase
|| channel
O active transporter

lumbar puncture (spinal tap) CSF	
cell numbers:	0-3 lymphocytes per cu mm
protein:	15-45 mg per 100 ml
chloride:	720-750 mg per 100 ml
glucose:	50-85 mg per 100 ml
appearance:	clear, colorless

CSF characteristics

condition	appearance	Pressure mmH$_2$O
normal	clear	70-100
encephalitis	clear	normal
brain abscess	cloudy(?)	very high
brain tumor	bloody(?)	high
poliomyelitis	clear or yellow	high

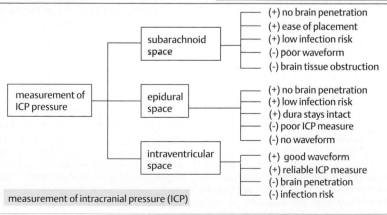

measurement of ICP pressure

subarachnoid space
(+) no brain penetration
(+) ease of placement
(+) low infection risk
(-) poor waveform
(-) brain tissue obstruction

epidural space
(+) no brain penetration
(+) low infection risk
(+) dura stays intact
(-) poor ICP measure
(-) no waveform

intraventricular space
(+) good waveform
(+) reliable ICP measure
(-) brain penetration
(-) infection risk

measurement of intracranial pressure (ICP)

Blood–Brain Barriers

The **blood–brain barrier** is a collective term referring to a complex system of metabolic, physical, and transport filters or barriers that control access of blood-borne chemicals to the brain. These barriers maintain an optimal and stable physicochemical environment within which the CNS can operate. The blood–brain barrier consists, broadly, of two main compartments: the **choroid plexus**, and the **CNS capillary bed**.

The choroid plexus (see also p. 16) serves as a blood–CSF barrier through the specialized structure of the ependymal cell lining of the plexus. The endothelial cells are bonded by **tight junctions** that bar the passage of high molecular weight substances. This is what is generally meant by the blood–brain barrier. Unlike the capillaries of the general circulation, choroid plexus cells have no intercellular pores and fenestrations. Instead, there are numerous **microvilli**, and the cells contain several enzymes that transport ions, such as Na^+ and K^+, and metabolites, such as glucose.

The endothelial cells of **brain capillaries** lie on a **basement membrane** (basal lamina), which is surrounded by **end feet** of the **astrocytes**. Endothelial cells, like those of the choroid plexus, are joined by tight junctions and possess the same ion and metabolite transport systems. There are very few pinocytotic vesicles in these cells, and no fenestrations. The brain capillary bed is enormous, and has been estimated to cover the area of a tennis court. The CNS capillary bed is also sometimes referred to as the blood–ECF (extracellular fluid) barrier, while the choroidal plexus is the blood–CSF barrier.

The tight junctions may break down or be breached under certain pathological conditions. Tumor development may be accompanied by the formation of new capillaries at the site of the lesion. These capillaries are not closely apposed to astrocytes, and they have intercellular pores and fenestrations that permit substances to pass through that are not normally allowed. This is of diagnostic value; if a tumor is suspected, the patient is injected with a radioactive amino acid that penetrates to the tumor and can be visualized there by scanning techniques. Tight junctions may be forced open in patients with hypertension, leading to cerebral edema and headaches, and, in severe cases, coma.

The brain is not uniformly impermeable to blood-borne components. Circulating macromolecules can breach the blood-brain barrier at the **circumventricular organs**. These are seven areas at the ependymal border of the third and fourth ventricles, where hydrophilic solutes can pass through capillaries. The **pineal body** makes melatonin, and is thought to be involved in certain brain rhythms. The **neurohypophysis** or posterior pituitary gland releases vasopressin and oxytocin into the peripheral blood stream. The **median eminence** is where brain neuropeptides such as CRF and GnRH are released in the portal system (see pp. 301, 303). The **area postrema**, which lies at the caudal end of the fourth ventricle, is in close contact with the nucleus of the tractus solitarius (solitary tract). This site allows passage of chemical stimuli that trigger, for example, the vomiting reflex. The **organum vasculosum of the lamina terminalis** (**OVLT**) lies in the wall of the third ventricle, and seems to mediate water balance through vasopressin. The **subfornical organ** in the dorsal wall of the third ventricle mediates drinking behavior via angiotensin signals. The **subcommissural organ** lies close to the pineal body.

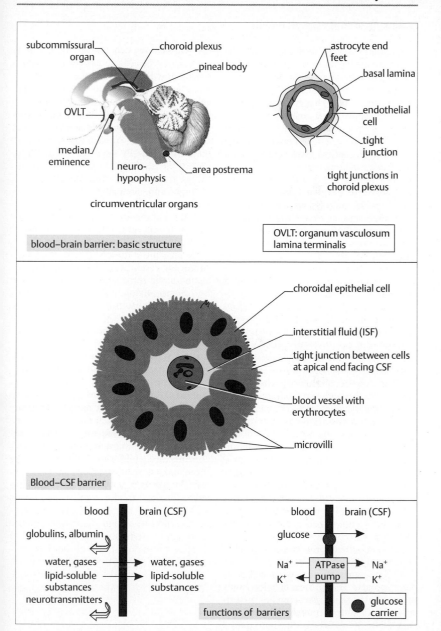

subcommissural organ
choroid plexus
pineal body
OVLT
median eminence
neuro-hypophysis
area postrema

circumventricular organs

blood–brain barrier: basic structure

astrocyte end feet
basal lamina
endothelial cell
tight junction

tight junctions in choroid plexus

OVLT: organum vasculosum lamina terminalis

choroidal epithelial cell
interstitial fluid (ISF)
tight junction between cells at apical end facing CSF
blood vessel with erythrocytes
microvilli

Blood–CSF barrier

blood | brain (CSF)

globulins, albumin
water, gases → water, gases
lipid-soluble substances → lipid-soluble substances
neurotransmitters

blood | brain (CSF)

glucose →
Na^+ → Na^+
ATPase pump
K^+ ← K^+

functions of barriers

● glucose carrier

Summary of Brain Development

The nervous system develops from the **neural plate**, which is an ectodermal thickening in the floor of the amniotic sac. During the third week, the plate forms paired neural folds that fuse to form the neural tube and neural canal. By the end of the fourth week, the open ends, the neuropores, become fused at either end and close. The formation of the neural tube is termed neurulation.

Even before neurulation begins, the brain starts to develop from the rostral (front) end of the tube, which expands to form three vesicles termed the forebrain, or **prosencephalon**, the midbrain or **mesencephalon**, and the hindbrain, or **rhombencephalon**. These three form the embryonic **brain stem**. During the fifth week, the prosencephalon divides further to form the **telencephalon** and **diencephalon**. The telencephalon is comprised of the cerebral hemispheres. The rhombencephalon also divides to form the **metencephalon** and **myelencephalon**. After these divisions, the embryonic brain now consists of five vesicles. Towards the end of the fourth week, the neuroepithelium of the neural tube begins to differentiate into the neuroblasts, glioblasts, and ependymal cells of the central nervous system. The neuroblasts will migrate to form the mantle zone, which will ultimately form the gray matter. The neuroepithelium proliferates beneath the mantle zone in the region of the brain stem and the spinal cord to form a ventricular zone, while migrating neuroepithelial fibers begin to form the marginal zone, which will become the white matter.

As development proceeds, between the fourth and eighth weeks, the embryonic brain undergoes flexion, or bending, at three points. The prosencephalon folds under the brain at the cranial (mesencephalic) flexure. A **pontine flexure** occurs in the area of the future pons, and a cervical flexure occurs between the spinal cord and the hindbrain. The myelencephalon will give rise to the medulla oblongata, the brain area most similar to the spinal cord in structure, while the metencephalon will give rise to the **pons**. The cerebellum develops from the end of the sixth week from the rhombic lips of the metencephalon. By the middle of the third month the cerebellum starts to bulge dorsally, forming a swelling at the cranial end of the rhombencephalon.

Within each of the brain vesicles the neural canal expands into a cavity termed the primitive ventricle. In the rhombencephalon this will become the fourth ventricle and in the mesencephalic cavity becomes the cerebral aqueduct (aqueduct of Sylvius). The third ventricle forms within the diencephalon, while paired lateral ventricles form within the cerebral hemispheres.

At 14 weeks the **lobes** of the cerebral hemispheres are defined; they are the **frontal**, **parietal**, **temporal**, and **occipital** lobes. The structures within the hemispheres, too, are forming. At 16 weeks, the **corpus callosum** is formed, as is the **optic chiasm**, where the optic nerves decussate on their way to the occipital lobe from the eyes. The basal ganglia are defined, as are the thalamus, hippocampus, **anterior commissure**, and fornix. At 28 weeks, the three major cortical **sulc**i are visible. These are the **central**, **lateral**, and **calcarine sulci**.

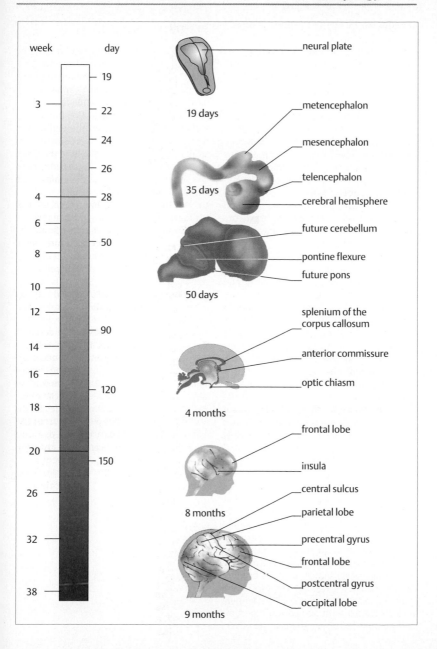

week | day

19

3 — 22

24

26

4 — 28

6

8 — 50

10

12

14 — 90

16

18 — 120

20 — 150

26

32

38

neural plate

19 days

metencephalon

mesencephalon

telencephalon

cerebral hemisphere

35 days

future cerebellum

pontine flexure

future pons

50 days

splenium of the corpus callosum

anterior commissure

optic chiasm

4 months

frontal lobe

insula

8 months

central sulcus

parietal lobe

precentral gyrus

frontal lobe

postcentral gyrus

occipital lobe

9 months

Development of the Peripheral Nervous System

The **peripheral nervous system** develops into **somatic** and **autonomic** divisions. The somatic division is sensorimotor, carrying conscious sensory inputs to the brain, which replies with motor output to the striated (voluntary) musculature. The autonomic nervous system (ANS) is almost entirely motor, carrying impulses from the CNS to the involuntary effector organs such as heart and sweat glands. The ANS develops into two main divisions, **sympathetic** and **parasympathetic**.

Neurons grow out from three principal embryonic tissues: the **neural crest**, the neuroepithelium that lines the neural canal, and from ectodermal placodes, which are specialized areas of ectoderm in the neck and head. **Dorsal root ganglia** develop in register with the somites, and contain cells that relay sensory inputs to the brain. Chains of **sympathetic ganglia** develop bilaterally along the spinal cord, and **parasympathetic ganglia** develop in the walls of the visceral target organs innervated by the ANS. At the same time, **motoneuron** axons grow out from the basal columns of the cord. They form ventral roots at the level of each somite, and grow to innervate their striated target muscles. Motoneurons are the first axons that sprout from the spinal cord. They originate in the ventral gray columns of the cord, and first appear at about day 30 at the **cervical level**, and thereafter appear in a craniocaudal sequence.

While the ganglia are developing, the sympathetic central neurons develop in the thoracolumbar region of the spinal cord, in the intermediolateral cell columns. Axons of the central sympathetic neurons leave the cord in the ventral roots, and immediately branch to form a white ramus, which enters the corresponding ganglion in the chain. Some of these fibers form synapses with sympathetic peripheral neurons in the ganglion, while others travel to other ganglia, thus expanding the chain of communication between the ganglia. Postganglionic sympathetic fibers of the ganglia re-enter spinal nerves through a branch termed a gray ramus.

The parasympathetic (craniosacral) division of the ANS is formed by the development of the brain stem and sacral spinal cord cell bodies that ultimately become the central nuclei. Their axons leave the brain through cranial nerves, and through sacral spinal cord from levels S2 to S4 (S = sacral). The cranial output will ultimately innervate parasympathetic ganglia in visceral organs of the head and trunk via the **vagus nerve**, while sacral fibers will innervate hindgut and pelvic visceral ganglia via the pelvic splanchnic nerves.

Spinal nerves are formed by the union of ventral and dorsal (also termed anterior and posterior) nerve roots where they make their exit from the vertebral canal. Put another way, it is a coming together of sensory fibers and the autonomic and somatic motor fibers leaving the CNS. Spinal nerves will ultimately supply somatic afferent fibers to the skin, and somatic efferent fibers to the skeletal muscles of the trunk and limbs. They will carry visceral efferent fibers and some visceral afferents as well.

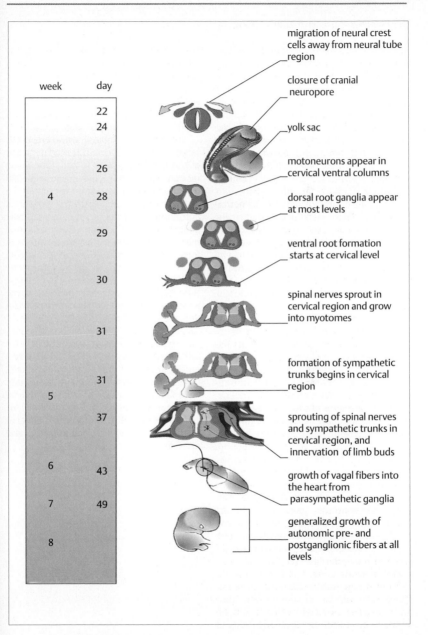

The Neural Plate and Neural Tube

Development of the central nervous system commences on day 18, with the formation of the **neural plate** in the ectoderm anterior to the **primitive pit**. The neural plate seems to be chemically induced by so-called inducing substances that are secreted by the **prechordal plate** and the cranial end of the **notochordal plate** in the underlying **mesoderm**. The cells in this area of ectoderm begin to differentiate into a thick plate of pseudostratified columnar neuroepithelium, forming the **neural groove** and the **neural folds**. The neural plate first appears at the cranial end, and develops in a craniocaudal direction. The plate is broad at the cranial end, and narrows caudally. The cranial end will expand into the brain, and even at this primitive stage can be differentiated visually into the fore-, mid-, and hindbrain. The caudal end of the neural plate, which lies above the notochord, develops into the spinal cord.

During the third week, the neural folds begin the process of neurulation. On day 22, the neural folds rise, their edges move in towards the midline and they fuse together to form the **neural tube**. This occurs in the region of the first five embryonic **somites**. (The somites are discrete blocks of segmental mesoderm running bilaterally alongside the notochord from the occipital area of the skull caudally to the embryonic tail.) Closure of the folds does not occur at the same time along the midline, but begins cranially, and subsequently continues in both cranial and caudal directions. When the two neural folds have almost completely fused with each other, there remain two openings of the neural tube where the fusing is delayed. These cervical and caudal openings of the neural tube are called **neuropores**. Formation of the neural tube creates a neural canal, which communicates directly with the amniotic cavity at either end. As neurulation proceeds, the cranial and caudal neuropores gradually shrink in size and finally close on the twenty-fifth and twenty-seventh days respectively. Closure of the caudal end is caused by a secondary neurulation that involves the mesoderm as well.

As the tube is closing, **neural crest** cells migrate from their origin at the lateral lips of the folds, and move in both lateral and medial paths. Those moving in a medial direction pass in between the neural tube and the somites and form the peripheral autonomic nervous system, dorsal root ganglia and the Schwann cells of spinal nerves. Those moving in a lateral direction form melanoblasts in the skin. The neural crest also gives rise to the ganglia of the peripheral nervous system. The neural tube itself moves and sinks deeper into the embryo as it differentiates into the brain and the spinal cord.

A failure of complete neural tube closure is termed **spinal dysraphism**. This will affect the induction of the vertebral arches and the differentiation of the CNS. Defects are most commonly associated with failure of closure of cranial or caudal neuropores. Failure or abnormalities of complete neural tube closure result in birth defects such as **spina bifida** and **anencephaly**.

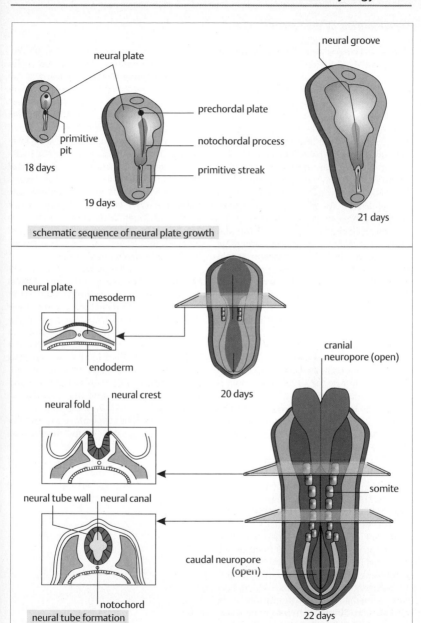

schematic sequence of neural plate growth

neural plate

primitive pit

18 days

neural plate

prechordal plate

notochordal process

primitive streak

19 days

neural groove

21 days

neural plate   mesoderm

endoderm

20 days

cranial neuropore (open)

neural fold   neural crest

neural tube wall   neural canal

notochord

neural tube formation

somite

caudal neuropore (open)

22 days

Development of the Spinal Cord

The **spinal cord** is formed from the **neural tube** caudal to the fourth pair of somites. During the closure of the tube the neuroepithelial cells multiply and increase the thickness of the wall. Once the neuropores are closed, some of the neuroepithelial cells differentiate into **neuroblasts**. These cells form a mantle layer around the outside of the neural tube, which is the precursor for the **gray matter** of the spinal cord. Nerve fibers from these neuroblasts will ultimately form the **white matter** of the spinal cord. Growth of the neuroblasts occurs in three main areas. These are: (i) the dorsal thickenings, known as the **alar plates**, which form the sensory areas; (ii) the ventral thickenings, known as the **basal plates,** which form the motor areas; to a smaller extent (iii) the **intermediate horn,** which only runs in the thoracic and upper lumbar parts of the cord and forms the sympathetic part of the autonomic nervous system. Axons from the basal plate pass directly through the **marginal zone**, but when axons from the alar plate enter the marginal zone they ascend or descend to a different level and are known as association neurons.

When neuroblast formation has ceased, the neuroepithelial cells begin to differentiate into glioblasts. These migrate into the **mantle layer** and the marginal zone where they become astrocytes and supporting CNS cells, which are responsible for CNS myelination. This process starts in the fourth month but may not be completed until the first year postnatally. When glioblast formation ceases, the remaining neuroepithelial cells become ependymal cells, which line the central canal as ependyma. Microglia, derived from mesenchymal cells are also present.

Some neural crest cells, which have moved medially during the fusion of the neural tube, differentiate into neuroblasts that form the **dorsal root ganglia**. These cells develop processes centrally and peripherally. Centrally-directed processes may either enter the **dorsal horn** of the spinal cord or ascend the marginal layer headed for a higher one. Peripherally-directed processes join paths with fibers from the **ventral horn** to form the spinal nerve trunk. Neural crest cells also form Schwann cells, which myelinate peripheral nerves by forming a neurilemmal sheath around them. The neural tube is covered with layers of mesenchyme. The outermost layer becomes the dura mater while the inner layer becomes the pia-arachnoid (or leptomeninges) connected by arachnoid trabeculae, and contains the fluid-filled subarachnoid space.

During the embryonic period, the spinal cord spans the length of the vertebral **canal**. The vertebral column grows faster than the cord, and the caudal end of the cord ascends cranially. At six months gestation, the caudal end of the cord lies at the first sacral vertebra, and at birth it lies at the second or third lumbar vertebra. The spinal nerve roots consequently run obliquely downwards as to exit at the corresponding vertebral level and become the cauda equina.

Failure of caudal spinal column closure results in spina bifida. If few vertebrae fail to fuse, there may be no defect. But if more do not fuse, the meninges alone, or the meninges and cord may protrude. These defects are termed meningocele and meningomyelocele, respectively.

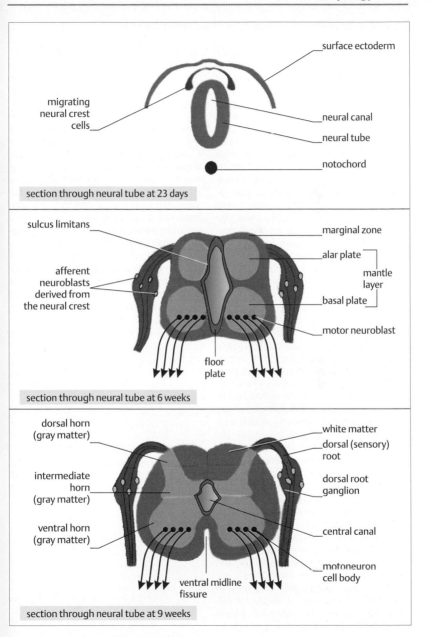

section through neural tube at 23 days

section through neural tube at 6 weeks

section through neural tube at 9 weeks

Development of the Rhombencephalon: Cranial Nerves

The **rhombencephalon** consists of the **myelencephalon** and the **metencephalon**. The myelencephalon lies caudally and forms the **medulla oblongata**. The metencephalon runs from the pontine flexure to the rhombencephalic isthmus, and forms the **pons** and the **cerebellum**.

The myelencephalon can be divided structurally into a caudal closed portion and a rostral open portion. The caudal closed portion resembles the **spinal cord**, as there is a small central canal. Neuroblasts from the alar plates migrate to the marginal zone where they form the cuneate nuclei laterally and the gracile nuclei medially, both of which form part of tracts linking the medullary spinal cord. Also in this area, but lying ventrally, are the pyramids, a pair of corticospinal fiber tracts originating from the cerebral cortex. With the development of the **pontine flexure**, the rostral portion of the myelencephalon and the metencephalon undergo a structural change that can be likened to a butterfly opening its wings. The lateral walls move outward, stretching and thinning the ependymal roof plate. The resultant cavity forms the **fourth ventricle**. The basal and alar plates split into three and four cell columns respectively, which form the basis for the development of the **cranial nuclei** and their nerves.

During the sixth week after fertilization, the **olfactory nerve** (**I**) develops from bipolar neurons in the epithelial lining of the olfactory pit. At the same time, the **optic nerve** (**II**) grows towards the brain from the retina, while the **oculomotor** (**III**) and **trochlear** (**IV**) nerves grow out from the midbrain. The **abducens** (**VI**) arises in the pons, and **nerves III, IV**, and **VI** migrate to innervate the extrinsic eye muscles. The **trigeminal nerve** (**V**) develops as three main divisions, which migrate peripherally to supply sensory innervation for the teeth, the mucous membranes of the oronasal cavity, and the skin of the scalp and face. A **motor trigeminal** root gives rise to nerves that drive mastication. The **facial nerve** (**VII**) grows out to the facial muscles that enable facial expression, and the **vestibulocochlear** (**VIII**) nerve will innervate the organs of balance and hearing. The **glossopharyngeal** (**IX**) is a complex cranial nerve that will supply sensory fibers to the oropharynx. The **vagus nerve** (**X**) is another complex nerve that supplies sensory fibers to the mucous membranes of the digestive tract and parasympathetic motor fibers to the heart and gastrointestinal tract. The **cranial accessory nerve** (**XIc**) travels with the vagus to the muscles of the pharynx and larynx, and the **spinal accessory nerve** (**XIs**) will innervate the trapezius and sternomastoid muscles. The **hypoglossal nerve** (**XII**) will innervate the muscles of the tongue.

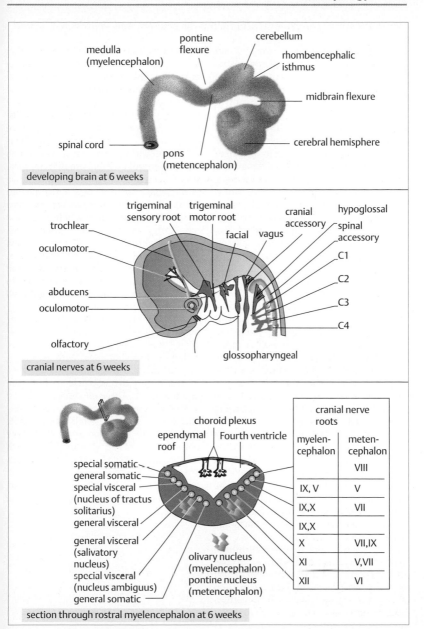

developing brain at 6 weeks

cranial nerves at 6 weeks

section through rostral myelencephalon at 6 weeks

Labels for developing brain at 6 weeks:
- medulla (myelencephalon)
- pontine flexure
- cerebellum
- rhombencephalic isthmus
- midbrain flexure
- cerebral hemisphere
- spinal cord
- pons (metencephalon)

Labels for cranial nerves at 6 weeks:
- trochlear
- oculomotor
- abducens
- oculomotor
- olfactory
- trigeminal sensory root
- trigeminal motor root
- facial
- vagus
- glossopharyngeal
- cranial accessory
- hypoglossal
- spinal accessory
- C1
- C2
- C3
- C4

Labels for section through rostral myelencephalon at 6 weeks:
- choroid plexus
- ependymal roof
- Fourth ventricle
- special somatic
- general somatic
- special visceral (nucleus of tractus solitarius)
- general visceral
- general visceral (salivatory nucleus)
- special visceral (nucleus ambiguus)
- general somatic
- olivary nucleus (myelencephalon)
- pontine nucleus (metencephalon)

cranial nerve roots	
myelen-cephalon	meten-cephalon
	VIII
IX, V	V
IX,X	VII
IX,X	
X	VII,IX
XI	V,VII
XII	VI

Development of the Rhombencephalon: Cerebellum and Ventricular System

The **cerebellum** develops from dorsal thickenings of the alar plates in the rostral metencephalon. These extensions of the alar plates are called the rhombic lips. With the combined effects of their growth and the deepening of the pontine flexure, they approach each other in the midline overlying the **fourth ventricle**. Fusion of the rhombic lips results in the formation of the cerebellar plate. The developing cerebellum becomes separated into cranial and caudal parts by the formation of a groove, termed the posterolateral fissure. The **flocculus** and the **nodule** develop into the flocculonodular lobes, which function in association with the vestibular apparatus. The flocculonodular nodes are the most phylogenetically ancient and primitive parts of the cerebellum.

The **vermis** is a narrow median swelling that connects the **cerebellar hemispheres**. The vermis and anterior part of the cerebellar hemispheres develop into the anterior lobe, which plays a role in the interpretation of sensory data from the limbs. The anterior lobe (also called the cranial lobe) grows more rapidly than the flocculonodular lobe and will eventually dominate cerebellar function. During development, the vermis and the cerebellar hemispheres fold extensively. By the end of the third month, a deep primary fissure has developed that divides the cranial part into an anterior lobe and a middle lobe. These subdivide further through the appearance of more transverse fissures. The thin gyri produced by this folding are termed folia, from their leaf-like appearance.

The posterior lobe is derived from the posterior part of the hemispheres and controls limb movement. Development begins at about the end of the sixth week, and continues to grow after birth. Nevertheless, the gross morphology at birth is the same as in the adult.

Histologically, the developing cerebellum comprises three layers, the neuroepithelium, the mantle, and the marginal layer. The neuroepithelium of the rhombic lips proliferates initially, and forms the three layers. In the third month, the ventricular layer produces a further layer, the external germinal layer, and the original forms the inner germinal layer. This inner layer will differentiate into the cerebellar nuclei, and will produce primitive Purkinje neuroblasts that will migrate into the cerebellar cortex. It will also produce Golgi neuroblasts, which will differentiate into Golgi cells.

The external layer will give rise, via basket, granule, and stellate neuroblasts, to basket, granule, and stellate cells. The granule cells and some of the other two types will eventually form the granular layer of the cortex.

The roof of the **fourth ventricle**, composed of a layer of vascular pia mater overlying the ependymal layer, is collectively called the tela choroidea. With growth of the pia mater, invaginations of the roof protrude into the ventricle to form the choroid plexus. These plexuses are formed in the third ventricle and the lateral ventricles and produce cerebrospinal fluid. Growth of the pia mater also causes three outpouchings of the tela choroidea, which rupture to form two **foramina of Luschka**. These foramina serve as a communication point between the central **foramen of Magendie**, subarachnoid space, and the ventricle.

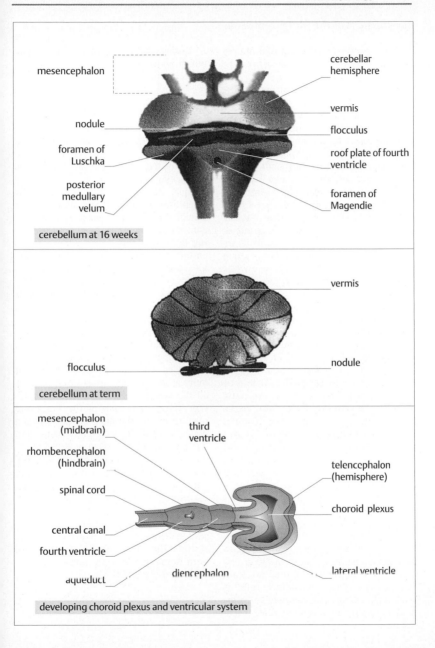

cerebellum at 16 weeks

cerebellum at term

developing choroid plexus and ventricular system

Development of the Mesencephalon

The **mesencephalon** is composed mainly of dense tracts of neurons passing from the forebrain to the spinal cord, but it also contains the nuclei of three cranial nerves. The mesencephalon contains nuclei of the **trochlear nerve (IV)**, the **oculomotor nerve (III)**, and the **trigeminal nerve (V)**. The trigeminal nuclei and the trochlear nuclei arise from metencephalic **alar** and **basal** neuroblasts respectively but migrate into the midbrain. There are two nuclei of the oculomotor nerve, which are both derived from neuroblasts of the basal plate of the mesencephalon: the **Edinger-Westphal nucleus** and the **somatic nucleus**. The Edinger-Westphal nucleus controls accommodation and pupillary constriction through parasympathetic pathways while the somatic nucleus controls most of the extrinsic ocular muscles.

Neuroblasts derived from the alar plates give rise to structures such as the **substantia nigra**, the **aqueductal gray matter**, and the **stratified nucleus of the inferior colliculus**. Those from the basal plates give rise to structures such as the **red nuclei,** the **mesencephalic nucleus of the trigeminal nerve (V)**, and the **somatic motor nucleus of the oculomotor nerve (III)**. This area in the mesencephalon is known as the **tegmentum**. Ventral to this area, cerebral fibers descending to the spinal cord and the brain stem pass through the mesencephalon in the **cerebral peduncles**.

The proliferation and migration of alar neuroblasts into the roof of the midbrain form **the inferior** and **superior colliculi**. This area is known as the **tectum**. A longitudinal midline groove, the **corpora bigemina**, separates adjacent colliculi. The inferior colliculi receive information from the cochlea and mediate auditory reflexes while the superior colliculi receive information from the retina and mediate visual reflexes.

During development, the neural canal, which widened to form the fourth ventricle in the rhombencephalon, narrows throughout the mesencephalon to form the cerebral aqueduct (aqueduct of Sylvius). This meets the third ventricle rostrally in the diencephalon. Abnormalities of the cerebral aqueduct can lead to a condition known as **hydrocephalus**. Hydrocephalus describes enlargement of the ventricular system of the brain caused by unequal absorption and production of cerebrospinal fluid (CSF), and can be classified into **communicating** and **noncommunicating** types. **Noncommunicating hydrocephalus** occurs when there is an obstruction in the ventricular system, for example, in the cerebral aqueduct or in the foramina of Luschka or Magendie. Obstruction of the cerebral aqueduct results most frequently from fetal infection with *Toxoplasma gondii* or cytomegalovirus, but aqueductal stenosis can also be transmitted as an X-linked recessive trait. This causes dilatation of the lateral and third ventricles, whereas blockage of one or more of the foramina causes dilatation of all the ventricles. The ventricular dilatation causes expansion of the brain and may result in thinning of the calvaria bones, atrophy of the cerebral cortex and basal ganglia compression.

The **Arnold-Chiari** malformation describes the herniation of the cerebellum and the medulla through the foramen magnum. This interferes with and reduces the absorption of the CSF causing a **communicating hydrocephalus**, which results in distension of the whole ventricular system. The malformation is associated with spina bifida with myelomeningocoele (see also p. 58).

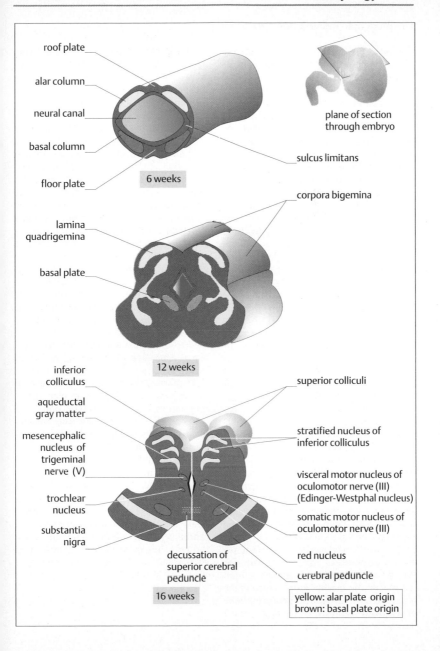

roof plate

alar column

neural canal

basal column

floor plate

6 weeks

plane of section through embryo

sulcus limitans

corpora bigemina

lamina quadrigemina

basal plate

12 weeks

inferior colliculus

aqueductal gray matter

mesencephalic nucleus of trigeminal nerve (V)

trochlear nucleus

substantia nigra

superior colliculi

stratified nucleus of inferior colliculus

visceral motor nucleus of oculomotor nerve (III) (Edinger-Westphal nucleus)

somatic motor nucleus of oculomotor nerve (III)

red nucleus

cerebral peduncle

decussation of superior cerebral peduncle

16 weeks

yellow: alar plate origin
brown: basal plate origin

The Diencephalon and Pituitary Gland

The **diencephalon** is the medial part of the prosencephalon. It differs from vesicles described previously in that the roof plate and the basal plates are not distinguishable. Important structures that develop in the diencephalon are the **thalamus**, a relay for sensory information, the **hypothalamus**, which controls endocrine and autonomic function, and the **pituitary gland**, which is involved in endocrine function. The cavity of the diencephalon forms the **third ventricle**.

By the sixth week of development, a groove is visible running across the center of the diencephalic walls (derived from the alar plates) which separates two swellings. The groove is the hypothalamic sulcus and the swellings are the thalamus and the hypothalamus. The **mamillary body** is a visible swelling on the ventral surface of the hypothalamus. By the seventh week of development the **epithalamus** is visible in the dorsal area of the diencephalon and is separated from the thalamus by the epithalamic sulcus. The thalami grow quickly, and in about 70% of brains, meet in the midline forming the interthalamic adhesion. The epithalamus later develops into the trigonum habenulae and the posterior and anterior commissures.

As in the mesencephalon, the roof plate in the diencephalon is composed of two layers, the ependymal layer and the vascular pia mater, which form the choroid plexus of the third ventricle. An epithelial thickening appears caudally in the roof plate, which invaginates in the seventh week. The structure formed is called the **epiphysis**, or the **pineal gland**.

The **pituitary gland** develops from two distinct ectodermal sources. The **anterior lobe or adenohypophysis** is formed from the roof of the **stomodeum**, which is the primitive oral cavity. The **posterior lobe or neurohypophysis** is formed from a downgrowth of the diencephalon.

Rathke's pouch, from the stomodeum, develops during the fourth week and passes between the basisphenoid and presphenoid bones of the skull. The connection of the oral cavity to Rathke's pouch usually degenerates during the sixth week; persisting remnants of the pouch are known as pharyngeal hypophysis. Within the pituitary, Rathke's pouch derivatives are the anterior lobe, the pars intermedia, and the pars tuberalis, which grows around the infundibular stem. **Craniopharyngiomas** are remnants of Rathke's pouch that form tumors usually situated in or above the **sella turcica**. (The sella turcica is a depression in the body of the sphenoid bone in which the pituitary gland lies.) Symptoms develop before the age of 15 years and are similar to those resulting from anterior lobe tumors. The remainder of the pituitary develops from the **infundibulum**, an outpocketing of the third ventricle in the diencephalon. The median eminence, the infundibular stem, and the posterior lobe are formed from this structure.

Tumors of the pituitary gland can lead to hormonal imbalances due to the inappropriate secretion of trophic hormones such as luteinizing hormone, follicle-stimulating hormone, and adrenocorticotropic hormone (ACTH). These tumors can therefore cause sterility and symptoms of Cushing's disease, among others. When possible, the tumor, or the entire pituitary, is removed surgically. During development of the diencephalon, retinal fibers from the primitive optic cup run centrally. Just before they enter the brain, the optic fibers meet to form the **optic chiasm**.

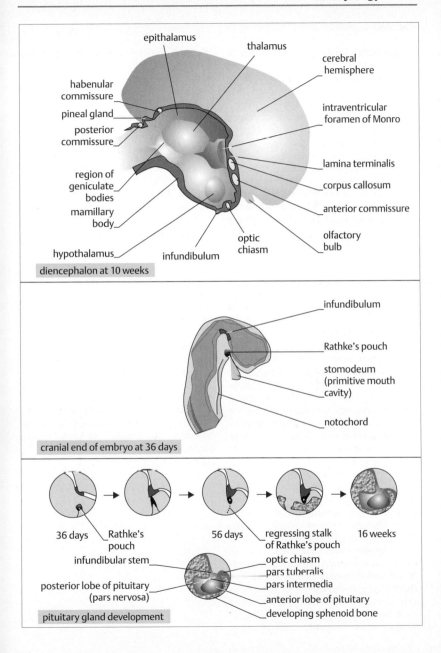

diencephalon at 10 weeks

cranial end of embryo at 36 days

pituitary gland development

The Telencephalon

The **telencephalon** is the rostral part of the prosencephalon. This vesicle gives rise to the **cerebral hemispheres**, which contain most of the brain cortex. It also differentiates into the **hippocampus**, which is involved in memory, and the **olfactory bulb**, which is part of the olfactory system. The telencephalon also gives rise to the basal ganglia, which consist of several large gray matter structures that are embedded deeply in the white matter of the cerebrum. These include the **caudate** and lenticular **nuclei** (together known as the **corpus striatum**; see below). These nuclei play an important role in motor function. The lenticular nucleus consists of the putamen and the globus pallidus (see also p. 34). The telencephalon also differentiates into the commissures, which connect the two opposite sides of the brain.

The precursors of the cerebral hemispheres are the cerebral vesicles, which appear as lateral outgrowths of the telencephalon at the end of the fourth week of gestation. Subsequent gross development of the vesicles is bilaterally symmetrical. The cavity of the vesicle and the subsequent hemisphere forms the **lateral ventricle** and communicates with the third ventricle through the **interventricular foramen of Monro**. The medial wall of the developing hemisphere runs along the diencephalon roof along the choroid fissure. In this area of the telencephalon, the hemisphere is composed only of ependymal cells and vascular pia mater and forms the **choroid plexus** of the lateral ventricle. The hemisphere grows rapidly and caudally, covering the mesencephalon and the rhombencephalon. The caudal part of the hemisphere grows in a ventral and rostral direction forming the temporal lobe whose cavity becomes the inferior horn with its own choroid plexus. A structure called the **corpus striatum**, a swelling in the floor of the hemisphere appearing in the sixth week, grows more slowly than the hemisphere and this results in the curvature of the hemispheres. The corpus striatum becomes divided by the **internal capsule**, which contains fibers running to and from the cerebral cortex, into the **caudate nucleus** and the **lentiform nucleus**. The head and body of the caudate nucleus lie in the floor of the lateral ventricle while its elongated tail lies in the roof of the inferior horn. The hippocampus develops from a thickening of the hemisphere just above the choroidal fissure.

Of the **commissures** that develop the four most prominent are found in the lamina terminalis, which is the midline portion of the telencephalon flanked by the cerebral vesicles on either side. The **anterior** and **hippocampal commissures** are the earliest to develop and they connect the olfactory bulbs and hippocampi respectively. The largest commissure is the **corpus callosum**, connecting the neocortices, whose growth extends beyond the lamina terminalis over the roof of the diencephalon. The **optic chiasm**, in the ventral area of the lamina, is a crossover point for fibers from the retina. The sulci and gyri, which are distinguishing furrows and elevations of the developed brain, are formed so that the massive growth of the cerebral cortex can be contained in the limited space of the cranium.

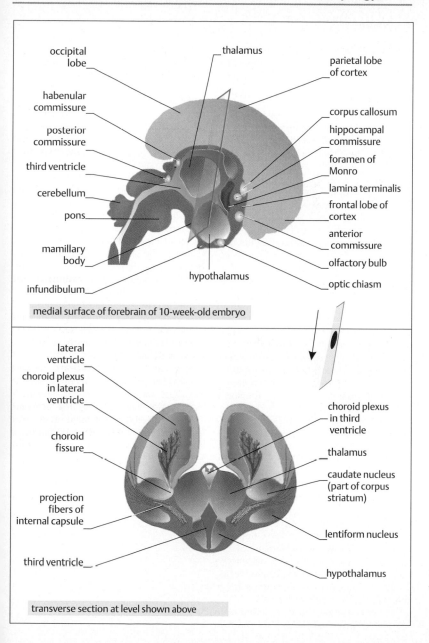

occipital lobe

thalamus

parietal lobe of cortex

habenular commissure

corpus callosum

posterior commissure

hippocampal commissure

third ventricle

foramen of Monro

cerebellum

lamina terminalis

pons

frontal lobe of cortex

mamillary body

anterior commissure

infundibulum

olfactory bulb

hypothalamus

optic chiasm

medial surface of forebrain of 10-week-old embryo

lateral ventricle

choroid plexus in lateral ventricle

choroid fissure

choroid plexus in third ventricle

thalamus

caudate nucleus (part of corpus striatum)

projection fibers of internal capsule

lentiform nucleus

third ventricle

hypothalamus

transverse section at level shown above

The Neuron

The nervous system is built up of nerve cells, or **neurons**, and their supporting cells, or glia. Neurons are electrically excitable, capable of generating and propagating action potentials.

The neuron consists of a cell body, also called a perikaryon or **soma**, from which processes radiate. These processes include **dendrites**, which may branch to form dendritic 'trees', whose large surface area facilitates the reception of multiple signals from other neurons. They also include the main process, or **axon**, which conducts the nerve impulse from the soma to other cells. The axon, too, may give off branches, or **collaterals**, which extend the potential complexity of information transmission through the nervous system.

The neuronal cell body, when stained, shows a large **nucleus** with a prominent **nucleolus**. The cytoplasm contains numerous **mitochondria**, which are necessary for the generation of ATP, free **ribosomes** and **rough endoplasmic reticulum** (rER), which synthesize proteins, and the **Golgi apparatus**, which modifies and packages newly synthesized proteins. The **axon hillock** is the part of the soma where the axon leaves it.

Neurons contain a cytoskeleton consisting of neurofibrils, which determine the shape of the soma and the various processes extending from it, and which transport substances through the neuron. There are three main types of neurofibrils:

(i) Actin, or microfilaments, present in high concentrations as a meshwork beneath the membrane in the axon. Actin is an important protein in axon development, and causes the movement of the growth cone (see p. 385). Actin appears to be present in all cells which can move, including muscle. Actin is also important in maintaining the shape of the cell;

(ii) microtubules and microtubule-associated proteins (MAP) are narrow longitudinal tubes present in all neuronal processes. The tubes maintain shape, and also transport molecules such as neurotransmitters from the soma to the axon terminals (anterograde transport), or from the terminals to the soma (retrograde transport). There are at least two types of axonal transport: (a) rapid, at about 400 mm per day, and (b) slow, at less than 1 mm per day;

(iii) neurofilaments, also called intermediary filaments, are the most abundant of the fibrillar elements in the neuron, and form the 'bones' of the cytoskeleton.

Axons conduct electrical impulses, the speed of conduction depending on fiber diameter (see also p. 78). Efficiency of conduction also depends on good insulation, which is achieved by the **myelin sheath**. The myelin sheath coats the axonal membrane, or axolemma. Myelin is composed mainly of lipids and proteins and, in the peripheral nervous system, is made by the **Schwann cells**. In the CNS, myelin is made by oligodendrocytes (see p. 76). Microscopic examination reveals that the myelin sheath is arranged in spiral lamellae round the axon, and that the myelin is actually part of the Schwann cell. The Schwann cells are covered by the connective tissue **endoneurium**, while several bundles of fibers are covered by the **perineurium**. Larger bundles may be covered by yet another layer, the epineurium. In general, in physiology, a bundle of fibers, for example nerve or muscle, is termed a **fasciculus**.

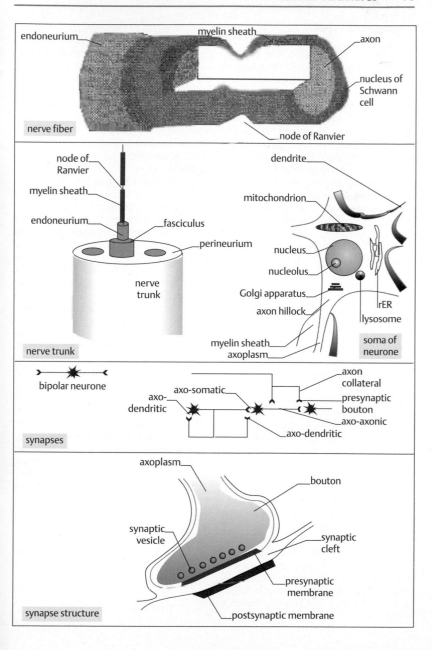

Neuronal Cell Types

The structure of a neuron may provide valuable information about its function. Not only is its anatomical location important, but also its size, origin and destination of the axon and dendrites. The connections made with it may provide clues about its function. The degree of branching, or arborization of neuronal processes, particularly the dendrites, gives some indication of the complexity of information processing. Small neurons with short axons, such as those found in the cerebral cortex and in the spinal cord, clearly service a local network, which integrates information. Neurons, such as the spinal motoneuron, may have long axons, which convey messages over long distances.

Early workers on the nervous system had physically to dissect out neurons, since many of the available cell-staining methods stained all neurons, which produced indecipherable images. The Golgi stain, which uses silver deposition was used to great effect by the Spanish neuroanatomist Ramón y Cajal to demonstrate neurons. The stain for some reason selectively stains only certain neurons, and is deposited selectively in the nerve cells but not in myelin. Myelin can be stained using the Weigert method, in which myelin is visualized by treating it with potassium dichromate, which renders myelin dark blue with hematoxylin. The Nissl method preferentially stains neuronal nuclei. Neurons can now be visualized with immunocytochemical and biochemical techniques, which may identify specific neurotransmitters, hormones, enzymes and other neurochemicals. Formaldehyde-induced fluorescence can be used to distinguish between different neurotransmitters; norepinephrine (noradrenaline) neurons fluoresce pale green under UV light, while serotonin (5-HT) neurons fluoresce yellow.

Neuronal axons can be traced using degeneration techniques. Destruction of the soma of the neuron results in gradual axonal degeneration and, by following the path of degeneration of the axon, its course and ultimate connections may be ascertained. The origin of an axon or its destination may be discovered using retrograde or anterograde axonal transport respectively, in which a substance that can be visualized (for example radioactive amino acid, or the enzyme horseradish peroxidase) is applied to the soma or axon terminal, respectively. With the advent of electron microscopy, it became possible to visualize the subcellular organelles and observe the detailed structures of myelin, and of the synaptic contacts between cells.

Design of neuronal arrangement is best exemplified by that of the cerebellum (see also p. 21). The cerebellum, which is concerned with the regulation of movement and which is the largest part of the hindbrain, has specific neuronal cell types, namely basket, stellate, Golgi, and granule cells (see opposite), and these are all in direct or indirect contact with the Purkinje cell. The different cell types lie in different layers, and send their processes to other layers. Purkinje fibers are excited by, for example, afferent inputs from (excitatory) granule cells or mossy and climbing fibers, and inhibited by the basket, stellate granule and Golgi cells, which are cerebellar interneurons, whose processes do not leave the cerebellum. The Purkinje axons are efferents, which leave the cerebellum, and project to intracerebellar nuclei or relay stations, which in turn send projections to the cerebral cortex and brain stem which modify muscular activity.

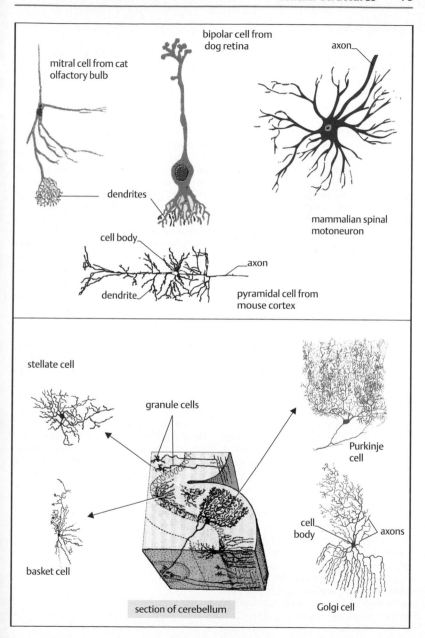

bipolar cell from dog retina

axon

mitral cell from cat olfactory bulb

dendrites

cell body

axon

dendrite

pyramidal cell from mouse cortex

mammalian spinal motoneuron

stellate cell

granule cells

Purkinje cell

cell body

axons

basket cell

section of cerebellum

Golgi cell

Neuroglia (Glia)

Neuroglia occur in both the central and peripheral nervous systems. They surround and invest virtually every exposed surface that is not occupied by blood vessels and neurons. There are far more glial cells than neurons. They may support neurons, form **myelin sheaths** around them, and may provide nutritional, ionic, and mechanical support. They may regulate neuronal shape and synaptic connectivity. Neuroglia have been classified into two major classes, namely microglia and macroglia, which are in turn subclassified as **astrocytes** (astroglia), **oligodendrocytes** (oligodendroglia) and Schwann cells.

Astrocytes are CNS stellate (star-shaped) cells with many processes. On the basis of the length of the processes they are subclassified as protoplasmic or fibrillary, respectively. These processes spread out to make 'feet' along the surfaces of the capillaries and around the surfaces of neurons except where the boutons make contact with other neurons. Astrocytes may provide a structural 'scaffolding' for developing nerve cells. Astrocytes form continuous sheets, called limiting membranes, and contribute to the blood–brain barrier between CNS and other tissues.

Astrocytes may exchange substances between capillaries and neurons. They may regulate extracellular concentrations of K^+, which is particularly important in the brain, where the extracellular space is relatively small. K^+ may increase rapidly due to neuronal excitation. Astrocytes may also mediate the removal and breakdown of neurotransmitters.

Oligodendrocytes have relatively few processes. They are central nervous glia which form the myelin sheaths around axons and are analogous to peripheral Schwann cells. They are often found close to the cell bodies of central neurons and for this reason are sometimes referred to as satellite cells. During development, the oligodendrocyte sends out processes; when a process encounters an axon, it wraps itself round the axon to form the myelin sheath. Thus, one oligodendrocyte may provide myelin sheaths for many axons, whereas in the peripheral nervous system, one Schwann cell is dedicated to one neuron. The **node of Ranvier** is formed by myelin-free regions between two neighboring glial cells. Most sodium ion channels occur at the nodes of Ranvier. There is virtually no current flow across myelin sheaths. Action potentials are generated at the nodes and seem to jump from one node to the next, so-called saltatory conduction. Therefore the oligodendrocyte plays a vital role in the propagation of impulses through its structural association with the neuron. Astrocytes appear to have limited phagocytic activity, and appear to form a sort of scar tissue at sites of CNS injury.

Microglia are the phagocytes of the nervous system and may be derived from the bone marrow. They express a common leukocytic antigen, CD45, which to date has only been described on cells derived from bone marrow. Microglia enter the brain during development, become uniformly distributed through it, and may form 5–20% of all CNS glial cells. During injury to the CNS, monocytes and macrophages migrate into the brain. Ependymal cells are cylindrical glial cells that line the ventricles.

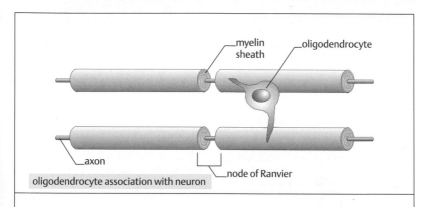

oligodendrocyte association with neuron

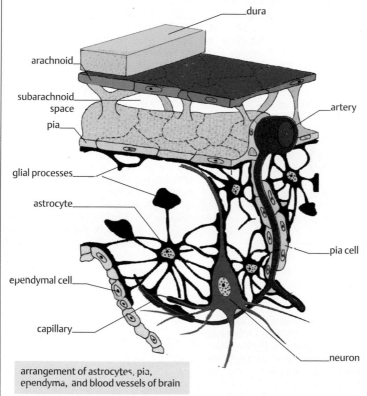

arrangement of astrocytes, pia, ependyma, and blood vessels of brain

Electrical Properties of Nerves I

Nerves transmit information as electrical signals. The nerve consists of an **axon** core, which is covered with the **axon membrane**, and a lipid bilayer, which allows the passage of ions across its surface through integral membrane **ion channels**. The lipid bilayer acts as an insulator between the intracellular and extracellular solutions of conducting ions, and therefore serves as a good **capacitor**, i.e. a reservoir of stored charge, which can be dissipated through the ion channels. These ion fluxes constitute the electrical current.

The nerve offers **resistance** to current, both longitudinally along the nerve axoplasm (R_L), and transversely, across the membrane (R_M), and can be thought of a set of units offering both transverse and longitudinal resistance. If the nerve were a passive conductor (e.g. copper wire), then the application of a voltage (V_o) would cause a current to flow along the nerve, and the voltage at increasing distance would fall off exponentially due to resistance, and to leakage of current across the axon membrane. Diameter influences this phenomenon. Doubling the diameter of the nerve halves R_M and reduces R_L to one quarter of its original value.

The rate of decay of V with distance along the cable is exponential, and depends on the ratio R_M/R_L. The rate of dissipation of the voltage, and its value at a given distance (x) after application can be calculated from the decay curve obtained. V is given by $V_o e^{-x/\lambda}$, where e is a constant of value 2.718, and λ is the **space constant**, defined as the distance from the point of application of V_o such that V_o has fallen to λ/e of its original value. In fact, l is equal to $\sqrt{(R_M/R_L)}$. From the above, it is readily apparent that the more the membrane leaks current, the smaller will be R_M, and the shorter the space constant.

In reality, however, an applied voltage that is above a threshold value is not dissipated by resistance and leakage, but generates an **action potential** whose amplitude, shape and rate of travel along the nerve are all at a rate independent of the original applied voltage. The independence of the properties of the action potential from those of the original stimulus constitutes what is called the all-or-none rule.

The mechanism whereby the nerve is able to initiate and propagate the action potential depends on the setting up of a local circuit around the area of the original applied stimulus. The first response is the passive spread of current (see above), which in turn sets up small local depolarizations in the nerve. These in turn increase the permeability of the membrane by opening ion channels, and the movement of the ions causes a larger depolarization. This depolarization sets up yet more local current flow and the action potential is generated, causing depolarization of the next part of the nerve. Movement of ions across the axon membrane is affected by the concentration gradients of the ions, and the voltage differences. Membranes with more ion channels will be more conductive to the ions, and the resistance of the membrane will be inversely proportional to the numbers of ion channels per unit area. The role of the ion channels in the propagation of the action potential and the nature of those ion movements are dealt with next.

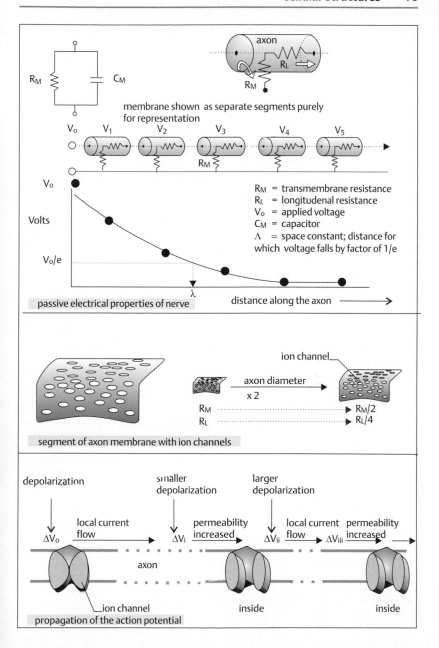

membrane shown as separate segments purely for representation

R_M = transmembrane resistance
R_L = longitudenal resistance
V_o = applied voltage
C_M = capacitor
Λ = space constant; distance for which voltage falls by factor of 1/e

passive electrical properties of nerve

distance along the axon

segment of axon membrane with ion channels

ion channel

axon diameter × 2

$R_M \dashrightarrow R_M/2$
$R_L \dashrightarrow R_L/4$

depolarization   smaller depolarization   larger depolarization

ΔV_o local current flow ΔV_i permeability increased ΔV_{ii} local current flow ΔV_{iii} permeability increased

axon

ion channel   inside   inside

propagation of the action potential

Electrical Properties of Nerve II: Generation of the Membrane Potential

The membrane potential is an electrical potential difference across the membrane. The ionic concentration is different on each side and the membrane is selectively permeable to certain ion species, which results in an ionic imbalance across the membrane.

The transmembrane potential is zero when concentrations of negatively and positively-charged ions are equal on each side of the membrane. When the K^+ channels open, K^+ ions, which occur in higher concentrations in the cytoplasm, diffuse down their concentration gradient through the membrane. However, negatively-charged counterbalancing anions, such as proteins, other organic anions and chloride, cannot cross through the K^+-selective ion channels. This imbalance of charge creates a negative electrical potential on the cytoplasmic side. This negative potential drives K^+ ions back across the membrane into the cytoplasm. When K^+ influx and efflux are in equilibrium, then the net movement of K^+ ions becomes zero, even though the K^+ channels are open. The resulting electrical potential is called the equilibrium potential for potassium (E_K). The value of E_K for a particular ion can be calculated using the **Nernst equation**:

$$E_K = \frac{RT}{zF} \cdot \ln \frac{[K^+]_o}{[K^+]_i}$$

where R is the gas constant, T is the absolute temperature in degrees Kelvin, F is Faraday's constant, z is the valency of the ion species, $[K^+]_o$ is the molar concentration of the ion outside the membrane, and $[K^+]_i$ the concentration inside. From the equation it is clear that when K^+ concentrations are equal across the membrane, then E_K will be zero. The membrane, however, contains ion channels specifically permeable not only to K^+ but to other ions, notably Na^+, and the equation has been modified to accommodate this:

$$E = \frac{RT}{zF} \ln \frac{P_K[K^+]_o + P_{Na}[Na^+]_o + P_{Cl}[Cl]_i}{P_K[K^+]_i + P_{NA}[Na^+]_i + P_{Cl}[Cl]_o}$$

where P is the permeability of the membrane to the specified ion. This equation, called the constant field equation, differs from the Nernst equation in that the relative permeabilities dictate the relative influence of the ion on the value of E. These permeabilities reflect the numbers of open ion channels for the ion. If P for one ion, say Na^+, is negligible at a given moment, then E will approximate more closely to the value of E for K^+ given by the Nernst equation. Therefore, the membrane potential is dictated by the changes in transmembrane concentrations to the most permeable ion at any given moment. The measured resting potential of neurons (typically –50 to –75 mV,) indicates that at rest the membrane is preferentially permeable to K^+ rather than to Na^+.

In **voltage clamp** experiments, ion permeabilities across the membrane are measured during potential changes. The membrane potential of an isolated nerve is clamped at a constant value by a negative feedback loop; changes in the potential are sensed and current flow to the nerve automatically altered to restore the potential to the desired value. The current (I) required to clamp the membrane will be equal to the sum of currents carried by Na^+ and K^+. If the membrane is depolarized by altering the set voltage, then a current flow is measured, which reflects the transient inward flow of Na^+ and outward flow of K^+.

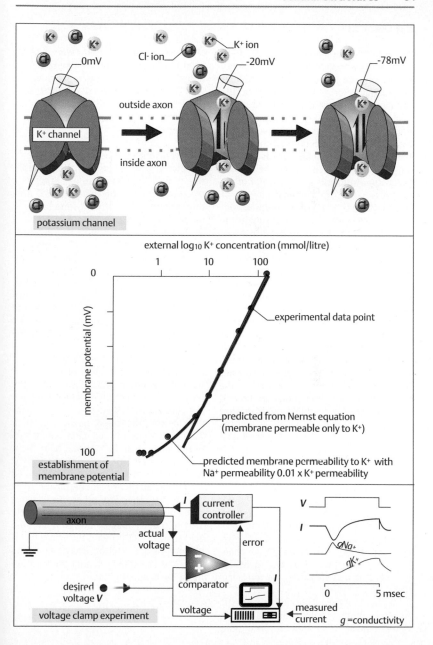

potassium channel

external log$_{10}$ K$^+$ concentration (mmol/litre)

membrane potential (mV)

experimental data point

predicted from Nernst equation
(membrane permeable only to K$^+$)

predicted membrane permeability to K$^+$ with
Na$^+$ permeability 0.01 x K$^+$ permeability

establishment of
membrane potential

voltage clamp experiment

g =conductivity

Ion Channels

The nerve cell is bounded by the cell membrane, which provides structural integrity for the cell and regulates the intracellular and extracellular ionic environment. The cell membrane consists basically of a lipid bilayer, composed of **phospholipids**, which are dipolar molecules. The molecules are arranged so as to present their hydrophilic **polar heads** to the aqueous environment, and their **nonpolar lipophilic tails** to the interior of the membrane. The hydrophobic interior of the bilayer acts as a barrier to the uncontrolled movement of ions through the membrane, and acts as a capacitor, since this thin non-polar layer (about 1.5-3 nm) separates unlike charges, thus storing electrochemical energy. Some of the phospholipids themselves can act as substrates for membrane-associated enzymes that transduce messages across the membrane.

Ion channels are integral membrane proteins that make possible the transfer of ions across the membrane, down their electrochemical transmembrane gradients. The channel achieves ion transfer through a channel or aqueous pore. The pore contains charged or polar amino acid residues, forming so-called **coordination sites** (selectivity filters), which attract the ions away from their hydration shell, and thus allow them to enter and penetrate the membrane.

Channels can switch between two states, namely open (ion permeable) or closed (ion exclusive), or may be inactivated. These states are determined by changes in the conformation of the proteins that make up the ion channel. Regulation of ion movement through the channel occurs through at least two identified mechanisms, namely gating and ion selectivity.

Gating is achieved through changes in channel protein conformation. These changes can be increased in probability by two main stimuli: voltage or stereospecific ligand-binding second messenger cascades. Sodium and calcium channels, which are essential for the properties of the action potential and for nerve conduction, are gated by changes in voltage across the membrane.

The ligand may be, for example, a neurotransmitter or hormone to a specific receptor region of the channel. Epinephrine (adrenaline), for example, binds to a receptor linked to the membrane **G protein** system. The G protein stimulates the membrane enzyme **adenylate cyclase** (AC). AC in turn catalyzes the conversion of **ATP** to **cyclic AMP**, which triggers a **phosphorylation cascade** resulting in the phosphorylation of the voltage-gated Ca^{2+} **channel**, which alters its conformation. Some channels, for example the Ca^{2+}-activated K^+ **channel** are both voltage- and ligand-gated, and are opened when Ca^{2+} ions bind to the cytoplasmic side of the channel.

Selectivity of channels may be determined by sign, or by size of the ion, or both. Generally, channels will allow the passage of positively or negatively charged ions, but not both. Voltage-gated Na^+ channels permit the rapid passage of both Na^+ and Li^+ ions (crystal radii about 0.05 nm). Rubidium and K^+ (crystal radii about 1.4 nm) pass through more slowly. Nevertheless, all K^+ channels so far studied are at least 50 times more permeable to K^+ than to Na^+. Therefore other mechanisms independent of size must operate as well. This selectivity may be due to the amino acid sequence of proteins lining the channel pore, since altering even one amino acid experimentally can alter the selectivity of the channel.

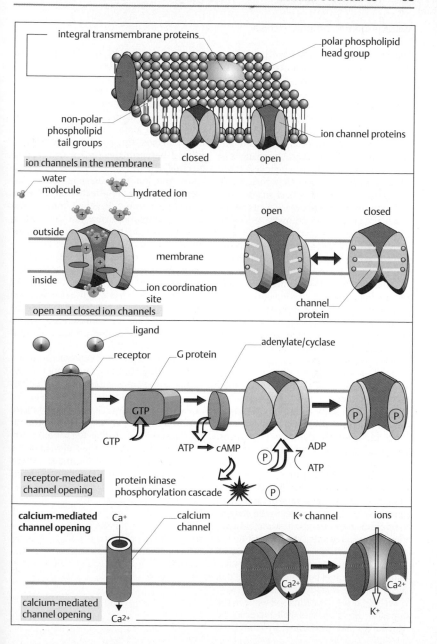

integral transmembrane proteins

polar phospholipid head group

non-polar phospholipid tail groups

ion channel proteins

closed   open

ion channels in the membrane

water molecule

hydrated ion

open   closed

outside

membrane

inside

ion coordination site

channel protein

open and closed ion channels

ligand

receptor   G protein

adenylate/cyclase

GTP

GTP

ATP → cAMP

protein kinase phosphorylation cascade

ADP

ATP

P   P

P

P

receptor-mediated channel opening

calcium-mediated channel opening

Ca⁺

calcium channel

K⁺ channel   ions

Ca²⁺   Ca²⁺

Ca²⁺   K⁺

calcium-mediated channel opening

Voltage-gated Sodium Channel

The **voltage-gated Na⁺ channel** is an allosteric, multi-unit integral membrane protein that selectively allows the passive diffusion of Na^+ ions through it. The direction and resulting equilibrium depend not on the application of energy but on the electrochemical driving force across the cell membrane. The channel is switched between open and closed state by changes in the state of membrane depolarization. These changes alter the conformation of the membrane, resulting in changes in ion permeability. The conductances of the individual channels can be measured using the technique of patch clamping.

Structurally, the functional unit of the voltage-gated Na⁺ channel is a single polypeptide chain arranged in the membrane as 24 transmembrane segments, forming four domains, each consisting of six transmembrane segments. Within each domain is the so-called **S4** region, whose amino acid sequence is highly homologous to that of the other S4 regions in the channel. The S4 region contains several positively charged amino acids, which detect membrane potential changes, and which then react to induce the conformational changes which cause activation. The **S5–S6** linking units within each domain are thought to form the pathway for the ions. Near the amino-terminus is the so-called **ball and chain** region, which can block the open channel to inactivate it.

The channel is switched between the probability of existing in one of three main functional states by changes in the state of membrane depolarization. More positive membrane potentials (**+V_m**) will shift the probability towards an **open activated state**. If the positive potential is maintained, the channel becomes inactivated in the open state. Negative membrane potentials (**-V_m**) drive the gating sequence in the opposite direction, and will increase the probability that the channel will shift from the open, inactivated state to the **open activated state**, and then to the **closed resting state**.

Patch clamping techniques can be used to study the state of the ion channel. An area of the membrane is gently sucked up against a glass microelectrode with a heat-polished tip. A very tight bond is formed between the surface of the glass electrode and the membrane that does not allow any ion flow between them. The piece of membrane attached to the electrode may become detached from the rest of the membrane, hence the name *patch*, which refers to the piece of membrane being studied. A very high electrical resistance, measured as high as 10^{11} ohms, is generated between the inside of the electrode and the extracellular fluid of the membrane, which is why the seal between the two is sometimes referred to as the *gigaohm seal*. Leakage from the electrode tip is negligible, and so the voltage inside the electrode can be clamped.

If the piece of membrane sucked up includes an **ion channel**, the channel affords virtually the only means of current flow when it opens, because it offers the lowest resistance. Therefore, if the channel opens due to a change in the applied voltage, the current flow can be detected using a sensitive amplifier. Several trials of the current flow measurement can be made using a single channel, and the results summed and averaged.

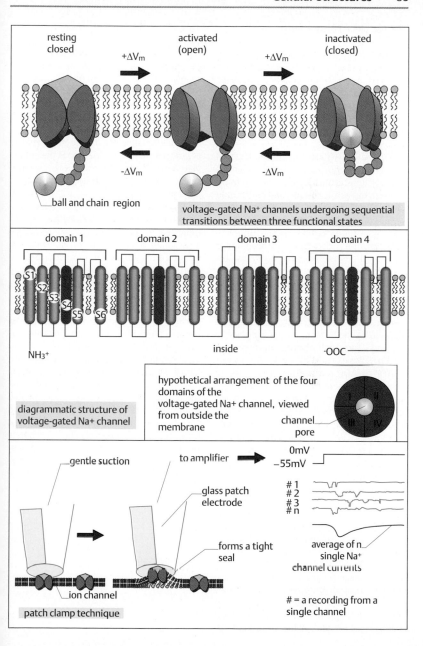

resting
closed

activated
(open)

inactivated
(closed)

$+\Delta V_m$

$+\Delta V_m$

$-\Delta V_m$

$-\Delta V_m$

ball and chain region

voltage-gated Na^+ channels undergoing sequential transitions between three functional states

domain 1

domain 2

domain 3

domain 4

S1
S2
S3
S4
S5
S6

NH_3^+

inside

^-OOC

diagrammatic structure of voltage-gated Na^+ channel

hypothetical arrangement of the four domains of the voltage-gated Na^+ channel, viewed from outside the membrane

channel pore

I   II

III   IV

gentle suction

to amplifier

0mV

−55mV

1
2
3
n

glass patch electrode

forms a tight seal

average of n single Na^+ channel currents

ion channel

patch clamp technique

= a recording from a single channel

The Na⁺/K⁺ ATPase Pump

External energy sources are required in addition to the selective opening of ion channels to maintain concentrations of ions in extracellular and intracellular compartments against their concentration gradients. Energy is supplied as ATP, which is used by ion pumps, such as the **Na⁺/K⁺ ATPase pump**.

The Na⁺/K⁺ ATPase pump is an integral membrane protein consisting of α and β chains. The α chains have ATPase activity on the cytoplasmic surface, and commonly have eight transmembrane segments. The pump actively translocates Na⁺ to the extracellular fluid, and K⁺ in the opposite direction. The β chains, which have **sugar units** on their external surface, do not appear to be necessary for ion transport. Subtle changes in conformation of the transport protein may be involved in ion translocation. In one state, the protein appears to possess three high-affinity binding sites for the Na⁺ ion on the cytoplasmic side, and two high-affinity binding sites for K⁺ on the extracellular side. Hydrolysis of **ATP** to **ADP** and inorganic phosphate (P_i) provides energy to alter the conformation of the protein, and to drive the pumping of the ions in opposite directions (the so-called 'antiport' action). ATP phosphorylates the ATPase on a specific aspartate residue on the enzyme. Once through the pump, Na⁺ ions are discharged into the extracellular fluid and K⁺ into the cytoplasm since the binding sites for them on these sides of the pump are of lower affinity for the ions. Sequentially, it is believed that the ATPase switches between at least two conformations, called E_1 and E_2. Therefore there may be at least four different conformations: E_1, E_1-P, E_2, and E_2-P.

Ion transport by the Na⁺/K⁺ ATPase pump (and other pumps) is much slower than through ion channels. Up to 10^6 Na⁺ ions can be transported through an ion channel per second, whereas about 10^3 Na⁺ions are transported through the pump per second.

For the Na⁺/K⁺ ATPase pump to work, it requires energy in the form of ATP, which is hydrolyzed to ADP and P_i by an ATPase on the cytoplasmic surface of the a chain. As much as a third of all body utilization of ATP may be allocated to the maintenance of pump function. The ATPase is phosphorylated provided that Na⁺ and Mg^{2+} are present, and then dephosphorylated if K⁺ is present.

Pharmacological agents can inhibit the action of the pump. The ATPase activity is inhibited, for example, by the vanadate ion, which binds to the phosphorylation sites on the cytoplasmic side and thus inhibits enzyme phosphorylation. The drug was used to localize the site of phosphorylation to the cytoplasmic side of the pump. The cardiotonic steroids digoxin and **digitoxigenin** are inhibitors of the pump. Digoxin binds to specific sites on the extracellular surface of the α subunits and blocks pump action, apparently by stabilizing the pump in the E_2-P configuration. Inhibition of the pump leads to higher intracellular Na⁺ concentrations, which diminishes the Na⁺ gradient, and this in turn slows the rate of extrusion of Ca^{2+}ions from the cell by the Na^+/Ca^{2+} exchange pump. The raised intracellular Ca^{2+} increases the force of concentration of cardiac cells in conditions such as congestive heart failure.

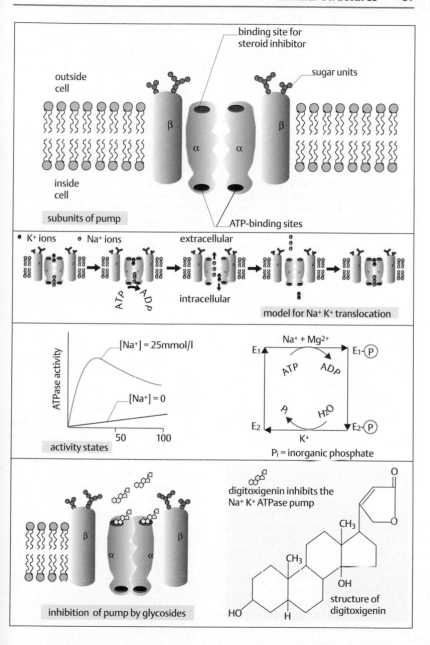

binding site for steroid inhibitor

sugar units

outside cell

β α α β

inside cell

subunits of pump

ATP-binding sites

• K⁺ ions • Na⁺ ions extracellular

ATP ADP

intracellular

model for Na⁺ K⁺ translocation

$[Na^+] = 25\,mmol/l$

ATPase activity

$[Na^+] = 0$

50 100

activity states

$Na^+ + Mg^{2+}$

E_1 → E_1-$\textcircled{P}$

ATP ADP

P_i H_2O

E_2 ← E_2-$\textcircled{P}$

K^+

P_i = inorganic phosphate

β α α β

inhibition of pump by glycosides

digitoxigenin inhibits the Na⁺ K⁺ ATPase pump

CH_3

CH_3

OH

HO H

structure of digitoxigenin

The Action Potential

The **action potential (AP)** is a single, transient reversal of membrane polarity. It is a regenerative impulse, which is rapidly carried, unattenuated, over long distances in the nervous system. The AP is an explosive all-or-nothing event with a distinct threshold. The initiating current does *not* determine the duration and amplitude of an AP, and the AP does not decline in amplitude or duration as it is propagated along the axon. The sequence of events of an AP must be completed before another AP can be initiated. Immediately after the AP is completed, that portion of the nerve is temporarily unable to initiate another AP. This period is called the refractory period. The nerve must be repolarized before another AP can be generated in that region. But if the nerve is depolarized again beyond threshold for a period longer than the refractory period, another AP may be initiated in that region of the nerve.

The AP has several phases or components. The earliest is (i) a rapid (within less than 1 msec) **depolarization** or reversal of membrane polarity to become positive in sign, to attain a maximum reversal at just below the equilibrium potential for sodium (E_{Na}). Reversal beyond 0 mV is termed the **overshoot**. This is followed by (ii) **repolarization**, when the membrane potential returns to negative values, and may become, briefly, more negative than the resting potential of the axon membrane. This is termed the **hyperpolarizing** afterpotential. The AP is triggered by changes in potential, caused by changes in the permeability of the membrane mainly to Na^+ and K^+, in a region of the membrane that expresses voltage-gated Na^+ and K^+ channels. Ca^{2+} also plays a role in determining changes in membrane **permeability** to the other two ions.

At rest, the membrane is normally more permeable to K^+ than to Na^+. During the initial depolarization phase of the AP, before threshold is reached, Na^+ channels open more rapidly than do K^+ channels. Therefore permeability to Na^+ increases relative to permeability to K^+. Thus, Na^+ ions move rapidly into the cell, down their concentration gradient, driven by the negative intracellular electrical potential. This influx of Na^+ further depolarizes the membrane, opening yet more voltage-gated ion channels, until a critical threshold potential is reached, when Na^+ influx exceeds K^+ efflux, and there is an explosive positive cycle of opening of Na^+ channels, with a concomitant leap of the polarity reversal. This sudden peaking results in an AP (often called a 'spike'). At peak positive level, membrane permeability to Na^+ (P_{Na}) may be up to 50x that to K^+ (P_K). Note, however, that during the depolarization phase, the voltage-gated K^+ channels are also opening, but at a much slower rate than the Na^+ channels. At the peak depolarization, P_K is well above its resting value, which approaches that of P_{Na}.

During repolarization, the increased P_K means that the **membrane potential** (E_M) begins to return to a voltage which is between E_{Na} and E_K. Also, P_{Na} declines because of E_M and inactivation of voltage-gated Na^+ channels. With depolarization, Na^+ channels become inactivated and non-conducting. As a result, K^+ channels dominate electrical determinants of the E_M, which will move closer to E_K than to E_{Na}. This explains after-hyperpolarization. However, as more K^+ channels become inactivated, E_M returns to the resting value for the membrane.

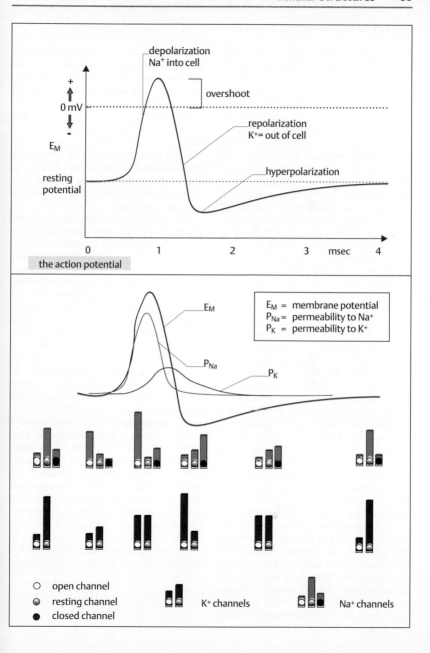

the action potential

Conduction of the Action Potential

Capacitance is the ability to store charge. The membrane is a resistor. But, through its unequal distribution of ions on two sides, the membrane also acts as a capacitor, with a capacitance C_M of about 1 $\mu F/cm^2$. If a current is passed through a resistor, e.g. an ion channel, the voltage across it *immediately* becomes $V = IR_M$, where V = voltage, I = current, and R = resistance. But because of the capacitive properties of the membrane, it takes longer to reach the new voltage, since time is required to charge it up to the new level. Thus, the voltage rises more slowly, and not in a stepwise fashion. The time course is exponential, given by $V = IR_M(1-e^{-t/\tau})$, where τ = the time constant for passive impulse propagation along the axon. The time constant can be defined as the time taken for the discrepancy of (IR_M-V) to fall by the factor e, and in this case is equal to R_MC_M. For axons the time constant may be a few milliseconds, which is important in limiting the rate at which the membrane can generate a voltage in response to local currents. The space (λ) and time (τ) constants can be combined to give a measure of the speed of passive electrical disturbance along an unmyelinated axon = λ/τ. Note, however, that λ but not τ (i.e. R_MC_M) varies with fiber diameter.

Myelin is interrupted along the axon at intervals of 1-2 mm, to reveal the **nodes of Ranvier**. Voltage-gated Na^+ channels are concentrated at the nodes, so an AP can be generated only at this region. Myelin greatly increases the membrane resistance R_M, while decreasing conductance C_M. Because capacitance is reduced, this reduces the amount of charge required to depolarize the internodal regions. The main advantage of myelin is that the space constant is enormously increased. External local currents have to travel further to reach the nodes where they gain access to the axoplasm. Effectively, impulses jump from node to node, a process called **saltatory conduction**, and, unlike conduction in unmyelinated fibers, velocity rises directly in proportion to fiber diameter. Velocity of conduction can be given, approximately, by

$$\text{velocity} = \lambda/\tau + T$$

where T = the time taken for the fiber to regenerate itself, and can be affected by several factors, such as anaesthetics, anoxia, density of ion channels, temperature, and pressure.

The **relative refractory period** is the period between stimuli when the threshold for firing is raised relative to the previous threshold. The period between stimuli when a second firing becomes impossible is termed the **absolute refractory period**. The absolute refractory period is determined mainly by Na^+ channels, which are inactivated after the peak of the spike, and need time to become activated. The relative refractory period seems to be determined by the delayed closing of K^+ channels after the AP peak. The refractory period is physiologically important since it prevents travel of the impulse backwards.

The **compound action potential** is due to the presence of fibers of several different diameters in a whole nerve. A **monophasic** action potential will be recorded with an internal electrode, but two external electrodes will produce a **biphasic recording**, as the impulse passes each electrode in turn. **Crushing** the nerve between the two abolishes the biphasic potential. Expansion of an action potential to produce the **dispersed compound action potential** reveals different fiber conduction velocities.

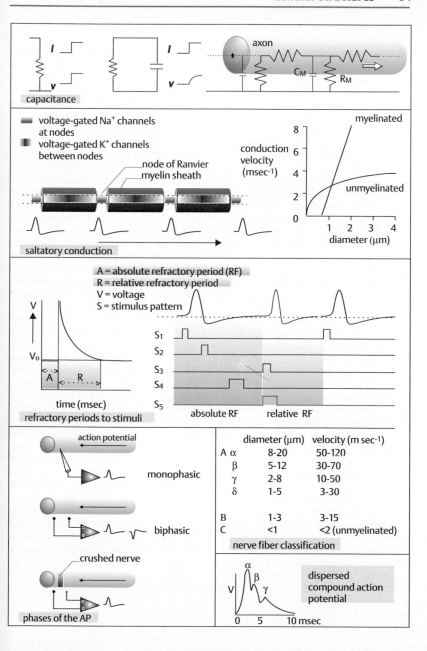

capacitance

- voltage-gated Na⁺ channels at nodes
- voltage-gated K⁺ channels between nodes

node of Ranvier
myelin sheath

myelinated
unmyelinated

conduction velocity (msec⁻¹)

diameter (μm)

saltatory conduction

A = absolute refractory period (RF)
R = relative refractory period
V = voltage
S = stimulus pattern

time (msec)
refractory periods to stimuli

absolute RF   relative RF

action potential
monophasic
biphasic
crushed nerve
phases of the AP

	diameter (μm)	velocity (m sec⁻¹)
A α	8-20	50-120
β	5-12	30-70
γ	2-8	10-50
δ	1-5	3-30
B	1-3	3-15
C	<1	<2 (unmyelinated)

nerve fiber classification

dispersed compound action potential

Communication between Neurons: Electrical Synapses

Neurons communicate with each other through **synaptic transmission**. Synaptic transmission may be **electrical** or **chemical**. The term **synapse**, introduced by Charles Sherrington at the beginning of the 20th Century, refers to the junction where communication occurs between two excitable cells. This section deals purely with electrical synapses.

Electrical synapses have been found not only in nervous tissue, but also between cardiac and smooth muscle cells, and between epithelial liver cells. At electrical synapses, the cytoplasm of the pre- and postsynaptic cells is continuous, connected by gap junctions formed by pores in the cell membrane, and the gap between the cells is about 3.5 nm. Since synaptic transmission is through ionic current, the synaptic delay is virtually non existent, compared with the delay through chemical synapses. The presynaptic fiber needs to be large to generate sufficient current, using its voltage-gated channels, for the current to be able to flow through the gap junction and generate an action potential in the postsynaptic cell, which should be smaller.

Current flow through an electrical synapse can be studied using the **giant motor synapse** of the **crayfish**, where the **presynaptic** fiber is indeed very much larger than the **postsynaptic** fiber. Pre- and postsynaptic stimulating and recording electrodes can be used to study the properties of transmission. Using this model, it was found that the latency for transmission is very brief, which is incompatible with chemical transmission. Surprisingly, current flow through the crayfish electrical synapse is unidirectional, or **rectifying**. This is probably because of the voltage sensitivity of the cells in this model. Usually, however, in electrical synapses of most other organisms studied, current is bidirectional i.e. **non-rectifying**,

and the synapse behaves like a pure resistor, which passes the current in either direction. In these synapses, unlike the case at chemical synapses, changes in potential in pre-and postsynaptic cells are very similar, and even subthreshold currents are conducted. This is a phenomenon that is reminiscent of the passive propagation of subthreshold impulses in nerve tissue. For this reason, impulse transmission at non-rectifying electrical synapses is sometimes referred to as **electrotonic transmission**. Note, also, that in some non-rectifying electrical synapses, pre- and postsynaptic cells may be of similar size, and that in some organisms (see below) more than two cells may be interconnected by gap junctions.

The obvious advantages of an electrical synapse are the very brief delay in transmission, and the combination of a group of neurons into an electrical unit. This property is exploited by organisms that need rapid escape mechanisms in time of danger. For example, the marine snail *Aplysia* is able to explosively release a cloud of purple ink when it encounters a noxious stimulus. This is because it has three cells interconnected by electrical synapses, which produce a synchronized discharge to the ink gland if the creature's tail is irritated by any noxious or rough physical stimulus. Another example is provided by the goldfish, which can flip its tail rapidly to move away from danger. In the goldfish, sensory inputs that alert it to danger make electrical synapses with the giant brain stem Mauthner neuron, which in turn transmits impulses to the tail motoneurons through chemical synapses.

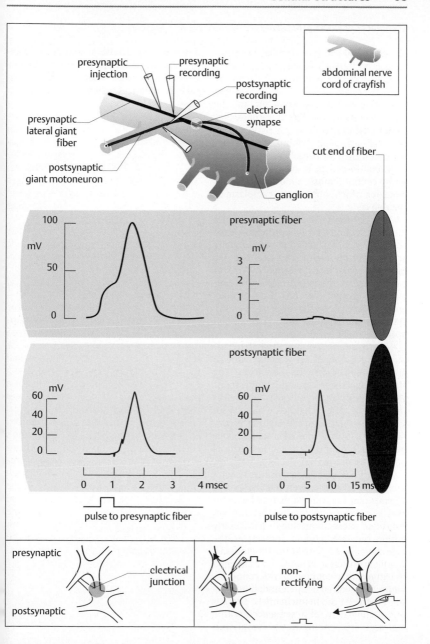

abdominal nerve cord of crayfish

presynaptic injection

presynaptic recording

postsynaptic recording

electrical synapse

presynaptic lateral giant fiber

postsynaptic giant motoneuron

ganglion

cut end of fiber

presynaptic fiber

postsynaptic fiber

pulse to presynaptic fiber

pulse to postsynaptic fiber

presynaptic

electrical junction

postsynaptic

non-rectifying

The Electrical Gap Junction

The **electrical gap junction** has been isolated from nervous tissue and characterized. All gap junctions studied consist of pairs of protein cylinders called **connexons**. One connexon is presynaptic, and the other is postsynaptic. The two connexons meet in the extracellular gap between the two cells, through homophilic interactions, and the two hemichannel cylinders align end-to-end to form a hollow tube, with a central channel, about 1.5-2.0 nm in diameter, which connects the cytoplasm of the two cells.

The connexon itself consists of six identical subunits, called **connexins**, each about 7.5 nm long, which are hexagonally arranged in the cell membrane. The gap junction brings cells relatively close to each other; at the gap junction the pre- and postsynaptic cells are about 3.5 nm apart, whereas usually and at chemical synapses the neurons are about 20 nm apart.

The channels may open through the rotation of the connexins, which creates an open pore through the connexon. The channel may close through the tilting of the connexins at the cytoplasmic end as they slide against each other, which causes a clockwise rotation of the base of the connexon. This form of conformational change may be a common feature of ion channel opening generally.

From gene cloning experiments with samples from heart, liver and the lens, it appears that the connexons may be members of a larger gene family. There are regions of close homology, particularly within the hydrophobic domains of the connexons that span the cell membrane, as well as within sequences corresponding to extracellular domains of the connexon, which are involved in the homophilic reactions between the hemichannels. There is less homology within sequences within regions corresponding to the cytoplasmic domain of the connexon, and this may explain partly why gap junctions vary between tissues with respect to their sensitivity to chemical mediators.

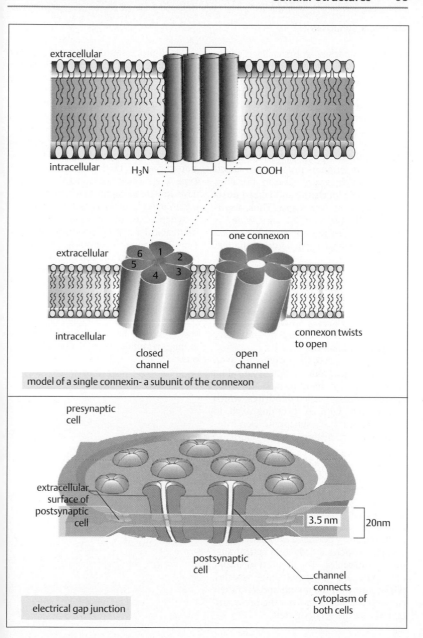

extracellular

intracellular   H₃N ——— COOH

extracellular   one connexon

intracellular

closed channel   open channel   connexon twists to open

model of a single connexin- a subunit of the connexon

presynaptic cell

extracellular surface of postsynaptic cell   3.5 nm   20nm

postsynaptic cell

channel connects cytoplasm of both cells

electrical gap junction

Chemical Synapses

Chemical synapses are specialized structures that enable the chemical transfer of information from one cell to another. They may occur between nerves, as happens most frequently in the central nervous system, or between nerves and effector tissues, such as muscle, glands, and sensory organs. At a typical chemical synapse, a branch of the afferent or **presynaptic** axon swells at its terminus to form a so-called **bouton**, which is very close to, but does not physically touch, the specialized **postsynaptic** side of the synapse. Thus, a **synaptic cleft,** typically 20 nm wide, is formed between the two communicating cells. The fluid-filled gap between the two cells prohibits the direct transfer of electrical current from one cell to the next. Transfer is effected instead through the rapid diffusion of a chemical substance called a neurotransmitter across the gap to the postsynaptic cell, where it may produce either an excitatory or inhibitory postsynaptic potential.

A synapse between presynaptic axon and postsynaptic soma (cell body) is called axosomatic; most neurons have fine cytoplasmic processes called **dendrites**, which may synapse with an incoming axon, to form axodendritic synapses. Dendrites from different neurons may synapse to form dendrodendritic synapses. Axons may synapse with axons from other neurons; these are called axoaxonic synapses (see also p. 73).

There are very pronounced thickenings or increased densities of the membrane on both sides of the synapse; the presynaptic thickening may be due to the clustering of synaptic **vesicles** filled with neurotransmitter molecules. The neurotransmitter molecules are packaged into vesicles, which fuse with the membrane, and their contents are extruded from the presynaptic cell into the synaptic cleft.

Small processes, or **spines**, are formed on dendrites, and these **dendritic spines** form synapses with other dendrites. From electron microscope studies of synapses on spines, synapses have been classified by the width of the synaptic cleft and the distribution of synaptic density. **Type 1 synapses**, for example, are characterised by a wider synaptic cleft and a denser region of synaptic thickening than occurs at **Type 2 synapses**. The classification may have functional significance, since in the pyramidal cells of the cerebral cortex, Type 1 synapses occur on spines projecting from apical or basal dendrites, whereas Type 2 synapses occur on the soma of the pyramidal cells of the cerebral cortex.

Synapses may also be complex, where a single spine may form several synapses with an incoming axon, as occurs most commonly in certain cell types in the central nervous system; complex synapses of this type have been described in, for example, pyramidal cells of the hippocampus.

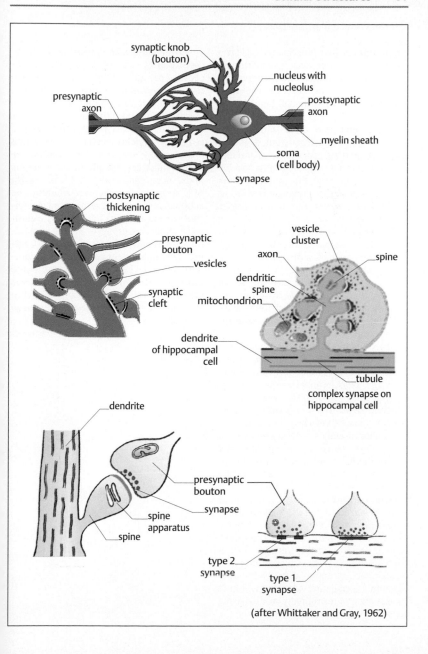

(after Whittaker and Gray, 1962)

The Neuromuscular Junction

The **neuromuscular junction** (NMJ) is the **synapse** where electrical information is chemically transmitted from nerve to skeletal muscle. The nerve is the **motoneuron**, which has its cell body in the spinal cord, and whose axon terminates at the **motor end plate** of the muscle. The NMJ has been extensively studied. It was one of the first synapses to be characterized anatomically, physiologically, and biochemically, because the muscle cell is large enough to take several electrodes, and because the NMJ can be seen under the light microscope.

The electrical information (action potential) is transduced to a chemical signal in the form of a neurotransmitter, **acetylcholine** (ACh; see also p. 101), which is transduced back to an action potential in the muscle. The action potential is then transduced to mechanical work as a muscle twitch. Usually, one axon innervates one fiber.

Shortly before the **axon** arrives at the end plate, it loses the **myelin sheath** and forms several thin branches. At the end plate, the axon terminal swells into the bouton, which is covered by a layer of **Schwann cells**. The presynaptic bouton contains synaptic **vesicles**, filled with ACh. The bouton occupies a depression in the muscle fiber surface. The **postsynaptic membrane** lies approximately 50 nm opposite, and is extensively **folded** opposite the bouton, with a high density of **acetylcholine receptors**. ACh receptors have been visualized at the NMJ using autoradiography. ACh receptors were labeled with radioactive antibodies to the receptors, or with a snake venom, α-bungarotoxin, which binds ACh receptors irreversibly. (ACh receptors at the NMJ and at autonomic ganglia are termed 'nicotinic', because they were originally studied using the partial agonist, nicotine.)

At the crest of the junctional fold, the density of ACh receptors is about 10^4 receptors per μm^2. There is a connective tissue layer over the muscle, the basement membrane, or basal lamina, consisting of glycoproteins and collagen. The basement membrane contains a high density of the enzyme **acetylcholinesterase**, one of the fastest-acting enzymes secreted from the postsynaptic cell, mainly in the synaptic folds. Acetylcholinesterase breaks down ACh and is the mechanism whereby the action of ACh is rapidly terminated. Acetylcholinesterase can be inhibited by a clinically important group of enzyme inhibitors called anticholinesterases. Short-acting anticholinesterases, such as edrophonium can be used to diagnose the muscle-weakening disease myasthenia gravis, while longer-acting anticholinesterases, such as neostigmine, are used in treatment.

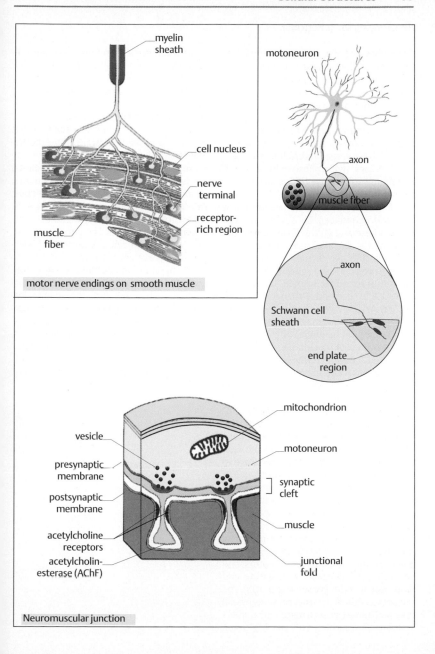

motor nerve endings on smooth muscle

Neuromuscular junction

Neuromuscular Junction II

Acetylcholine (ACh) is the neurotransmitter at the neuromuscular junction. Chemically, it is a choline ester. ACh is synthesized at the **cholinergic** nerve terminal from **choline** and **acetyl coenzyme A** (acetyl CoA). The reaction is catalyzed by the enzyme **choline acetyltransferase** (also referred to sometimes as choline acetylase). Newly synthesized ACh is packaged into **vesicles**, which fuse with the cell membrane and release their contents into the synaptic cleft.

ACh release from the nerve terminal at the NMJ is effected by several mechanisms. These are: (i) the formation of the vesicles; (ii) the presence of the active zone, which is the region of nerve membrane proteins specialized for neurotransmitter release, and (iii) the voltage-gated Ca^{2+} channels. Release occurs in quanta, or packages, each of which involves several thousand molecules of ACh. Release occurs spontaneously at a relatively low rate. A much larger quantal release of ACh occurs in response to the arrival at the nerve terminal of the **impulse**, or action potential (AP). The AP causes the influx of Ca^{2+} ions through voltage-gated channels into the nerve terminal, and intracellular Ca^{2+} triggers the fusion of vesicles with the nerve terminal membrane. The released ACh diffuses across the synaptic cleft to **nicotinic ACh receptors** in crests of the folds of the postsynaptic muscle membrane. Two ACh molecules bind to one receptor, and this results in the opening of the receptor channel to Na^+. The resultant stimulation of the muscle end plate is called an **end plate potential** (EPP; see also p. 105). One vesicle delivers one quantum of ACh to the receptors, and one quantum generates a miniature end plate potential (MEPP; see also p. 105). The release of ACh from the nerve terminal may be blocked by pharmacological intervention. Ions such as Co^{2+} and Mg^{2+}, and neurotoxins such as botulinum toxin will prevent fusion of the vesicles with the membrane.

Important pharmacological and therapeutic agents, such as **tubocurarine** and **suxamethonium** reduce the effects of ACh on the receptors by blocking the binding and effects of the neurotransmitter on the receptor.

Inactivation of ACh as a neurotransmitter is rapidly accomplished through the action of the enzyme **acetylcholinesterase**. This enzyme inactivates ACh by hydrolyzing it to choline and acetate. Choline is taken up by the nerve terminal for recycling in the ACh synthetic pathway, and the uptake process can be blocked by the compound **hemicholinium**. Although interesting as an experimental tool, hemicholinium has no use therapeutically. Acetylcholinesterase occurs mainly on the postsynaptic side in the muscle; it is known to be secreted into the cleft from the basement membrane of the end plate. The enzyme can be blocked by a series of important chemicals, the anticholinesterases.

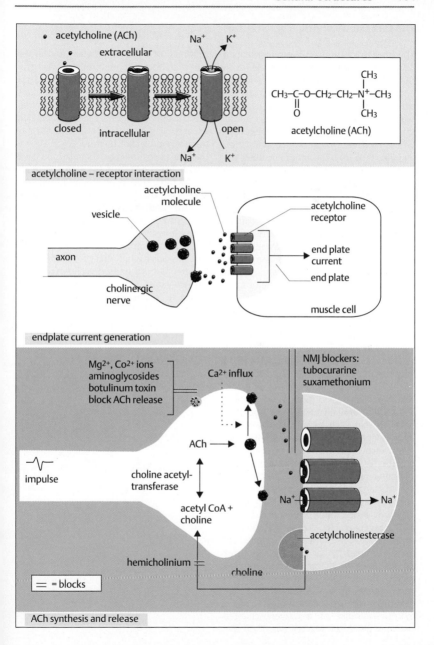

acetylcholine (ACh)

extracellular

closed   intracellular   open

$$CH_3-C-O-CH_2-CH_2-N^+-CH_3$$
$$\quad\;\; \| \qquad\qquad\qquad\quad |$$
$$\quad\;\; O \qquad\qquad\qquad\quad CH_3$$

acetylcholine (ACh)

acetylcholine – receptor interaction

acetylcholine molecule

vesicle

acetylcholine receptor

end plate current

end plate

axon

cholinergic nerve

muscle cell

endplate current generation

Mg^{2+}, Co^{2+} ions
aminoglycosides
botulinum toxin
block ACh release

Ca^{2+} influx

NMJ blockers:
tubocurarine
suxamethonium

impulse

ACh

choline acetyl-transferase

acetyl CoA + choline

Na^+ Na^+

acetylcholinesterase

hemicholinium

choline

= blocks

ACh synthesis and release

The Nicotinic Acetylcholine Receptor

The **nicotinic acetylcholine receptor** is a ligand-gated ion channel that mediates the action of ACh at several sites in the body, including the ganglia and at the neuromuscular junction. The receptor has been extensively characterized biochemically, largely through studies of the receptors of electric organisms such as *Torpedo* and *Electrophorus*. The genes encoding the receptor have been sequenced, and the amino acid sequence of the receptor has been determined. From knowledge of the amino acid sequence, the secondary and tertiary structures of the receptor can be predicted. The receptor has been visualized using the electron microscope.

The nicotine ACh receptor is a glycoprotein of molecular weight about 275 000, and spans the cell membrane. The ACh receptor in electric organs of fish consists of four separate **subunits** termed α, β, δ, γ. In adult mammals, the receptor has an e subunit instead of γ. There are two subunits that have a high affinity for ACh, and one molecule of ACh must bind to each subunit for the receptor channel to open. The ACh-binding site occurs extracellularly near two cysteine residues on a hydrophilic domain of the subunit. It is believed that each subunit contains four hydrophobic regions, and each of these regions forms an α-helix that spans the membrane. The four putative membrane-spanning regions have been labeled M1, M2, M3, and M4. The M2 region together with the region that connects M2 and M3 may provide the lining of the pore channel of the receptor. The channel exhibits cation selectivity ($K^+ > Na^+ > Li^+$), which may be determined by the presence of three rings of negative charge that flank the M2 region. This selectivity can be changed by point mutations in the central ring. The negative charge of each ring is determined by the presence of negatively charged amino acids in the M2 regions of all five subunits, of which glutamate and aspartate are the most predominant. One ring occurs in the cytoplasmic domain of the receptor, at the inner mouth of the channel, and is formed by amino acids linking the M1 and M2 regions. There is a centrally situated ring consisting of amino acids of the M2 region, and the third ring in the extracellular region consists of amino acids which link the M2 and M3 regions. The internal and external rings may function as anion-blocking sites at both funnel mouths, and the central ring within the membrane may act as a filter that determines ion selectivity.

The receptor has been visualized, and is shaped somewhat like a funnel that widens at both ends (2.5-3 nm), with a very narrow, short central membrane-spanning region of 0.6-0.8 nm diameter.

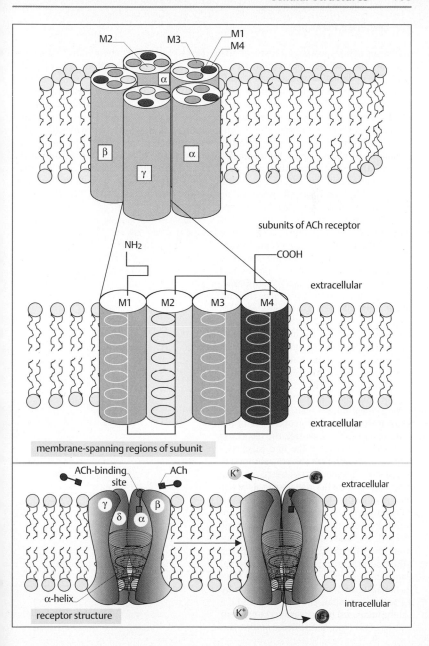

M2   M3   M1
            M4

α

β
γ

subunits of ACh receptor

NH$_2$

COOH

extracellular

M1   M2   M3   M4

extracellular

membrane-spanning regions of subunit

ACh-binding
site   ACh   K$^+$ extracellular

γ
δ   α   β

α-helix   intracellular

receptor structure   K$^+$

The End Plate Potential

When an action potential arrives at the nerve terminal of the motoneuron, it triggers the opening of voltage-gated Ca^{2+} channels, Ca^{2+} influx, and thus an increase in intracellular Ca^{2+}. This in turn causes the fusion of ACh-containing **vesicles** at the active zone in the presynaptic membrane. This results in the release into the synaptic cleft of about 2.5×10^7 molecules of ACh. The neurotransmitter takes less than a millisecond to diffuse across the cleft to the postsynaptic membrane, where it combines with the ACh **receptors**. The binding of two ACh molecules with the ACh receptor causes the opening of the cation-selective ACh receptor **channel**. Due to the high electromotive force for Na^+, there is an influx of Na^+, which depolarizes the postsynaptic membrane. This sequence of events produces the **end plate potential** (EPP). The EPP in turn opens voltage-gated Na^+ channels to cause the action potential to fire off. If the release of ACh from the nerve terminal is blocked, then it is no longer possible to measure the EPP from the end plate after stimulation of the nerve.

The end plate potential can be seen during recordings taken from the end plate as the initial portion of the rise of the action potential. If, however, the recording is made from outside the end plate, the EPP is not observed. Even in the absence of nerve stimulation it is possible to measure continual, relatively small potentials at the end plate when the muscle is mechanically at rest. These small potentials are termed **miniature end plate potentials** (MEPP). The MEPP has the same approximate shape as the EPP but is smaller. The MEPP occurs because the nerve terminal continuously releases quanta of ACh even in the absence of electrical stimulation by an action potential. The size of the MEPP can be increased by increasing the concentration of Ca^{2+} ions at the nerve ending (i.e. by increasing the rate of ACh release). The EPP is therefore a summation of many MEPPs.

The EPP differs from the action potential in that it is just subthreshold. This can be explained in terms of membrane capacitance, which is discharged during the initial current flow. The membrane capacitance recharges slowly through the resting membrane potential, until equilibrium is finally restored when the membrane capacitance is fully recharged to the resting potential E_R.

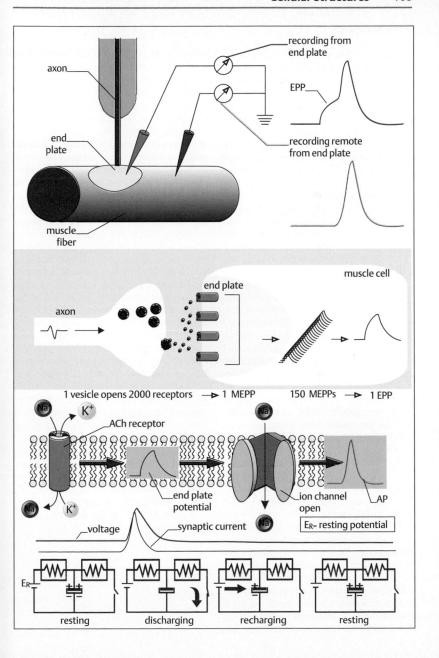

recording from
end plate

EPP

recording remote
from end plate

axon

end
plate

muscle
fiber

muscle cell

end plate

axon

1 vesicle opens 2000 receptors → 1 MEPP   150 MEPPs → 1 EPP

Na   K⁺

ACh receptor

Na

end plate
potential

ion channel
open

AP

E_R= resting potential

Na   K⁺

voltage   synaptic current

Na

E_R

resting   discharging   recharging   resting

GABA Receptors

GABA (γ-aminobutyric acid) is the most widely distributed inhibitory neurotransmitter in the vertebrate CNS, and is believed to be responsible for at least 40% of all CNS inhibitory processes. GABAergic neurons are found in large abundance in the cerebellum and neocortex, although their distribution is widespread in the CNS, including the **spinal cord**, mainly in **interneurons**. GABA is formed by the action of glutamic acid decarboxylase (GAD). GABA appears to be stored in vesicles in the nerve terminal, and is released through a Ca^{2+}-sensitive mechanism. Following its release into the synaptic cleft, GABA binds to postsynaptic receptors, of which there are at least three subtypes, termed **GABA$_A$**, **GABA$_B$**, and **GABA$_C$**.

The **GABA$_A$** receptor is a ligand-gated chloride channel. It is a pentamer, composed of several subunits, namely α, β, γ, and δ, and there are several different forms of the subunits as well. There are at least 13 different subtypes of the receptor, depending on the nature of the various subunits in the receptor. The α, β, and γ subunits need to be present for the GABA$_A$ receptor to function properly. The receptor binds the agonists **GABA** and muscimol, and the antagonist bicuculline on the α and β subunit. In addition, there are binding sites on the receptor for **barbiturates** (which are sedative-hypnotic), **ethanol**, and on the α subunit for the **benzodiazepines**. All of these substances potentiate the channel-opening action of GABA on the GABA$_A$ receptor.

The **GABA$_B$** receptor has seven membrane-spanning domains and is coupled to a **G protein,** which inhibits the formation of cyclic AMP. This causes the closing of Ca^{2+} channels and the opening of K^+ channels. (The adrenergic α_2 and dopaminergic D_2 receptors have a similar action on these ionic channels.) The GABA$_B$ receptor binds **GABA** and also the muscle relaxant baclofen (β-chlorophenyl GABA), which does not bind to GABA$_A$ receptors. GABA$_B$ receptors appear to occur mainly on nerve terminals or axons, therefore mediating presynaptic influences on neurotransmitter discharge.

GABA$_C$ receptors are a more recent discovery, and appear to occur predominantly in the vertebrate **retina**. The receptor binds GABA, muscimol and the agonists *cis*- and *trans*-4-aminocrotonic acid (CACA, TACA, respectively), and is insensitive to baclofen and bicuculline. Structurally, the receptor consists of so-called ϱ subunits, which have now been cloned from a human cDNA library. The ϱ subunits form homo-oligomeric chloride channels, which are sensitive to picrotoxin but not to bicuculline. Apart from the retina, receptors are also significantly expressed in the hippocampus and neocortex. When GABA or other agonists bind to the GABA$_C$ receptor, it activates a chloride ionophore. There is evidence that binding of 5-HT or glutamate to their receptors activates the protein phospholipase C (**PLC**) through a G protein to increase intracellular diacylglycerol (**DAG**). DAG enhances phosphorylation of the GABA$_C$ receptor by protein kinase, which results in the inhibition of the GABA$_C$ receptor.

GABA is inhibitory in the CNS in the reciprocal inhibition of extensor and flexor **motoneurons** in the spinal cord. GABA interneurons are activated by incoming afferents from stretch receptors in skeletal muscle, and these inhibit the firing of the appropriate motoneurons.

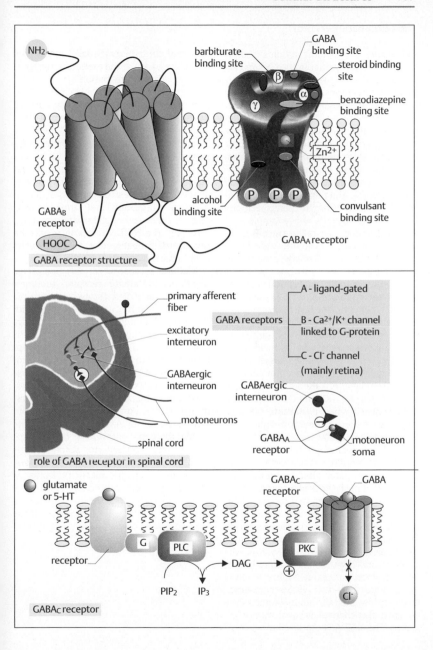

GABA receptor structure

role of GABA receptor in spinal cord

GABA$_C$ receptor

The Glutamate Receptor

Glutamate is the most abundant excitatory neurotransmitter in the CNS and activates a variety of specific receptors. Many glutamate receptor subtypes have been reported, but it is possible to categorize glutamate receptors into two basic types: **ligand- or directly-gated ion channels,** sometimes referred to as ionotropic receptors, and **G protein-coupled 'metabotropic' glutamate (mGlu) receptors.**

The various **ligand-gated ion channel receptors** for glutamate were differentiated originally through their specificity for different ligands. For example, the **NMDA receptor** is so-called since it binds the glutamate-like synthetic agonist N-methyl-D-aspartate. Similarly, other glutamate receptors were discovered, which bind other ligands, notably **kainate** and **kainate-quisqualate-A (AMPA)** – binding receptor subtypes. The NMDA receptor can be distinguished from the other subtypes using the antagonists APV (2-amino-5-phosphonovalerate, or the hallucinogenic drug PCP (phenylcyclidine; 'angel dust'). Functionally, the NMDA receptor contains a high conductance cation channel that is permeable to Na^+, K^+, and Ca^{2+}. The channel is opened when **glutamate** binds to the receptor site, and neurotransmitter action is modulated by a number of other agents. Glutamate requires glycine, which binds to its own site on the receptor. Glutamate action is potentiated by polyamines, and the channel is blocked by extracellular Mg^{2+} at !65 mV, the normal resting membrane potential, and by dizolcipine, Zn^{2+}, and H^+ which all bind to unique sites on the receptor. When the cell membrane is depolarized, Mg^{2+} is driven out of the channel, and if glutamate is bound to its receptor, then the channel opens to allow Na^+ and Ca^{2+} into it. If glycine concentrations are low, then the ability of glutamate to open the channel is significantly reduced. The NMDA receptor-channel complex may contribute virtually exclusively to the late phase of the excitatory synaptic current. This contribution is revealed through the use of APV. At a membrane potential of !80 mV, little if any current flows through the NMDA channel, but when the membrane is depolarized to 20 mV, a large, late AMP-sensitive component is revealed.

Physiologically, NMDA receptors are believed to be involved in neural signaling, neural gene expression, and in synaptic plasticity, outgrowth, and survival. Also, massive excitation of glutamate receptors, especially the NMDA receptor, results in cell death, probably due to excessively high intracellular levels of Ca^{2+}.

Kainate receptors. At least two other ionotropic glutamate receptor subtypes have been identified through the use of selective agonists, antagonists, and through the cloning of cDNAs that encode pharmacologically distinct receptors. It was discovered that the neurotoxin kainate binds to glutamate receptors, and that certain of these kainate receptors are antagonized by the drug AMPA and others not. For example, primary afferent C-fibers in the spinal cord are depolarized by kainate but not by AMPA.

Metabotropic glutamate (mGlu) receptors are coupled to second messengers, and are believed to have important roles in synaptic plasticity, learning, memory, and neuroprotection.

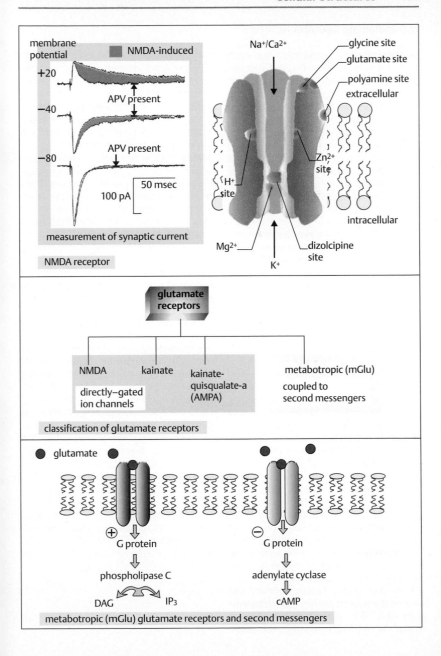

membrane
potential

NMDA-induced

Na⁺/Ca²⁺

glycine site
glutamate site
polyamine site
extracellular

+20

APV present

−40

APV present

−80

Zn²⁺ site

H⁺ site

50 msec

intracellular

100 pA

measurement of synaptic current

Mg²⁺

dizolcipine site

NMDA receptor

K⁺

glutamate receptors

NMDA   kainate   kainate-quisqualate-a (AMPA)   metabotropic (mGlu)

directly–gated ion channels

coupled to second messengers

classification of glutamate receptors

glutamate

$\oplus$
G protein

$\ominus$
G protein

phospholipase C

adenylate cyclase

DAG   IP₃

cAMP

metabotropic (mGlu) glutamate receptors and second messengers

Catecholamine Neurotransmitters

Norepinephrine, a **catecholamine**, (called **noradrenaline** in the UK) is the principal neurotransmitter of the adrenergic nervous system. **Epinephrine** (**adrenaline**), another catecholamine, acts both as a neurotransmitter and a hormone. **Dopamine**, also a catecholamine, is an important neurotransmitter, especially in the CNS, where it is the most abundant catecholamine neurotransmitter. These neurochemicals bind to specific receptors, which may be ligand-gated ion channels or linked to intracellular second messenger systems.

Catecholamines are **synthesized** at the nerve terminal and stored in **vesicles**. Dietary phenylalanine is converted to **tyrosine**, which is taken up into the cytoplasm of the nerve terminal and hydroxylated to form **DOPA** by **tyrosine hydroxylase**. This is the rate-limiting step of catecholamine biosynthesis. Tyrosine hydroxylase requires iron, molecular O_2 and tetrahydrobiopterin as cofactor. The cofactor helps to keep TH active in a reduced state. When NE or dopamine accumulate in the cytoplasm they inhibit the action of the cofactor. Thus the neurotransmitters control the action of TH by end-product inhibition. DOPA is converted to **dopamine**, which enters the vesicle and is converted to norepinephrine (**NE**). NE is stored in the vesicle in association with ATP, Ca^{2+}, neuropeptide Y as cotransmitter, and a protein called chromogranin. In the adrenal medulla, NE is subsequently methylated to form epinephrine (**EP**). EP is also formed in several CNS nerve terminals.

NE is **released** from the nerve terminal when an action potential arrives and mobilizes Ca^{2+} stores, which enable the vesicles to fuse with the cell membrane and release the neurotransmitter into the synaptic cleft. The neurotransmitter diffuses across the cleft and binds to its **receptors**.

Catecholamine receptors occur as several different subtypes depending on the affinity for NE, EP or dopamine. The major NE/EP subtypes are α_1, α_2, β_1, and β_2. The α_1 and β receptors occur predominantly postsynaptically, while the α_2 receptor occurs mainly presynaptically in the CNS and acts as an autoreceptor limiting the release of NE and other neurotransmitters such as 5-HT and glutamate. Autoreceptors regulate the release of the neurotransmitter. There is now evidence that there are many different subtypes of α_1 and α_2 receptors in the CNS, but the significance of this variation is not known.

The action of the catecholamine neurotransmitters is terminated by their uptake into the nerve terminal by active transport, which requires ATP. This transport mechanism is called **uptake 1**. There is another uptake mechanism into the postsynaptic cell, called **uptake 2.** Once in the nerve terminal, NE may enter a vesicle or the mitochondrion where it is metabolized by **monoamine oxidase** (MAO). MAO is an important metabolic enzyme, found principally in neural and glial cells and in liver, glandular tissue, and the gut. There are two forms of MAO, MAO-A and MAO-B. MAO oxidizes the catecholamines to their corresponding aldehydes. The enzyme is an important target for inhibitors, the **MAOI** drugs, which are used to keep biological concentrations of catecholamines high. MAOI drugs have been used to treat clinical depression, for example. The catecholamins are metabolized also by a cytoplasmic enzyme, **catechol-*O*-methyltransferase (COMT)**, which occurs in high concentrations in liver and kidney.

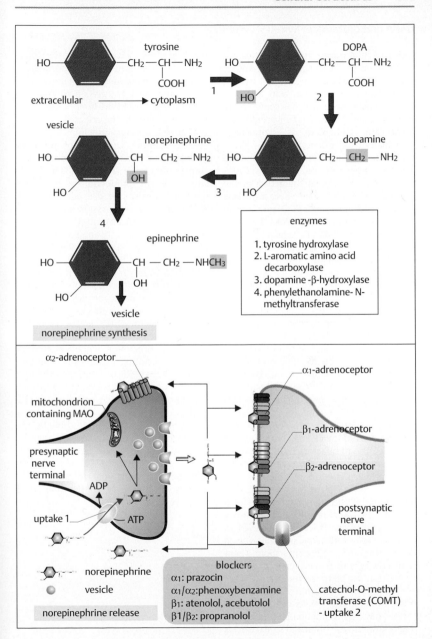

tyrosine

DOPA

extracellular ⟶ cytoplasm

vesicle

norepinephrine

dopamine

epinephrine

enzymes

1. tyrosine hydroxylase
2. L-aromatic amino acid decarboxylase
3. dopamine-β-hydroxylase
4. phenylethanolamine-N-methyltransferase

norepinephrine synthesis

α₂-adrenoceptor

α₁-adrenoceptor

mitochondrion containing MAO

β₁-adrenoceptor

β₂-adrenoceptor

presynaptic nerve terminal

ADP

ATP

uptake 1

postsynaptic nerve terminal

norepinephrine

vesicle

catechol-O-methyl transferase (COMT) - uptake 2

blockers
α₁: prazocin
α₁/α₂: phenoxybenzamine
β₁: atenolol, acebutolol
β₁/β₂: propranolol

norepinephrine release

GABA and Glutamate: Synthesis and Role

GABA and **glutamate** are both synthesized and broken down in pathways linked to the **citric acid cycle** (Krebs cycle), and the GABA shunt. The citric acid cycle is powered by glucose, which is converted to **pyruvate**, which in turn is converted to **oxaloacetate**. Glutamate is synthesized principally from α-ketoglutarate or from the amino acid aspartate, although it can also be synthesized from glutamine. GABA is synthesized through the action of the enzyme **glutamic acid decarboxylase** (**GAD**), which removes a COO$^-$ group from glutamate. GABA is broken down by **GABA transaminase** (**GABA-T**), which regenerates glutamate through the formation of **succinic semialdehyde**. Thus the metabolism of the principal CNS excitatory and inhibitory neurotransmitters is intimately linked. Both GABA and glutamate are present in relatively huge concentrations in the brain. GABA, for example, is present in concentrations at least 1000-fold higher than those of the catecholamines.

Glutamate pathways appear to be the major form of excitatory output, or efferents, from the cortex and cerebellum to other brain areas. These include the **corticostriatal**, bulbar, pontine, and thalamic pathways. Glutamate may be the neurotransmitter of the cerebellar mossy fiber afferents, and of olfactory bulb pathways.

The major concentration of **GABAergic innervation** occurs in the brain, spinal cord, and retina (in the form of inhibitory interneurons), and mainly within localized sites where GABA is a local modulatory neurotransmitter. There is, however, a relatively long GABAergic projection from the striatum to the substantia nigra. There is also thought to be a projection from hypothalamic nuclei to the forebrain.

The high concentration of these neurotransmitters in the CNS renders it difficult to determine their functions. However, the role of GABA in the brain and spinal cord is being gradually elucidated. In the spinal cord, for example, GABA interneurons modulate transmission of pain impulses to the brain, and transmission to opposing skeletal muscles. In the brain, GABA interneurons modulate the release of peptides that govern pituitary function.

For example, the **anterior pituitary gland** secretes the hormone adrenocorticotropic hormone (**ACTH**), which in turn stimulates the production of the stress hormone cortisol by the adrenal gland. ACTH release is enhanced by **stress** and by excitatory neurotransmitters such as 5-HT; GABAergic neurons inhibit the release of ACTH, perhaps by inhibiting 5-HT release.

Similarly, GABA inhibits the release of the anterior pituitary hormone **prolactin**. Prolactin release is controlled by the hypothalamus, which releases a prolactin-inhibiting factor (**PIF**), and a prolactin-releasing factor (**PRF**). The major PIF appears to be dopamine, while a number of peptides, including angiotensin II and substance P, act as PRF. In addition, GABAergic terminals have been found in the median eminence, and they do appear to release GABA into the pituitary blood portal system (see p. 299). Thus, GABA could be acting as another PIF. Since stress is a potent cause of both ACTH and prolactin release, this suggests that GABA, and possibly glutamate, have a role to play, either directly or indirectly, in the release of stress-related hormones.

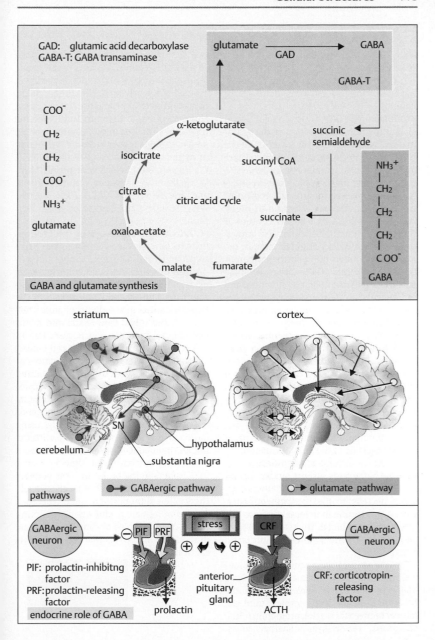

GAD: glutamic acid decarboxylase
GABA-T: GABA transaminase

glutamate $\xrightarrow{\text{GAD}}$ GABA

GABA-T

$$
\begin{array}{l}
\text{COO}^- \\
| \\
\text{CH}_2 \\
| \\
\text{CH}_2 \\
| \\
\text{COO}^- \\
| \\
\text{NH}_3^+
\end{array}
$$

glutamate

α-ketoglutarate

isocitrate

succinyl CoA

citrate

citric acid cycle

oxaloacetate

succinate

malate

fumarate

succinic semialdehyde

$$
\begin{array}{l}
\text{NH}_3^+ \\
| \\
\text{CH}_2 \\
| \\
\text{CH}_2 \\
| \\
\text{CH}_2 \\
| \\
\text{C OO}^-
\end{array}
$$

GABA

GABA and glutamate synthesis

striatum

cortex

SN

cerebellum

hypothalamus

substantia nigra

pathways

●→ GABAergic pathway

○→ glutamate pathway

GABAergic neuron → ⊖ PIF PRF

stress ⊕ ⊕

CRF ⊖ ← GABAergic neuron

PIF: prolactin-inhibitng factor
PRF: prolactin-releasing factor

anterior pituitary gland

prolactin

ACTH

CRF: corticotropin-releasing factor

endocrine role of GABA

Catecholamine Pathways in CNS

Norepinephrine, **epinephrine**, and **dopamine** are important CNS neurotransmitters, and their pathways and receptors have been mapped and localized to a large extent.

Dopamine (**DA**) is the major catecholamine neurotransmitter of the mammalian CNS, comprising at least 50% of the total CNS catecholamine content. There are four major dopaminergic pathways in the brain. The **mesolimbic** pathway originates in the **ventral tegmental region** of the midbrain, near the **substantial nigra**, and projects to several higher centers of the limbic system, including the **amygdala**, the **frontal** and **cingulate cortex**, the nucleus acumbens, the olfactory tubercle, and the **septum**. These areas mediate mood changes and cognitive function, and are believed to be the sites where drugs such as cocaine and amphetamines produce their stimulant effects. Other CNS drugs such as **antidepressants**, which block MAO, and **antischizophrenia neuroleptic** drugs, which block DA receptors, may act in these regions. The **nigrostriatal** pathway projects from the substantia nigra to the **corpus striatum**, and specifically to the putamen and caudate nuclei, which are implicated in the control of fine motor function. The **mesocortical** pathway projects from the ventral tegmentum to the frontal cortex, and the **tuberoinfundibular** pathway is a short but important DA projection from the hypothalamic arcuate nucleus to the median eminence, where the terminals release DA into the pituitary portal blood. The released DA has an hormonal role, suppressing prolactin release.

Noradrenergic innervation of the brain is diffuse, and projections are widespread. Major noradrenergic nuclei occur in the brain stem in the locus ceruleus and the **lateral tegmental nuclei**, projecting to the **thalamus**, **cerebellum**, olfactory lobes, and the **neocortex**. The precise functions of these projections are largely unknown, but may involve cognition, alertness, arousal and motivation. Noradrenergic innervation also appears to involve central components of autonomic and endocrine function. For example, noradrenergic pathways appear to coordinate the release of hypothalamic releasing factors such as CRF (see p. 301), which controls ACTH release from the anterior pituitary gland, and the release of GnRH (see p. 303), which controls the release of gonadotrophins.

Adrenergic pathways in the CNS appear to be restricted mainly to the brain stem and modulate autonomic and endocrine function. Adrenergic nuclei occur principally in the dorsal and ventral **tegmentum**, and ascend to terminate in the **hypothalamus** in the diencephalon. They descend the spinal cord to the intermediolateral cell column, which gives rise to the sympathetic preganglionic cell bodies.

The catecholaminergic innervation of the various CNS regions can be visualized by localizing the receptors the catecholamines act upon. This can be done by autoradiography, when radioactive ligands are attached to the receptors, or by using radioactive probes that hybridize with the mRNA that codes for the receptor. Thus, α and β receptors have been shown to occur very widely in the brain, and it is possible to distinguish between the localization of the various subtypes of α and β receptors. These findings are useful when attempting to discover the roles of catecholaminergic innervation in both normal and pathological brain function.

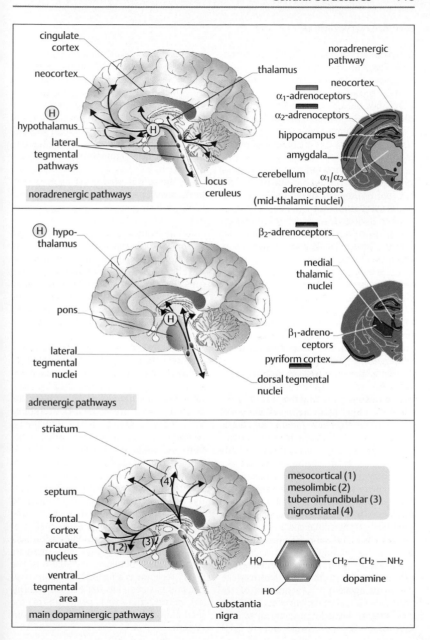

cingulate cortex
neocortex
(H) hypothalamus
lateral tegmental pathways

thalamus

noradrenergic pathway
neocortex
α_1-adrenoceptors
α_2-adrenoceptors
hippocampus
amygdala

locus ceruleus
cerebellum
α_1/α_2 adrenoceptors
(mid-thalamic nuclei)

noradrenergic pathways

(H) hypo-thalamus

pons

lateral tegmental nuclei

β_2-adrenoceptors

medial thalamic nuclei

β_1-adreno-ceptors

pyriform cortex

dorsal tegmental nuclei

adrenergic pathways

striatum
septum
frontal cortex
arcuate nucleus
ventral tegmental area

(4)

(1,2)
(3)

mesocortical (1)
mesolimbic (2)
tuberoinfundibular (3)
nigrostriatal (4)

HO — CH$_2$ — CH$_2$ — NH$_2$
HO

dopamine

substantia nigra

main dopaminergic pathways

5-Hydroxytryptamine

5-Hydroxytryptamine (**5-HT**; **serotonin**) is an indolamine neurotransmitter, and its pathways in the CNS parallel, approximately, those of norepinephrine. 5-HT is found not only in brain cells but also in blood platelets, enterochromaffin cells in the gut, and in mast cells. It also occurs in the pineal, where it is the precursor of melatonin.

5-HT is **synthesized** from the essential dietary amino acid **tryptophan**. In the neuron, tryptophan is hydroxylated to **5-hydroxytryptophan** by the enzyme **tryptophan hydroxylase**, which resembles tyrosine, since tryptophan hydroxylase also requires molecular O_2 and a tetrahydropteridine cofactor. Unlike tyrosine hydroxylase, whose activity is regulated by norepinephrine, 5-HT does not regulate the activity of tryptophan hydroxylase. Finally, 5-hydroxytryptophan is decarboxylated to **5-HT** by the enzyme **L-amino acid decarboxylase**. Once synthesized, 5-HT is stored in granules, or vesicles, in the nerve terminal.

There are several **serotonergic pathways** in the CNS. These originate in the **raphe nuclei** in the midline region of the pons and upper brain stem. Cell bodies of the 5-HT neurons have been grouped and classified as B1 through B9 serotonergic nerve groups. Groups lying more rostrally in the brain stem (B4-B9) innervate the higher centers i.e. cerebellum, the neocortex, thalamus, and the limbic system. The more caudally placed serotonergic nuclei innervate lower CNS centers, such as the medulla and the spinal cord.

What is known of 5-HT function in the CNS comes mainly from studies with drugs such as *p*-cholorophenylalanine, which inhibits tryptophan hydroxylase, and with agonists or antagonists of the various 5-HT receptors. Midbrain 5-HT nuclei have an intrinsic pacemaker activity blocked by norepinephrine and by 5-HT autoreceptors. Pacemaker activity is high during wakefulness, low during sleep, and cannot be recorded during REM (rapid eye movement) sleep. Various hallucinogenic drugs, such as lysergic acid diethylamide (LSD), are structurally similar to 5-HT, and may exert their effects through interactions with 5-HT receptors. 5-HT may mediate social interactions between individuals.

In the **spinal cord**, 5-HT neurons may be involved in a **central pattern generator** (CPG), which generates patterned motor output. The CPG regulates motoneuron excitability by means of a rhythmic lowering of the motoneuron membrane potential. This produces an alternating modulation of reflex inputs and outputs to opposing muscles. The motor behaviors associated with the CPG identified so far include swimming, walking, running, chewing, licking, biting, and grooming with the tongue in animals.

Multiple forms of 5-HT receptors exist. The receptors may be ligand-gated or coupled to G proteins and second messenger systems. Receptors may be excitatory or inhibitory. $5-HT_2$ receptors are generally excitatory, while $5-HT_1$ receptors are mainly inhibitory. $5-HT_{1A}$ and $5-HT_{1D}$ receptors are coupled to G_i transducer proteins and inhibit cyclic AMP production. $5-HT_{1A}$ receptors have been localized to raphe nucleus nerve cells, and appear to act as autoreceptors, to inhibit 5-HT activity. $5-HT_{1D}$ receptors have been localized to the basal ganglia, and may be involved in control of voluntary muscle. $5-HT_2$ receptors activate the phosphoinositol second messenger system and mediate depolarization of neocortical neurons. The $5-HT_3$ receptor is a ligand-gated ion channel, and has been localized to the entorhinal cortex, the area postrema of the medulla, and in the peripheral nervous system.

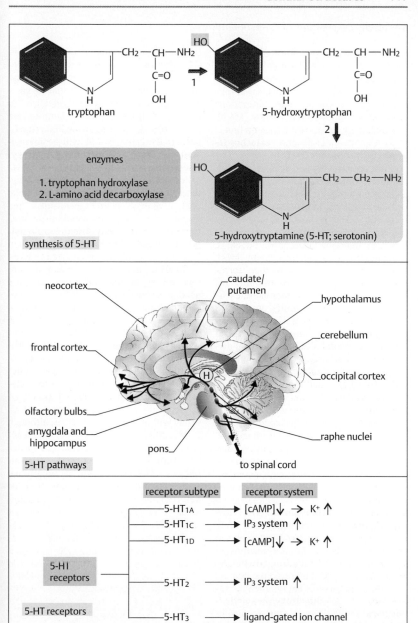

enzymes

1. tryptophan hydroxylase
2. L-amino acid decarboxylase

synthesis of 5-HT

5-HT pathways

5-HT receptors

Metabolic Disposition of Catecholamines

The actions of norepinephrine and epinephrine are terminated by uptake into the nerve terminal of other tissues, where they become subject to the actions of metabolizing enzymes. Two important enzymes are **monoamine oxidase** (MAO), of which there are at least two main types: MAO-A and MAO-B, and **catechol-O-methyltransferase** (COMT).

Both enzymes are widely distributed in the body. **MAO** occurs on the outer mitochondrial membrane in glial and neuronal cells, and in liver, kidney, gastrointestinal tract (GIT), and glandular cells. MAO is present in the nerve terminal where it metabolizes norepinephrine after uptake 1. Dopamine, too, is metabolized by MAO. MAO oxidizes the amines to their corresponding aldehydes. MAO is an important therapeutic target for the monoamine oxidase inhibitors (MAOI), which are used to treat clinical depression. The drugs may act to keep biogenic amines elevated and thus elevate mood. **COMT** is a widely distributed cytoplasmic enzyme found in highest concentrations in liver and kidney. COMT transfers a methyl group from S-adenosylmethionine to the 3-OH (hydroxyl) group on the catecholamine.

Some of the metabolic products of the two enzymes are important diagnostic tools. Most of the epinephrine and norepinephrine that enters the circulation after exocytosis from adrenergic nerve terminals, or from the adrenal medulla, or after administration, are first metabolized by COMT to **metanephrine** and **normetanephrine**, respectively. Any norepinephrine or epinephrine **released intraneuronally** will first be deaminated by MAO to **3,4-dihydroxyphenylglycoaldehyde** (DOPGAL). Within the neuron, DOPGAL may be reduced by aldehyde reductase to **3,4-dihydroxyphenylethyleneglycol** (DOPEG). In extraneuronal sites such as GIT or liver, if the catecholamine

has first been deaminated by MAO to DOPGAL, this metabolite is oxidized by aldehyde dehydrogenase to **3,4-dihydroxymandelic acid** (DOMA). Circulating catecholamines are preferentially oxidized to DOMA, while CNS catecholamines are preferentially reduced to DOPEG. Finally, both DOPEG and DOMA will be methylated by COMT to **3-methoxy-4-hydroxyphenylethyleneglycol** (MOPEG; also called MHPG) or to **3-methoxy-4-hydroxymandelic acid** (vanillylmandelic acid, VMA). Normetanephrine and metanephrine are both acted on by MAO to produce **3-methoxy-4-hydroxyphenylglycoaldehyde** (MOPGAL) which can then be reduced to MOPEG or oxidized to VMA.

MOPEG and VMA are major urinary metabolites of catecholamines, and are used as diagnostic indices of endogenous catecholamines. In humans, the normal twenty-four hour urinary excretion of MOPEG is 1.2-1.8 mg, and about 25% of this is thought to originate in the CNS. For VMA the normal urinary excretion is 2-4 mg. In addition, 100-300 mg of normetanephrine, 100 mg of metanephrine, 25-50 mg of norepinephrine, and 2-5 mg of epinephrine may be measured. MAOI drugs will increase these values, although COMT inhibitors will have no significant effect. Abnormal secretion of catecholamines, such as occurs in the rare condition of pheochromocytoma, an adrenal catecholamine-secreting tumor, will be detected by measuring urinary metabolites.

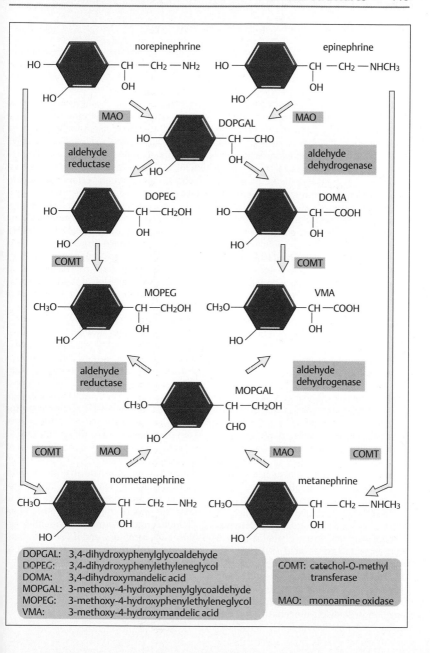

Metabolic Disposition of Dopamine and 5-HT

Dopamine is a major CNS catecholaminergic neurotransmitter, which has been implicated in certain diseases of the CNS, for example Parkinson's disease (see p. 370), and also in normal neuroendocrine function. Thus, dopamine has been identified as an important inhibitor of the release of prolactin from the anterior pituitary gland (see p. 112). Therefore, dopamine agonists and dopamine precursors have been developed to treat neuroendocrine disorders involving abnormal prolactin release, and to treat Parkinson's disease. It is therefore very important to be able to monitor the excretion of dopamine metabolites.

Dopamine is **metabolized** by **MAO** and **COMT**. The major urinary metabolites of dopamine are 3,4-dihydroxyphenylacetic acid (**DOPAC**) and 3-methoxy-4-hydroxyphenylacetic acid (**homovanillic acid, HVA**). Metabolism and excretion are very rapid, and at least 80% of an administered dose of dopamine is excreted in the urine within 20 minutes of administration of the dose. DOPAC and HVA account for about 50% of the metabolites of dopamine. Fecal excretion of dopamine metabolites is negligible. Lesser amounts of dopamine are metabolized directly by COMT to **methoxytyramine**, and to norepinephrine by **dopamine-β-hydroxylase**.

5-Hydroxytryptamine is widely distributed in the body, and is a CNS neurotransmitter. It is **metabolized** by oxidative deamination by the enzyme MAO to **5-hydroxyindoleacetaldehyde**, which is further oxidized by **aldehyde dehydrogenase** to the urinary metabolite **5-hydroxyindoleacetic acid** (**5-HIAA**). The normal adult human excretes about 2-10 mg of 5-HIAA due to metabolism of endogenous 5-HT. Relatively smaller amounts of 5-HT are reduced by the enzyme alcohol dehydrogenase to another urinary metabolite of 5-HT, 5-hydroxytryptophol (**5-HTOL**). The three enzymes that metabolize 5-HT are all present in the liver, and in other 5-HT-metabolizing tissues, including the CNS.

Patients with malignant carcinoid tumors, for example of enterochromaffin cells of the GIT, which normally synthesize 5-HT, will secrete significantly larger amounts of 5-HIAA. This makes measurement of this urinary metabolite of clinical importance, although certain amine-containing foods may also increase the urinary measurements of 5-HIAA. Consumption of ethyl alcohol will interfere with the normal pattern of metabolism of 5-HT. This occurs because ethyl alcohol ingestion results in elevated tissue levels of NADH. This suppresses the further oxidation of 5-hydroxyindoleacetaldehyde to 5-HIAA. Instead, the aldehyde is reduced to 5-HTOL.

The **ergot alkaloids**, found in ergot, a fungal contaminant of wheat, are in some respects structurally similar to endogenous dopamine and 5-HT. Thus their ingestion will interfere with normal metabolism of these substances. More importantly, some of these alkaloids compete with dopamine and 5-HT at their **receptor sites**. This has proven to be of importance both pathologically and therapeutically. 5-HT has been implicated in the dilatation of the cerebral arterioles that contributes to the pain of migraine, and an ergot alkaloid, **methysergide**, which acts as a partial agonist at 5-HT_1 receptors, has been used to treat the pain of migraine. Another ergot alkaloid, bromocriptine, is a dopamine agonist at D_1 receptors, and is used to inhibit the release of prolactin in the treatment of certain forms of infertility.

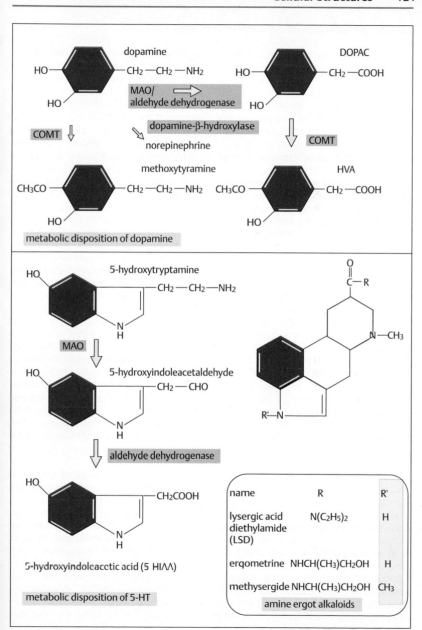

metabolic disposition of dopamine

metabolic disposition of 5-HT

name	R	R'
lysergic acid diethylamide (LSD)	N(C₂H₅)₂	H
ergometrine	NHCH(CH₃)CH₂OH	H
methysergide	NHCH(CH₃)CH₂OH	CH₃

amine ergot alkaloids

Cholinergic Pathways and Muscarinic Receptors

Cholinergic neuron systems occur in the peripheral and central nervous systems. In the CNS, they are widespread, and release ACh opposite **muscarinic** (**M**) and **nicotinic** (**N**) receptors. M receptors outnumber N receptors 10-100-fold in the CNS. In the CNS, major **cholinergic pathways** originate from cell bodies in the **septum**, **diagonal band of Broca**, and **basal nucleus** in the ventral forebrain, and project to **the hippocampus, interpeduncular nuclei**, and **neocortex**, respectively. Cortical cholinergic innervation appears to play a role in **memory**, and may be involved in the etiology of Alzheimer's disease (see p. 376). Within the **striatum** there are smaller cholinergic neurons involved in control of fine movement; blockade of these muscarinic receptors with atropine, a muscarinic antagonist, can be used to treat **parkinsonian tremor**. There are cholinergic cell bodies in the **brain stem tegmentum**, and these project to **hypothalamus** and thalamus. Cholinergic cell bodies of the **cranial parasympathetic outflow** occur in the brain stem, and lower down in the spinal cord in the **sacral region**. In the spinal cord are also the cholinergic cell bodies of the **thoracolumbar preganglionic sympathetic outflow** and those of the α-motoneurons.

The term **muscarinic** is derived from the poisonous mushroom *Amanita muscaria*, which contains muscarine. Muscarine produces parasympathomimetic effects after injection. A number of different **subtypes** of muscarinic receptors have been discovered, encoded by distinct but homologous genes. These receptors have been termed M_1-M_5, and different types are found in different proportions in different tissues. Despite their different genetic origin, the subtypes display remarkably similar patterns of affinity for various agonists and antagonists, and some, such as **zamifenacin**, an M_3 receptor antagonist, are being evaluated, for example, treatment of irritable bowel syndrome. The receptors transduce their ligand-activated signal through coupling to guanine nucleotide-binding regulatory proteins (**G proteins**).

There is evidence that in smooth muscle the **balance** between the contracted or relaxed state may depend on the relative activity of the sympathetic or parasympathetic drive to the muscle. The sympathetic drive to smooth muscle, mediated by the neurotransmitter **norepinephrine**, activates a G_s **protein**, which activates the enzyme **adenylate cyclase**. This results in increased **cAMP** production, and relaxation of the muscle. ACh is released by the **parasympathetic** nerve terminal and acts on M_2 **receptors**, which activate an **inhibitory G_i protein**, which in turn moves to and inactivates adenylate cyclase. Thus, synthesis of the second messenger cAMP is inhibited, and this increases muscle contractility. Also, ACh binds to an M_3 **receptor**, which activates a G_q **protein**, which activates the enzyme **phospholipase C** (**PLC**), which in turn activates the IP_3 **second messenger system**, which results in Ca^{2+} mobilization and increased contractility. A similar balance between noradrenergic and muscarinic inputs to neurons and glia may operate in the CNS.

Muscarinic receptors occur **presynaptically** as well as **postsynaptically** on CNS neurons, and the presynaptic receptors function as **autoreceptors** that, when activated by the released neurotransmitter, namely acetylcholine, modulate release of ACh. Both nicotinic and muscarinic receptors may occur at the same synapse. Recently, nicotinic autoreceptors have been found presynaptically in the substantia nigra, striatum, medial septum, hippocampus, and medial habenula, and may occur in other brain areas as well.

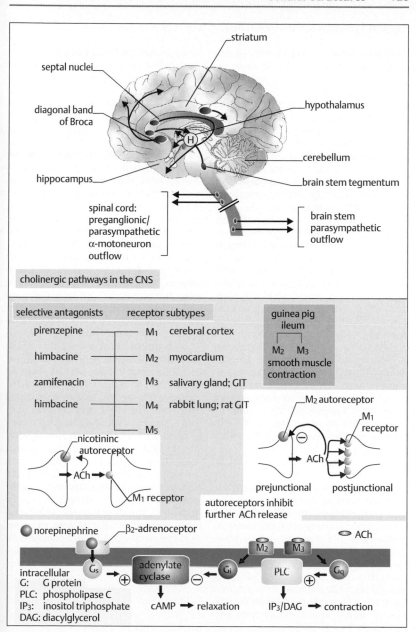

striatum

septal nuclei

diagonal band
of Broca

hippocampus

hypothalamus

cerebellum

brain stem tegmentum

spinal cord:
preganglionic/
parasympathetic
α-motoneuron
outflow

brain stem
parasympathetic
outflow

cholinergic pathways in the CNS

selective antagonists	receptor subtypes	
pirenzepine	M_1	cerebral cortex
himbacine	M_2	myocardium
zamifenacin	M_3	salivary gland; GIT
himbacine	M_4	rabbit lung; rat GIT
	M_5	

guinea pig
ileum

M_2 M_3
smooth muscle
contraction

nicotininc
autoreceptor

ACh

M_1 receptor

M_2 autoreceptor

M_1
receptor

ACh

prejunctional   postjunctional

autoreceptors inhibit
further ACh release

norepinephrine

β_2-adrenoceptor

ACh

M_2 M_3

intracellular
G: G protein
PLC: phospholipase C
IP_3: inositol triphosphate
DAG: diacylglycerol

G_s ⊕

adenylate
cyclase

⊖ G_i

PLC

⊕ G_q

cAMP → relaxation

IP_3/DAG → contraction

Central Synapses I: The Stretch Reflex

Synapses between cells in the central nervous system may be excitatory or **inhibitory**. Such duality of control is essential for integration and regulation of central control of sensory information and motor regulation. The **stretch reflex** is a powerful and easily understood example.

A monosynaptic reflex arc in the **spinal cord** consists, typically, of a sensory **afferent 1a fiber**, which synapses excitatorily with a **motoneuron** in the ventral horn of the spinal cord. The motoneuron's **axon** exits the cord and innervates the same muscle from which the afferent fiber came. When the afferent fiber is stimulated to release its excitatory transmitter onto the motoneuron, the motoneuron responds with an excitatory postsynaptic potential or **EPSP**. The excitatory neurotransmitter which causes an EPSP is most probably glutamate. The **tendon jerk response** is a well-known example of a monosynaptic reflex arc. The response is a simple test carried out to check for normal CNS-neuromuscular function. The **patellar tendon** of the muscle is tapped, which causes a brief stretch of the muscle and the muscle spindle. The intramuscular stretch receptor in turn fires off the 1a afferent, which excites the spinal motoneuron that innervates the same muscle, which twitches.

But innervation may also be inhibitory. A very good example is the reciprocal innervation of skeletal muscle. Muscles are often arranged in pairs, so that excitation and contraction of one are accompanied by inhibition and relaxation of an **antagonist** muscle. This is necessary for normal, coordinated movement. So, for the tendon stretch reflex and muscle response to occur, the flexor biceps muscle in the leg must relax while the quadriceps extensor contracts. This mechanism occurs because the 1a afferent from the quadriceps synapses in the spinal cord not only with the motoneuron that innervates the quadriceps, but also with an **inhibitory interneuron**, which in turn innervates the motoneuron that serves the biceps. Note that the same neurotransmitter (glutamate) that excites the motoneuron of the quadriceps also excites the inhibitory interneuron to the biceps.

The interneuron, however, must release a different neurotransmitter, which causes an inhibitory postsynaptic potential or **IPSP** on the biceps motoneuron, which is thereby prevented from sending excitatory messages to the biceps muscle. The identity of the inhibitory neurotransmitter is not known; but γ-amino butyric acid (GABA) and glycine are strong candidates. Both are powerful inhibitor neurotransmitters in the CNS. The inhibitory neurotransmitter released from the interneuron hyperpolarizes the motoneuron by binding to GABA or glycine receptors, which thus open their chloride (Cl-) channels. Note, however, that inhibition can also be mediated through activation of second messengers that open K^+ channels. The influx of Cl$^-$ adds to the negative charge inside the motoneuron cell, while the efflux of K^+ removes positive charge from inside the cell. Both theses events lead to an hyperpolarization.

The EPSP and IPSP can be characterized electrically through the experimental passing of currents into the afferents and the motoneuron, and the recording of potential changes. Ion fluxes, too, can be measured. The 1a afferent is readily accessible through the **dorsal root ganglion**, and the motoneuron is large enough to be penetrated by the electrodes for stimulation and recording.

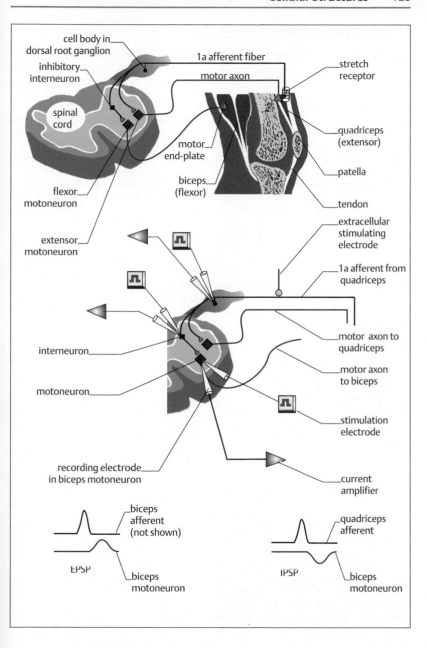

Central synapses II: Types of Synapse

Synaptic contact between cells in the CNS is made at several sites. Synapses may be **axodendritic**, **dendrodendritic**, **axoaxonic**, or **axosomatic**, the last indicating that an axon may synapse with the cell body. Dendrodendritic and axoaxonic synapses are relatively rare. This diversity of synaptic contact makes possible a vast array of control mechanisms for enhancement or inhibition of electrical activity and for integration and regulation (see also p. 97).

Central synapses may be one of two main types: **Type I** and **Type II**. Type I synapses are usually excitatory, and a very common example is the glutaminergic synapse. The synapse is characterized by a relatively **large active zone** (1-2 mm²), **prominent presynaptic density**, **round vesicles**, and a **dense basement membrane**. The synaptic cleft is about 30 nm wide. Type I synapses are frequently made on to the axon, or on to the main shaft of the dendrite, on a special dendritic apparatus called a **spine**. Spines are found, for example, on pyramidal cells in the CAI region of the hippocampus. Type II synapses, for example the glycine or GABAergic synapses, are usually **inhibitory**, and are characterized by **flattened vesicles**, a **smaller active zone** (less than 1 mm²), **less prominent presynaptic density**, a **less dense basement membrane** and a **narrow synaptic cleft** (about 20 nm wide). Type II synapses frequently occur on the soma of the cell. (In invertebrates there are many exceptions to the rule that GABAergic synapses are inhibitory.)

When an **excitatory synapse** releases its neurotransmitter, it binds to its receptor on the postsynaptic membrane, and this causes an inward flow of current in the form of Na^+ ions through cation-selective ion channels. This produces a large depolarizing synaptic potential at the site. An **inhibitory synapse**, on the other hand, causes an outward current in the form of Cl^- ions. This results in a large hyperpolarization at the initial segment. In the working cell, inhibitory and excitatory inputs operate simultaneously, and these generate inhibitory and excitatory postsynaptic currents. These summate to produce the postsynaptic potential, which may cause an action potential at the axon hillock.

The anatomical location of the excitatory and inhibitory synapses is important in determining their effectiveness. Excitatory inputs to dendrites result in depolarizations which must pass through the cell body before reaching the axon. Therefore, inhibitory synaptic currents that are concentrated at or near the initial axon segment will be most effective in shunting away much of the depolarizations caused by spreading excitatory currents.

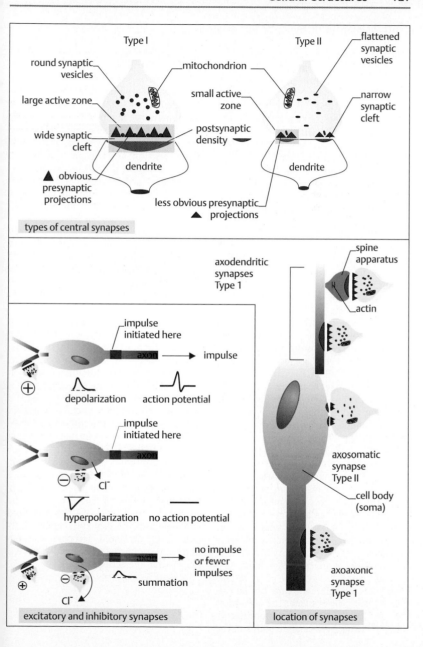

types of central synapses

excitatory and inhibitory synapses

location of synapses

Central synapses III: Synaptic Integration

When the neurotransmitter binds to its postsynaptic receptor on a CNS cell, it may initiate a **postsynaptic potential** (**PSP**). The PSP may be an **excitatory postsynaptic potential** (EPSP) if the membrane potential decreases, or an **inhibitory postsynaptic potential** (IPSP) if the membrane potential increases. The EPSP, like the EPP at the neuromuscular junction, is a local graded potential. For an EPSP, after an initial synaptic delay of around 0.5 msec, the membrane potential rises to its peak in about 1-2 msecs, and then decays exponentially to its resting value. The amplitude varies from excitation to excitation, and time constants vary from cell to cell, with values ranging, typically, from 100 µV to 2 mV for the amplitude change, and from 2 msec to several hundred msec for the time constant. Two important properties of EPSPs are (i) that they last longer than action potentials, and (ii) propagation along the membrane is **passive** (**electrotonic**). These two properties are crucial determinants of cellular electrical integration.

An **EPSP** may bring the membrane potential to threshold, depending on the amplitude and the threshold. A Type I synapse commonly evokes an EPSP. An **IPSP** resembles the EPSP in terms of voltage amplitude changes, and time constants, but works the opposite way, since it hyperpolarizes the membrane, and works to oppose the rise of the membrane potential to firing threshold. This system of the IPSP and EPSP enables an integration of inputs to any CNS excitatory cell, whose output therefore depends on the relative numbers and activity of the excitatory and inhibitory synapses at any given moment.

The size and direction of a voltage change on the cell membrane can be calculated using **Ohm's Law**. The law states that in a fixed metallic conductor the current (I) flowing between two points in the conductor is proportional to the potential difference (V) between these two points and indirectly proportional to resistance provided the temperature remains constant. According to this law V = IR, where R is the resistance in ohms. Two calculations are performed: (**1**) the current (I) flowing through channels across the cell membrane at an individual synapse is measured. I is the product of synaptic conductance (G) and the electrochemical driving force across the membrane ($V_m - E_{EPSP}$), or ($V_m - E_{IPSP}$), where V_m = the membrane potential, and E = synaptic reversal potential; (**2**) the membrane potential change (ΔV_m) in the postsynaptic cell due to *all* synaptic currents is calculated. The magnitude of the membrane potential change (ΔV_m) depends on the total synaptic current and the overall membrane conductance (G).

The multiplicity of inputs to the neuron requires integration of these inputs, and perhaps the most fundamental decision a neuron makes is an all-or-none one, namely whether or not to fire off an action potential down its axon. This integration is possibly achieved through the **spatial** and **temporal summation** of these inputs. In spatial summation, the individual EPSPs, which on their own are unable to generate an action potential, become added to each other as excitation spreads over the cell, until sufficient EPSPs are added to raise the neuron's membrane potential to firing threshold. Temporal summation is the adding of a rapid series of EPSPs generated by the neuron, until the cell membrane attains firing threshold. Temporal summation can occur because the EPSP lasts longer than the action potential.

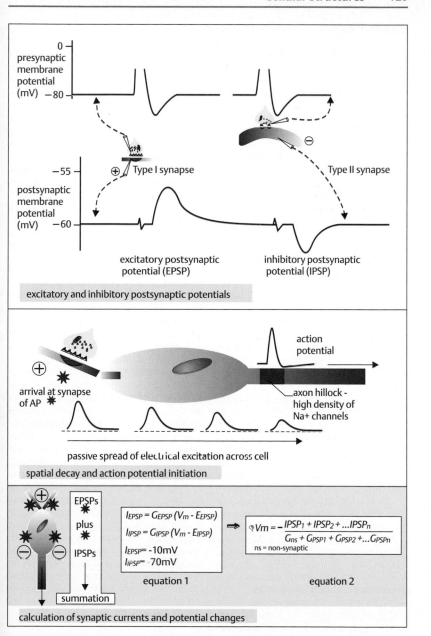

presynaptic membrane potential (mV)

0

−80

−55 Type I synapse ⊕

Type II synapse ⊖

postsynaptic membrane potential (mV)

−60

excitatory postsynaptic potential (EPSP)

inhibitory postsynaptic potential (IPSP)

excitatory and inhibitory postsynaptic potentials

⊕ arrival at synapse of AP ✳

action potential

axon hillock – high density of Na+ channels

passive spread of electrical excitation across cell

spatial decay and action potential initiation

⊕ EPSPs ✳

plus

⊖ ⊖ IPSPs ✳

summation

$$I_{EPSP} = G_{EPSP} (V_m - E_{EPSP})$$

$$I_{IPSP} = G_{IPSP} (V_m - E_{IPSP})$$

$$I_{EPSP} = -10mV$$

$$I_{IPSP} = -70mV$$

equation 1

$$V_m = -\frac{IPSP_1 + IPSP_2 + \ldots IPSP_n}{G_{ns} + G_{PSP1} + G_{PSP2} + \ldots G_{PSPn}}$$

ns = non-synaptic

equation 2

calculation of synaptic currents and potential changes

Synaptic Plasticity

Synaptic plasticity is the property of synapses to change their characteristics. These changes explain to some extent the ability of neurons to alter during development, disease, damage and **repair** processes, and during the processes of learning and **memory**. These changes may be pre- or postsynaptic, or both, and may be short or long lasting. The **structural changes**, **electrophysiology**, and **biochemistry** of synaptic plasticity are being intensely studied. An important impetus for the study of synaptic plasticity is **long-term potentiation** (**LTP**). LTP is an increase in synaptic transmission measured after tetanic stimulation of a synapse. Various types of LTP are recognized, but the most widely studied form is called **NMDA receptor-dependent LTP**.

LTP raises several questions. What mechanisms are involved in initiation and maintenance of LTP? Do pre- or post synaptic changes or both cause LTP? What determines the specificity of LTP development? In other words, how does the synapse 'know' what stimulus needs to be remembered? The mechanisms that keep the synapse firing long after stimulation are still unknown, but the initial events at the synapse are better understood. Initially, there is an influx of Ca^{2+} through **NMDA** receptor channels while the cell is depolarized by activation of **AMPA** receptors. If NMDA receptors in the rat brain are blocked with a specific antagonist, the rats largely lose spatial memory required to learn their way through a maze, without any impairment of visual discrimination.

The NMDA receptor alone is insufficient to maintain synapse firing for longer than an hour or so, and other receptors need to be involved, possibly the **metabotropic glutamate receptor**.

Metabotropic glutamate (**mGlu**) receptors are important in learning and memory, since they can theoretically generate long-lasting synaptic changes because they are coupled to second messenger cascades, which could reverberate in the cell for weeks and even months. Spatial learning in animals is particularly sensitive to blockers of mGlu receptors. It is also possible given the common neurotransmitter, i.e. glutamate, that both NMDA and mGlu receptors act in a coordinated fashion. This could be through short-term changes in neurotransmitter release, ionic permeabilities, membrane threshold properties, and longer term changes in second messenger activity and **protein synthesis** to mediate learning and memory. Longer term firing is blocked by interference with kinase activity and by interference with **transcription**. Gene products induced by tetanic stimulation of the synapse most probably include structural proteins, housekeeping proteins, and molecules such as cell adhesion molecules more commonly associated with neural development.

Presynaptic changes observed include quantal alterations in the synthesis and release of the neurotransmitter and in the numbers of presynaptic boutons. Post synaptic changes include alterations in receptor number and sensitivity and in the electrical properties of the cell membrane. It is possible that one active zone becomes split into two separate zones through structural changes at the synapse. Plasticity may be achieved through variations in the rate of release of quanta of neurotransmitters. The integrated end product of such interactions might be an altered PSP, altered in size and duration, or both. Synaptic plasticity could occur through changes in the inputs to the presynaptic or postsynaptic neuron from other neurons. Presynaptic inhibition or facilitation often modulate neurotransmitter release from CNS synapses.

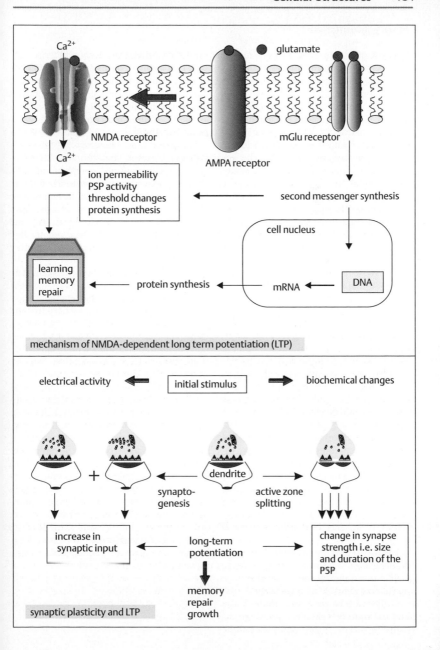

mechanism of NMDA-dependent long term potentiation (LTP)

synaptic plasticity and LTP

Sensory Information

Sensation and perception of the internal and external environments and the response of the organism are achieved through the integrated operation of the **sensory** systems. These share in common three basic features, namely (i) a **stimulus**, (ii) **transduction** of the stimulus into a train of **nerve impulses** which produce a **subjective experience**, and (iii) the **response**. One or more of the five senses may detect the stimulus.

The stimulus itself has attributes, namely **modality**, **duration**, **location**, and **intensity**, and all of these can be quantitatively correlated with the sensation experienced. The modalities are **sight**, **sound**, **touch**, **taste**, and **smell**, and each has **qualities** or submodalities. For example, sight has qualities of color and movement. Touch has qualities of flutter, vibration, vectorality, and duration of stimulus. Taste has qualities of sweet, sour, salt, and bitter.

Intensity is a measure of the strength of the stimulus. The sensory threshold is the lowest stimulus strength that can be detected by the organism, and is measured statistically. The relationship between stimulus intensity and the probability that an organism will detect 50% of a number of stimuli at a given intensity is termed the psychometric threshold. The theoretical absolute sensory threshold curve gives a relationship between stimulus intensity and probability of detection, but in reality detection can be influenced by factors such as fatigue and context. For example, pain thresholds are raised in sport, childbirth, and in conflict scenarios such as physical combat.

The **location** of the stimulus is defined and measured in terms of (i) the ability to localize precisely the site of the stimulus, and (ii) the ability to distinguish two anatomically closely applied stimuli. Some painful stimuli, for example those at the extremities, such as fingers and toes, can be localized relatively precisely, while visceral pain is often more diffusely perceived. The degree of ability to distinguish two closely applied stimuli is measured as the minimum distance between two points of the applied stimulus, and is termed the **two-point threshold**.

Duration can be expressed as the relationship between the stimulus intensity and the duration of perception of the stimulus. Some sensory receptors maintain impulse generation for the duration of the stimulus; these are slowly adapting receptors. Other receptors fire at the onset of the stimulus, but cease to fire even if the stimulus persists. These are **rapidly adapting** receptors.

Different receptor types subserve different sense modalities. Sight is the detection of a light stimulus by the retinal rods and cones (see p. 274), which transduce the light stimulus into trains of impulses. Similarly, hair cells in the cochlea (see p. 269) detect vibrations in the air, and transduce these into patterns of impulses whose frequency and amplitude are a function of the frequency and amplitude of vibration. In other words, the sense modalities of light and sound can interpret the intensity and nature of the original stimulus and convert this into a language of nervous impulses that the brain can decode and convert into a subjective experience. Similarly, the somatic nervous system detects chemical, thermal, and mechanical stimuli through (mainly) cutaneous receptors and can convert the original stimulus into a train of impulses whose intensity and frequency is eventually decoded by the brain into a subjective experience of (for example) heat, movement, or pain.

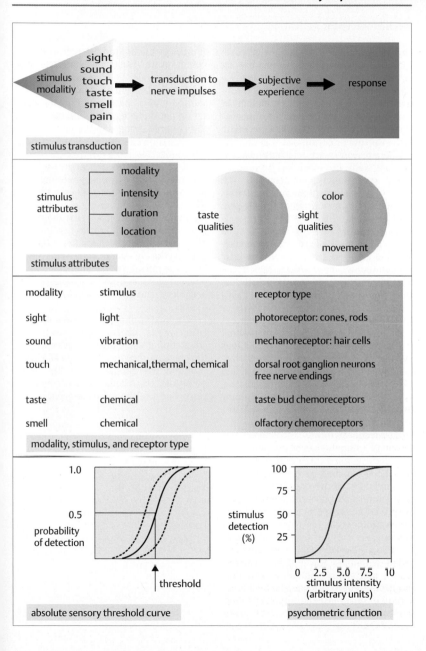

stimulus transduction

stimulus attributes

modality, stimulus, and receptor type

absolute sensory threshold curve

psychometric function

Mechanoreceptor Activation

Mechanoreceptors transduce a physical stimulus into an electrical impulse by means of which the organism is able to localize the stimulus and gain some perception of its intensity and duration. In humans, this is achieved through mechanoreceptors such as **Meissner's**, **pacinian**, and **Ruffini's corpuscles**. Vertebrate mechanoreceptors are relatively inaccessible for study, but much has been learnt about mechanoreceptors through the study of a small, transparent, free-swimming roundworm, *Caenorhabditis elegans*. In *C. elegans*, the external cuticle is coupled to the sensory neurons by a **mantle**. The mantle in turn is attached by a 'spring' gating system to the extracellular domain of an ion channel. When the cuticle is touched, the mantle is distorted, and this opens **mechanogated** (**MG**) membrane channels coupled to intracellular collagen **microtubules**. The mechanism includes a multi-unit ion channel that allows the influx of Na^+ and K^+ ions into the cell, resulting in the depolarization of the cell membrane and a so-called receptor potential. In the unstimulated, i.e. undistorted tissue, very few receptor channels are open, whereas after distortion many more ion channels open.

The response of the mechanoreceptor system to a stimulus can be measured, and is graded according to the degree of distortion. Increasing the degree of distortion results in greater **generator potentials**, and once a threshold generator potential is attained, an **action potential** is generated. An intriguing aspect of mechanoreceptor activation is the phenomenon of accommodation, or **adaptation**. Generator and action potentials may not be sustained with continuous stimulation. Some mechanoreceptors, such as the Meissner's corpuscle, adapt fast and stop responding, while the Merkel's cell adapts more slowly. Recordings reveal that even with a continuously applied stimulus such as skin indentation, the Meissner's corpuscle stops firing off, while the Merkel's cell sustains firing with continuous application of the same stimulus. The mechanism of adaptation is poorly understood, but may involve the possible changes in the rate at which ions are allowed through the ion channels with time.

Once an action potential has been generated by the mechanoreceptor, it is propagated along a nerve fiber to the central nervous system. Many of these fibers are **myelinated**, which speeds the rate of transmission of the message to the CNS. The **cell body** of the neuron lies in the ganglion on the dorsal root of the spinal nerve. Thus, the dorsal root ganglion has two axonal branches, one of which projects to the periphery, and another which projects to the CNS.

The quality of mechanoreceptor stimulation varies, depending on the rate of adaptation and the anatomical location of the mechanoreceptor. However, all have in common the property that the action potentials they generate are conducted along fibers of the same diameter.

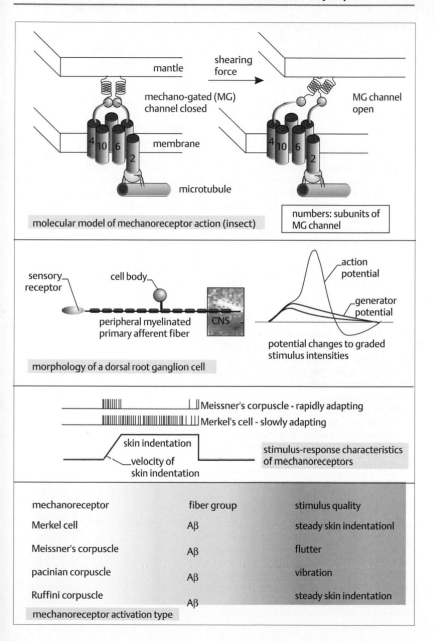

mantle

shearing force

mechano-gated (MG) channel closed

MG channel open

4 10 6 2

membrane

microtubule

molecular model of mechanoreceptor action (insect)

numbers: subunits of MG channel

sensory receptor

cell body

action potential

generator potential

peripheral myelinated primary afferent fiber

CNS

potential changes to graded stimulus intensities

morphology of a dorsal root ganglion cell

Meissner's corpuscle - rapidly adapting

Merkel's cell - slowly adapting

skin indentation

velocity of skin indentation

stimulus-response characteristics of mechanoreceptors

mechanoreceptor	fiber group	stimulus quality
Merkel cell	Aβ	steady skin indentationl
Meissner's corpuscle	Aβ	flutter
pacinian corpuscle	Aβ	vibration
Ruffini corpuscle	Aβ	steady skin indentation

mechanoreceptor activation type

Cutaneous Mechanoreceptors

The modality of **touch** is mediated by skin **mechanoreceptors**. These may be **slowly** or **rapidly adapting** to a constantly applied stimulus. Rapidly adapting mechanoreceptors may respond at the onset and possibly at the offset of the stimulus, while slowly adapting mechanoreceptors continue to respond throughout the duration of the stimulus.

Skin may be **glabrous**, i.e. smooth and hairless, or **hairy**, and this determines the distribution of mechanoreceptors. Each hair is innervated by a hair follicle receptor. In glabrous skin, the two main receptors are the rapidly adapting **Meissner's receptor**, and the slowly adapting **Merkel receptor**, also referred to as a 'cell' or 'disk'. Merkel's cells also occur in hairy skin. Both receptors have a relatively small receptive field of 2-4 μm. Therefore these receptors have a fine power of resolution, especially at the fingertips, where innervation is dense. The **receptive field** may be defined as the area of skin within which the adequate stimulus for a sensory receptor excites the sensory neuron. There are also **free nerve endings** that act as mechanoreceptors.

Below the skin, in the subcutaneous tissues, lie two other mechanoreceptors, namely the rapidly adapting **pacinian corpuscle**, and the slowly adapting **Ruffini's corpuscle**. These two receptors have relatively large receptive fields. In contrast to the Meissner's corpuscle and Merkel cell, spatial resolution is relatively coarse.

The **spatial and temporal resolving power** of the mechanoreceptors can be measured using a sinusoidal oscillating pattern of skin indentation. It has been found that pacinian corpuscles, which occur in the deeper subcutaneous layer, respond to higher frequency stimuli, and may be more sensitive to applied stimuli, while the more superficial Meissner's corpuscles respond to lower frequency stimu-

lation. Using this experiment, the threshold for the receptor may be found as the lowest stimulus intensity, i.e. degree of skin indentation, that evokes an action potential from one cycle of a sinusoidal stimulus.

Cutaneous receptors can be studied in humans using the technique of microneurography, in which a fine metal electrode is inserted percutaneously (i.e. through the skin) into a nerve, e.g. the radial nerve in the wrist, and recordings made from axons. The axons are stimulated electrically or a natural stimulus applied within the neuron's receptive field.

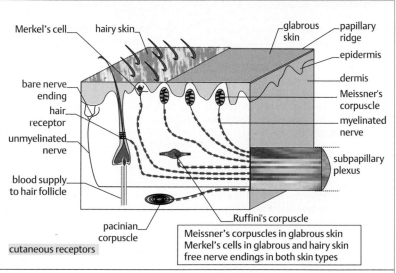

Merkel's cell — hairy skin —
glabrous skin — papillary ridge
epidermis
bare nerve ending
dermis
hair receptor
Meissner's corpuscle
unmyelinated nerve
myelinated nerve
blood supply to hair follicle
subpapillary plexus
pacinian corpuscle
Ruffini's corpuscle

cutaneous receptors

Meissner's corpuscles in glabrous skin
Merkel's cells in glabrous and hairy skin
free nerve endings in both skin types

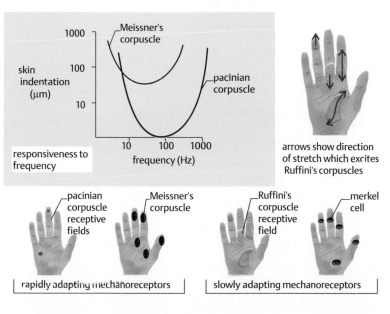

skin indentation (μm)

Meissner's corpuscle

pacinian corpuscle

responsiveness to frequency

frequency (Hz)

arrows show direction of stretch which excites Ruffini's corpuscles

pacinian corpuscle receptive fields

Meissner's corpuscle

Ruffini's corpuscle receptive field

merkel cell

rapidly adapting mechanoreceptors

slowly adapting mechanoreceptors

Thermoreceptor Action

Thermoreceptors are cutaneous receptors that detect changes in temperature. They fall into two main categories: those which are activated by cold, i.e. **cold** thermoreceptors, which respond to lower temperatures (~ 17-35 °C), and **warm** thermoreceptors, which are activated by heat (~ 30-45 °C), respectively. Cold and warm thermoreceptors are innervated by myelinated Aδ and unmyelinated C fibers. Cold and warm thermoreceptors do not respond to noxious hot and cold stimuli (see nociceptors, p. 166). It is now generally accepted that the thermoreceptors are free nerve endings. Temperature sensitivity in skin is described as being **punctate**, i.e. there are discrete, separate areas on skin, about 1 mm in diameter, each of which is innervated by a single nerve fiber.

Thermoreceptors respond to **changes** in skin temperature. At steady temperatures, the receptors transmit action potentials at a relatively low frequency. But even a small change in temperature will generate a marked increase in action potential transmission. A change as small as 0.2 °C will be detected by the thermoreceptors. The rate of increase is directly related to the speed with which the temperature is raised or lowered. For example, if one has cold hands and puts them into slightly warmed water, the water will feel hotter than if the hands were warm.

Thermoreceptors also produce so-called **paradoxical responses** to changes in temperature. This occurs when a cold stimulus is registered as heat, and *vice versa*. For example, if a temperature of 50 °C is applied to a cold spot, then the signal will be perceived (wrongly) as a cold stimulus. This phenomenon is an example of what is called **labeled line coding**; regardless of the nature of the stimulus, because the signals are carried in a cold-serving fiber, a sensation of cold will be experienced.

The responses of thermoreceptors to cold or heat are **graded**. The response is not all-or-none. The rate of firing of the receptor is a function of the temperature change of the applied stimulus. In the case of humans, the rate of change of response to cold is not as steep as that to a heat stimulus. The rate of firing may double when the stimulus temperature is raised from 38 °C to 40 °C.

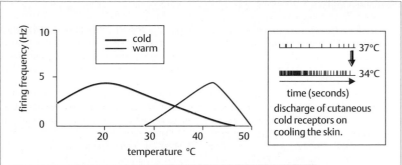

tonic firing frequencies of warm and cold cutaneous fibers (monkey)

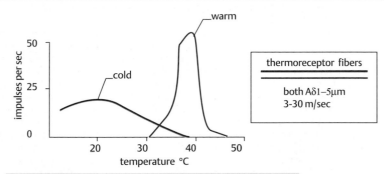

cutaneous cold and warm fiber response characteristics (human)

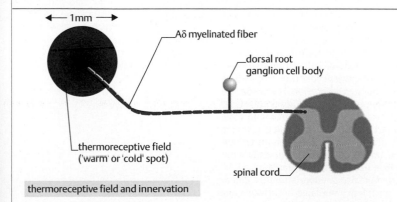

thermoreceptive field and innervation

Receptive Fields

The **receptive field** of a skin receptor is an area within which a **stimulus** must occur in order to activate the fiber which subserves that field. The size of the field depends on the type of receptor, the degree of spread of the stimulus over the skin, and on the degree of branching of the fiber. Thermoreceptors, for example, are punctate in nature, and have a relatively small receptive field. The receptive field of a mechanoreceptor such as a Ruffini's corpuscle may be much larger. A stimulus may be applied to a small area of skin, and yet elicit a widespread response. For example, an indentation of the skin at one point will result in skin indentation over a larger area, and this effectively enlarges the receptive field. Branching of free nerve endings, such as those that subserve thermoreception or pain (see p. 167), will also enlarge the receptive field for a given fiber. For example, one mechanoreceptor fiber may branch extensively to innervate more than one hundred hair follicles.

The larger the receptive field, the greater the possibility that **overlap** may occur. Overlap occurs when two or more receptive fields share the same area together or in part. Not only that, one follicle may receive innervation from several fibers. Overlap increases the complexity of stimulus detection and processing, and in many ways increases efficiency of detection and stimulus localization. For example, if a stimulus falls within two overlapping receptive fields, then both fibers will fire at rates proportional to the degree of influence of the stimulus within each receptive field. Thus the brain can localize the exact position of the applied stimulus more precisely than if the stimulus fell within one receptive field, especially if the receptive field is relatively large.

Overlap also renders stimulus detection much less vulnerable to surface damage, or nerve injury, or disease. For example, if a fiber is damaged, then overlap means that other fibers whose receptive fields overlap with that of the damaged fiber, will fire even if the damaged fiber does not. The degree of precision of localization and the intensity of the stimulus may not be accurately perceived, but there will nevertheless be an appreciation of the stimulus.

Overlap can result in blurring of stimulus appreciation, and this is countered through the mechanism of **lateral inhibition**. Typically, a sensory system may consist of the receptor and its associated fiber that relays impulses to a second order neuron. The receptor-associated fiber also innervates inhibitory interneurons that innervate second order neurons which receive impulses from neighboring receptive fields. Therefore, if a receptive field receives a powerful enough stimulus, this will result in the suppression of firing of adjacent second order neurons, which helps to sharpen the area of the receptive field stimulated. Lateral inhibition also sharpens the edges of receptive fields. For example, when one puts an arm or leg into very hot water, there is a clearly defined ring of the burning sensation where the surface of the water surrounds the limb. This is because the receptors which lie just within the edge of an extended uniform stimulus will receive less lateral inhibition than those lying further towards the middle of the field.

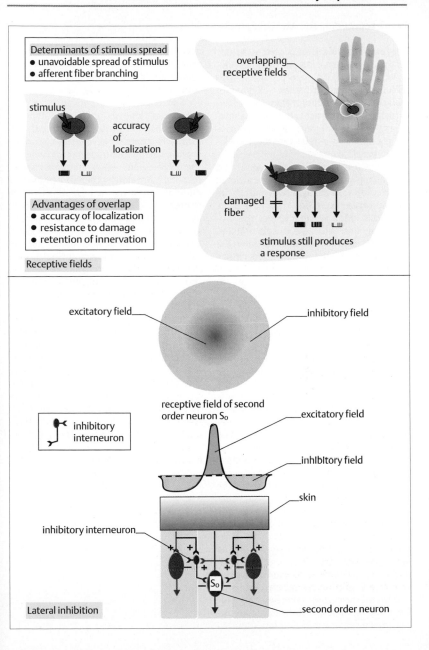

Determinants of stimulus spread
- unavoidable spread of stimulus
- afferent fiber branching

stimulus

accuracy of localization

overlapping receptive fields

damaged fiber

stimulus still produces a response

Advantages of overlap
- accuracy of localization
- resistance to damage
- retention of innervation

Receptive fields

excitatory field

inhibitory field

receptive field of second order neuron So

excitatory field

inhibitory field

skin

inhibitory interneuron

inhibitory interneuron

second order neuron

Lateral inhibition

Proprioceptors I: The Muscle Spindle

The term **proprioceptor** is used to include reception of sensation in the musculoskeletal system, i.e. deep sensation. This includes **joint capsules**, ligaments, **muscles** and **tendons**. These are low-threshold, stretch-activated mechanoreceptors, whose afferent signals are conducted centrally in relatively thick myelinated axons.

The **muscle spindle** is an elongated organ lying **in parallel** among the striated muscle fibers, attached at both ends to the muscle connective tissue. This means the spindle is indirectly attached to the tendons. Therefore when the muscle stretches this will stretch the spindle, and when the muscle contracts the spindle fibers will be passively shortened.

The spindle consists of specialized muscle cells enclosed for most of their length in a connective tissue capsule, and bathed in a gelatinous fluid that facilitates sliding of the fibers over each other. The spindle can be 4-10 mm in length, and about 0.2 mm in diameter. The muscle fibers of the spindle are called **intrafusal fibers** and are cross-striated only at the ends, as opposed to the normal muscle fibers, **extrafusal fibers**, which are cross-striated along their entire length. Therefore spindle fibers can contract only at the ends. There are two principal spindle fiber types: **nuclear bag fibers** and **nuclear chain fibers**. In nuclear bag fibers the cell nuclei are concentrated together in the middle of the fibers, whereas in nuclear chain fibers the nuclei are evenly distributed along the length of the fiber. In addition, nuclear bag fibers have been further subclassified into **dynamic** and **static** nuclear bag fibers, which have different innervation. Dynamic nuclear bag fibers are innervated by dynamic gamma motoneurons, whereas static nuclear bag and nuclear chain fibers are innervated by static gamma motoneurons. In addition, all spindle fiber types have primary afferent Ia innervation, while secondary afferent II innervation is absent from dynamic nuclear bag fibers.

The functional significance of this differential innervation is that dynamic nuclear bag fibers do not respond uniformly to stretch. The central region responds rapidly to muscle stretch, whereas the polar regions, which are more viscous, respond more slowly. Therefore primary Ia afferents fire off with high sensitivity to stretch. Also, differential innervation of dynamic nuclear bag fibers with dynamic gamma motoneurons enhances the sensitivity of the central fiber to stretch, because efferent stimulation during stretching produces more stretching of the central region of the dynamic nuclear bag fiber due to contraction at the polar region.

If action potentials are measured in primary and secondary fibers by recording in the dorsal roots of anesthetized animals, it is observed that the firing rate is increased in both types when the muscle (and hence the spindle) is stretched, and firing is decreased when the muscle contracts. When the muscle length is kept constant, the firing rate in both types of afferent remains constant. Therefore the spindle is able to inform the brain continuously of muscle length.

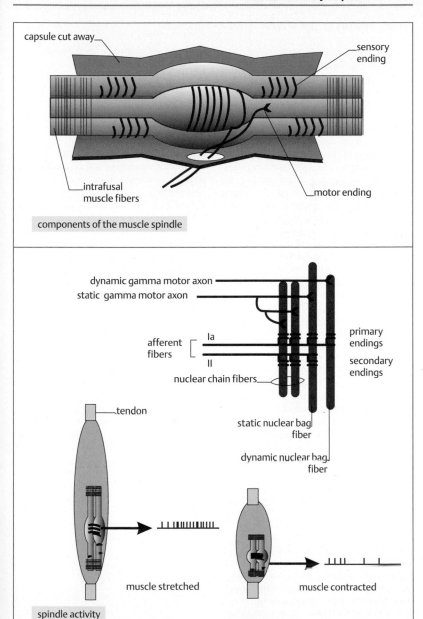

capsule cut away

sensory ending

intrafusal muscle fibers

motor ending

components of the muscle spindle

dynamic gamma motor axon
static gamma motor axon

afferent fibers
Ia
II

primary endings

secondary endings

nuclear chain fibers

static nuclear bag fiber

dynamic nuclear bag fiber

tendon

muscle stretched

muscle contracted

spindle activity

Proprioceptors II: The Muscle Spindle - Function

If action potentials are recorded from the **dorsal roots** of **Ia** and **II afferents** from the **muscle spindle**, we can study the roles of the **primary** and **secondary fibers** in the response of the **muscle spindle** to **stretch**. The role of the γ-**motoneuron** in the functioning of the muscle spindle can be studied by stimulating the neuron in the ventral horn of the spinal cord.

When the muscle is stretched, both primary and secondary fibers exhibit increased firing rates during the **static phase**. Conversely, when the muscle shortens, decreased firing rates are measured. Action potential may even cease to occur. When the muscle remains at a constant length (**static phase**), the rate of firing remains constant, i.e. the spindle afferents are slowly adapting, a phenomenon termed **static sensitivity**. Thus the CNS is kept constantly aware of the length of the muscle.

During periods of changing length (**dynamic phase**), however, primary (Ia) and secondary (II) fibers have different response patterns of firing rates. During the stretching phase, **Ia afferents** show a marked **increase** in firing rates, whereas secondary afferents do not. Also, the firing rate in Ia afferents increases as the rate of shortening increases. This is termed **dynamic sensitivity**. During the shortening phase, Ia fibers exhibit virtually no impulse traffic at all. Group II fibers, i.e. the secondary afferents, do not have the property of dynamic sensitivity. Therefore primary afferents inform on static and dynamic status, secondary fibers inform on only static status of the muscle.

The differential firing rates in Ia and II afferents is most probably due to differences in the nature of the intrafusal fibers they innervate. Primary afferents innervate dynamic nuclear bag fibers (see p. 142) whereas II afferents do not, and there is evidence that the dynamic nuclear bag fibers are responsible for dynamic sensitivity.

The role of the γ-**motoneuron**: Firing rates in Ia and II afferents shown on p. 145 were made in the absence of any γ-motoneuron activity. The γ-efferent motoneuron innervates the cross-striated ends of the muscle spindle fibers, and causes the ends to contract. This stretches the middle portion of the fiber where the sensory efferents originate. The γ-motoneurons also cause a change in the viscoelastic properties of the fiber, so that stretch of the intrafusal fiber is facilitated. Therefore the CNS, through its modulation of γ-motoneuron activity, can control muscle length and sensitivity to stretch.

Two types of γ-motoneuron have been described: **gamma dynamic** (γ_d) and **gamma static** (γ_s). Gamma dynamic motoneurons enhance the firing rate of Ia afferents during the dynamic phase in response to rapid stretch, whereas the firing rate during the static phase is not enhanced. This is useful when the body needs to respond quickly to altered posture or imbalance. Firing of the γ-static motoneuron, on the other hand, increases firing rates in both Ia and II afferents. This is probably functionally significant in maintaining signal passage from the spindle to the brain even when the muscle is not in a dynamic phase, which would facilitate fine or precise muscle movement and management. It is not certain whether γ_d motoneurons innervate dynamic nuclear bag fibers exclusively.

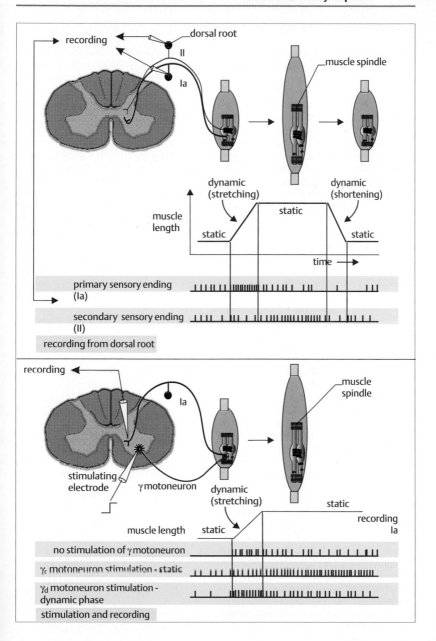

recording

dorsal root

II

Ia

muscle spindle

dynamic (stretching)

dynamic (shortening)

muscle length

static

static

static

static

time

primary sensory ending (Ia)

secondary sensory ending (II)

recording from dorsal root

recording

muscle spindle

Ia

stimulating electrode

γ motoneuron

dynamic (stretching)

static

recording Ia

muscle length

static

no stimulation of γ motoneuron

γ$_s$ motoneuron stimulation - static

γ$_d$ motoneuron stimulation - dynamic phase

stimulation and recording

Proprioceptors III: The Golgi Tendon Organ

The **Golgi tendon organ** is an elongated encapsulated structure typically found at the junction between the **tendon** and the **muscle** (the musculotendinous junction) where the extrafusal muscle fibers are attached to the collagen fibers of the tendons. It is about 1-1.5 mm long and about 0.5 mm in diameter at its midpoint. Each Golgi organ is innervated by a single **myelinated Ib axon** (thinner than Ia), that becomes unmyelinated after it penetrates the tendon organ. The nerve branches into several fine fibers that proliferate throughout the network of collagen fibers within the capsule. There is *no* efferent connection from the CNS to the tendon organ. There are usually almost as many tendon organs as **spindles** in a single muscle.

When the tendon organ is stretched through muscle contraction, the collagen fibers within the tendon organ become stretched and straightened, and this deforms the Ib nerve endings, which are intertwined between the collagen fibers. The nerve is extremely sensitive to deformation, and is depolarized and fires off action potentials. In other words, **contraction of the muscle** fires off the nerve of the tendon organ. (This is in direct contrast to the action of the muscle spindle, which fires off in response to *stretching* of the muscle.) The difference between the nature of the response of the spindle and tendon organs can be explained in terms of the different anatomical arrangements of the two proprioceptors. Spindles are arranged **in parallel** with extrafusal muscle fibers, whereas tendon organs are arranged **in series** with the extrafusal muscle fibers. Also, the collagen fibers of the tendon organ are less elastic than the intrafusal fibers spindles. Therefore the muscle fibers take up most of the stretch exerted. On the other hand, when the muscle fibers contract, they pull on the tendons directly.

Functionally, the tendon organ informs the CNS about **muscle tension**, whereas the spindle informs primarily about **muscle length**. Thus, both types of proprioceptor have complementary functions in informing the CNS about the mechanical status of the muscle at any given point or period of time. The Golgi tendon organ provides afferent inputs regarding muscle tension during, for example, gripping with hands and toes or tail in certain animals. It also enables the organism to compensate for muscle fatigue by adjusting the motor effort applied. The spindle is important for, for example, posture, since the length of the muscle will vary with the angle of the joint it is acting on, thus enabling the CNS to be aware of relative limb segment position.

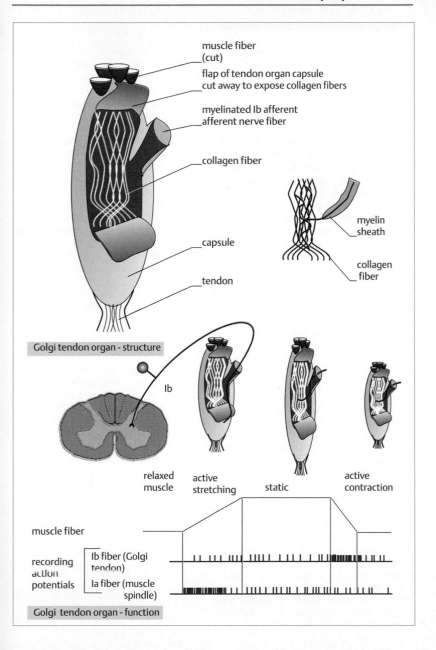

muscle fiber (cut)

flap of tendon organ capsule cut away to expose collagen fibers

myelinated Ib afferent afferent nerve fiber

collagen fiber

myelin sheath

collagen fiber

capsule

tendon

Golgi tendon organ - structure

Ib

relaxed muscle

active stretching

static

active contraction

muscle fiber

recording action potentials

Ib fiber (Golgi tendon)

Ia fiber (muscle spindle)

Golgi tendon organ - function

Proprioceptors IV: The Stretch Reflex

The **stretch reflex** is a monosynaptic spinal reflex that causes skeletal muscle to contract when it is stretched, and is mediated by the **muscle spindle**. The reflex was first characterized by Sherrington using decerebrate animals, in which the cerebrum is disconnected surgically from the spinal cord. This heightens the facilitatory brain stem influence on the reflex. The reflex circuit is completed through a single synaptic contact between the **Ia afferent** from the spindle and the α-motoneuron. Although not shown here, the Ia afferent excites not only its homonymous (same) muscle but synergist muscles as well. In addition, the Ia afferent synapses with inhibitory **interneurons**, which inhibit the α-motoneurons that innervate **antagonist** muscles.

The stretch reflex is produced when the muscle is stretched. This fires off the spindle Ia afferent, which in turn fires off homonymous and synergist α-motoneurons, which cause the muscle to contract. This reflex is a useful diagnostic test for the integrity of the motor system. The tendon knee jerk, for example, is a test in which a light blow to the tendon causes the leg to jerk upwards from below the knee. A hypoactive or flabby response could indicate a lesion to one or more component of the reflex arc. An exaggerated response could indicate a central lesion, which dampens inhibitory descending tone from the cerebrum. (Group II afferents operate within a polysynaptic reflex arc, which slows the response, and is more suited to a control system that modulates *tonic components* of the stretch reflex arc.)

The stretch reflex contributes to **muscle tone**, and is therefore an important modulator of steady-state muscle tension in sustained muscle work, for example during gripping and posture. Muscle tone can be defined as the force exerted by a muscle to *resist being lengthened*. The intrinsic viscoelastic properties of muscle together with the stretch reflex combine to exert this force. The property of elasticity enables the muscles to store energy, during locomotion, for example, and it contributes to posture, since the muscles resist stretching during movement, such as swaying, that can upset body balance.

The stretch reflex can be considered as a negative feedback loop that controls and maintains muscle length (the controlled variable). The set or desired value is determined by the sum of ascending and descending influences to the α-motoneuron. These influences could involve the γ-motoneuron to the intrafusal spindle fibers. Firing of the γ-motoneuron contracts the distal ends of the spindle fiber, which stretches the spindle. This fires the Ia afferent, and the α-motoneuron is excited to counteract the stretch. Thus a steady state of tension can be maintained. If the muscle is stretched through the application of any load, then the feedback system operates to restore the desired value. This can be achieved through firing of the Ia afferent, which causes the muscle to contract to the desired length.

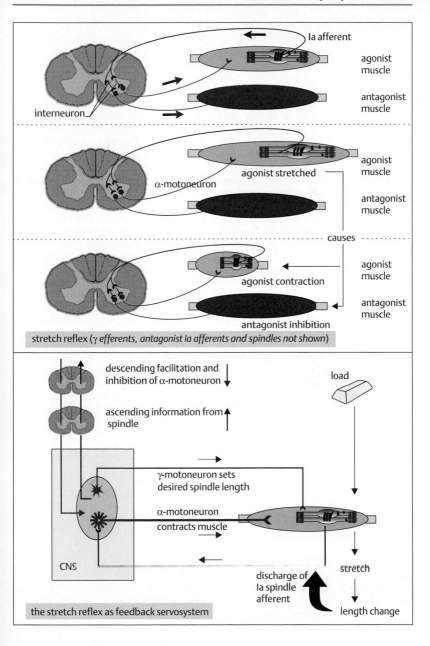

Ia afferent

agonist muscle

antagonist muscle

interneuron

α-motoneuron

agonist stretched

agonist muscle

antagonist muscle

causes

agonist contraction

agonist muscle

antagonist inhibition

antagonist muscle

stretch reflex (γ efferents, antagonist Ia afferents and spindles not shown)

descending facilitation and inhibition of α-motoneuron

load

ascending information from spindle

γ-motoneuron sets desired spindle length

α-motoneuron contracts muscle

CNS

stretch

discharge of Ia spindle afferent

length change

the stretch reflex as feedback servosystem

Sensory Fibers and Dorsal Roots

Sensory fibers, including those from the muscle spindle, pass into the **dorsal roots** and from there into the **spinal cord**. Once in the cord, the sensory fibers split into **ascending** and **descending** branches, and also give off **collaterals** that terminate in different areas of the **gray matter** of the cord.

The dorsal root fiber axons that leave the ganglion and enter the cord are of different diameters depending on function, and the diameter determines the speed of conduction. The myelinated fibers are classified as Group A, and Group C fibers are unmyelinated. Aα are the thickest and fastest of the myelinated afferent (sensory) axons, having a diameter ranging from around 12-20 mm and conduction velocities ranging from 70-120 m/sec. The Ia muscle afferents are an example of Aα fibers. The terminals of these fibers end relatively far down in **Rexed's laminae** VI and VII of the spinal gray matter and in the **ventral horn** in lamina IX.

The myelinated Aβ afferents range in diameter from 5-14 μm and have conduction velocities ranging from 25-70 m/sec. The Group II muscle mechanoreceptor afferents are an example of the Aβ afferent type, and appear to send terminals into spinal gray laminae III, IV, V and VI. Aδ are Group III afferents, and are the thinnest of the myelinated sensory afferents, having axon diameters ranging from 2-7 μm and conduction velocities of 10-30 m/sec. These afferents subserve temperature, pain, and crude touch and pressure. Their terminals end in the spinal cord mainly in laminae I and, to, a lesser extent, in lamina V.

Group IV fibers (C) are unmyelinated, have diameters ranging from 1-5 μm and conduction velocities of less than 2.5 m/sec. They subserve temperature and (together with Aδ) subserve afferent transmission of pain. The terminals of the Aδ and C afferent fibers are almost completely separate from those of the Aα and Aβ fibers. Most of their endings are in laminae I and II (marginal nucleus and substantia gelatinosa, respectively), although some of the Aδ fibers terminate in lamina V. It is likely that the differential termination of sensory inputs into the laminae of the cord has functional significance. For example, nociceptive inputs from skin terminate in laminae I, II, and V, whereas those from muscle and viscera end in I and V, i.e. not in the **substantia gelatinosa** (lamina II). Since nociceptive inputs from muscle and viscera are generally poorly localized while those from skin are better discriminated, it is possible that the distribution of endings in the cord may contribute to the ultimate degree of anatomical discrimination of pain.

As well as a differential topographical distribution of afferent fiber endings, there is also a differential distribution in the ventral horn of the gray matter of the cord of the motor outputs. For example, the axial musculature is supplied by medially located motoneurons, while limb musculature is supplied by motoneurons located laterally in the ventral horn.

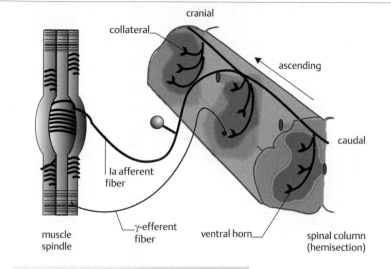

cranial

collateral

ascending

caudal

Ia afferent
fiber

γ-efferent
fiber

ventral horn

muscle
spindle

spinal column
(hemisection)

termination and branching of Ia afferent in spinal cord

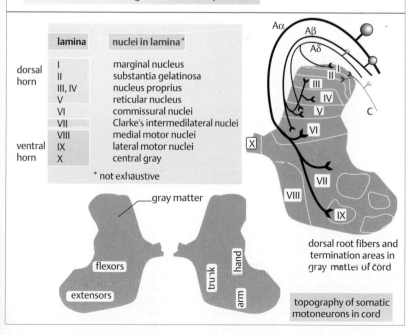

	lamina	nuclei in lamina*
dorsal horn	I	marginal nucleus
	II	substantia gelatinosa
	III, IV	nucleus proprius
	V	reticular nucleus
	VI	commissural nuclei
	VII	Clarke's intermedilateral nuclei
	VIII	medial motor nuclei
ventral horn	IX	lateral motor nuclei
	X	central gray

* not exhaustive

Aα
Aβ
Aδ
C

dorsal root fibers and
termination areas in
gray matter of cord

gray matter

flexors

extensors

trunk

hand

arm

topography of somatic
motoneurons in cord

Segmental Organization of Spinal Cord

In humans, the **vertebral column** serves as the central supporting pillar of the body, supporting the head and trunk. It also protects the **spinal cord**. It is made up of irregularly shaped bones called **vertebrae**, which are separated by fibrocartilaginous **intervertebral discs**. The vertebrae have been divided into five groups. There are seven **cervical**, 12 **thoracic**, and five **lumbar** vertebrae; five **sacral** vertebrae are fused to form the sacrum, and there are four **coccygeal** vertebrae, the lower three usually being fused.

In adults, the **spinal cord** begins rostrally above the foramen magnum, where it is continuous with the medulla oblongata and extends caudally as far as the level of the first or second lumbar vertebrae. The spinal cord possesses along its length 31 pairs of spinal nerves, each of which is attached to the cord through dorsal sensory roots and ventral motor roots. (There is evidence that there are some sensory fibers in the ventral roots as well.) The cord is a continuous structure, but is divided into segments through the spinal roots. A segment may be thought of as the area of spinal cord which possesses one pair of dorsal and ventral roots. Each segment may also have a pair of dorsal root ganglia. An exception is C1, which may have no dorsal root ganglion. The cervical segments (C1-C7) supply the face, the neck, the arms, and the trunk; the thoracic segments (T1-T12) supply the trunk and the sympathetic ganglia; the lumbar segments (L1-L5) supply the legs; the thoracolumbar segments also serve the sympathetic ganglia; the sacral (S1-S5) and coccygeal segments (one segment) supply the saddle region, the buttocks, and the pelvic organs. The sacral segments, together with the cranial nerves, also serve the parasympathetic ganglia. All sensory information to the CNS is relayed to the brain via the dorsal roots. Therefore the axons which arise in the dorsal root ganglia may be referred to as **primary afferent fibers**.

The sensory fibers that enter the CNS have traveled from receptors in the body. Many of these receptors are located in the skin, and the area of skin that is served by a particular dorsal root ganglion is termed a dermatome. The dermatomes have been mapped (see pp. 154), and it has been discovered that there is significant overlap between different dermatomes. Therefore, damage to any one dorsal root need not necessarily result in loss of sensation within the corresponding dermatome.

The ventral root axons arise almost exclusively from cell bodies in the ventral horn, and are mainly motor neurons supplying the peripheral skeletal musculature. The ventral root axons meet up with the peripheral fibers of the dorsal root ganglia to make up what is termed a spinal nerve. The spinal nerves ultimately merge to form the peripheral nerve.

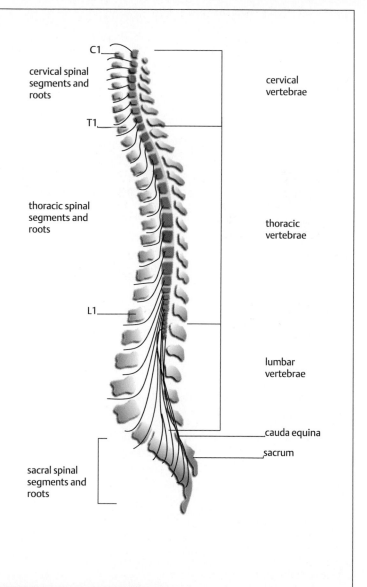

cervical spinal
segments and
roots

C1

T1

cervical
vertebrae

thoracic spinal
segments and
roots

thoracic
vertebrae

L1

lumbar
vertebrae

cauda equina

sacrum

sacral spinal
segments and
roots

organization of the spinal cord into segments

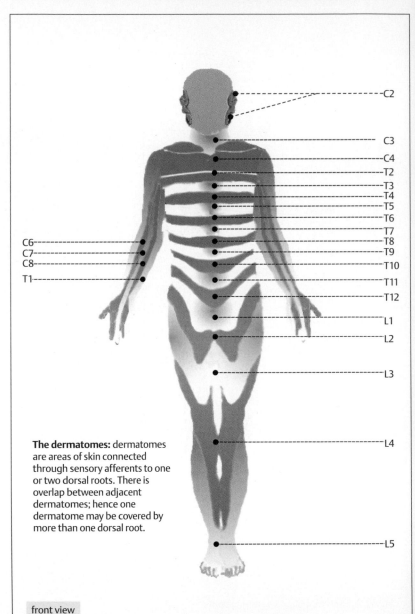

C2

C3
C4
T2
T3
T4
T5
T6
T7
T8
T9
T10
T11
T12

C6
C7
C8
T1

L1
L2

L3

The dermatomes: dermatomes are areas of skin connected through sensory afferents to one or two dorsal roots. There is overlap between adjacent dermatomes; hence one dermatome may be covered by more than one dorsal root.

L4

L5

front view

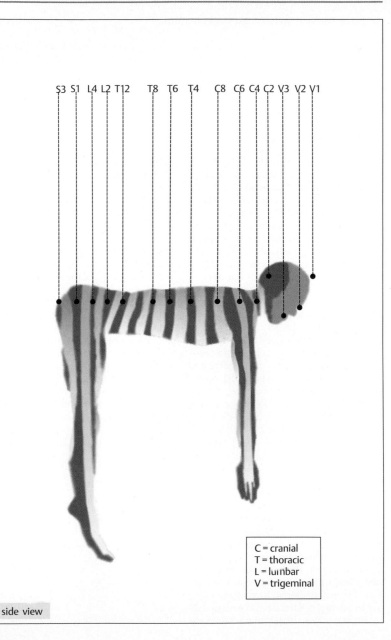

S3 S1 L4 L2 T12 T8 T6 T4 C8 C6 C4 C2 V3 V2 V1

C = cranial
T = thoracic
L = lumbar
V = trigeminal

side view

Sensory Tracts I: Spinal Cord Organization

The sensory input from the periphery to the CNS is highly organized in the **spinal cord** in order to transmit information about the different modalities to the brain, and to facilitate rapid execution of the spinal reflexes. The gray matter of the spinal cord is surrounded by the **white matter**, which consists of the ascending and descending pathways or tracts. The white matter has been arbitrarily divided into three main sections, namely the **dorsal**, **lateral**, and **ventral funiculi**. The white matter of the cord is organized into pathways that separate the transmission of different sensations. For example, conscious and non-conscious proprioception are separated, as are pain and light pressure. Information about conscious proprioception will ultimately reach the cerebral cortex, while non-conscious proprioception is carried by the cerebellum.

All sensory information enters the spinal cord through the dorsal roots. Where the dorsal root fibers enter the spinal cord at the dorsal root entry zone, these separate into two divisions, the **medial** and **lateral divisions**. The medial division contains fibers whose original receptors include those in skin, joints, and the spindles. The fibers are of relatively larger diameter than those in the lateral division, and carry information about muscle length and tension; they mediate spinal reflexes either through direct synapsis with motoneuron or through interneurons. They also transmit information to the ascending fiber tracts. Dorsal root fibers that target the local segment of entry will enter the gray matter through the dorsal horn and synapse with interneurons or with motoneurons at the same segmental level. These dorsal horn entry fibers and interneurons therefore constitute the central afferent arm of the reflex arc. Axons and collaterals of the medial division may enter the white matter in the dorsal funiculus and ascend the spinal cord where they will eventually synapse in relay nuclei.

Fibers that enter the white matter in the dorsal funiculus will displace more caudal inputs towards the medial part of the cord. Thus a sort of lamination of dorsal column pathways occurs, with sacral inputs more medially placed than lumbar inputs and so on.

The lateral division axons form a bundle of fibers called **Lissauer's tract**. Lateral division fibers contain smaller diameter non-myelinated and myelinated axons, and typically transmit responses to thermal and painful (nociceptive) stimuli in skin and the viscera. Axons in Lissauer's tract may descend or ascend through several segments of the spinal cord before entering the gray matter to synapse in one or more or more of the layers of the dorsal horn, for example the substantia gelatinosa or the marginal nucleus. These second order neurons of the dorsal horn, which receive information from the axons of Lissauer's tract, may transmit this information to the brain through axons which ascend to the brain in the ventral or lateral funiculi. (Note: in top diagram, C = cervical, Th = thoracic, L = lumbar, S = sacral.)

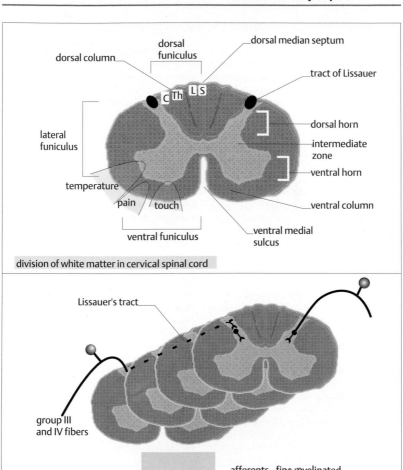

division of white matter in cervical spinal cord

dorsal column

dorsal funiculus

dorsal median septum

tract of Lissauer

lateral funiculus

dorsal horn

intermediate zone

ventral horn

ventral column

temperature

pain

touch

ventral funiculus

ventral medial sulcus

Lissauer's tract

group III and IV fibers

dorsal root fibers

lateral

afferents - fine myelinated and unmyelinated - nociception (pain) and thermal from viscera and skin

medial

afferents - larger myelinated from muscle, muscle spindles, joints, and skin

dorsal root entry zone

division of afferent axons in spinal cord.

Posterior (Dorsal) Column Medial Lemniscus Pathway

There are two main afferent sensory pathways which carry somatic sensation to the brain. These are the **posterior or dorsal column lemniscal pathway** and the **spinothalamic pathway**. Both pathways have several important features in common. (i) Both consist of first-, second-, and third-order sensory neurons. (ii) The cell bodies of the first-order neurons lie in the dorsal root ganglion, and those of the second-order neurons lie ipsilaterally in the gray matter of the spinal cord. (iii) The second-order neurons **decussate**, i.e. cross the midline of the cord, and ascend to terminate, ultimately, in the thalamus. The third-order neurons terminate in the somatosensory cerebral cortex. (iv) The gray matter of both pathways where neurons terminate can be shown to represent specific areas of the body, i.e. the pathways are **somatotopic**. (v) At these terminations, synaptic transmission can be stimulated or inhibited by other neurons.

The **dorsal columns** are made up chiefly of the thick, myelinated fibers that enter the cord and turn to travel rostrally towards the brain where they terminate in the **dorsal column nuclei** of the medulla. The more caudally derived **gracile fasciculus** terminates in the **gracile nucleus**, while the more rostrally derived **cuneate fasciculus** terminates in the **cuneate nucleus**. From there, the second-order fibers **decussate** to the contralateral side of the cord and ascend in the **medial lemniscus**. The medial lemniscus terminates, ultimately, in the lateral portion of the **ventral posterior nucleus** (ventral posterolateral nucleus) of the **thalamus**. From there, the third-order neurons project to the **somatosensory cortex**.

Functions of the dorsal column medial lemniscus system: The system subserves modalities of **conscious proprioception** and **discriminative touch**. These two modalities together inform the parietal lobe of the cortex about the position of the body at rest or when moving at any given moment of time. Damage to the medial lemniscus will impair, for example, the ability to grasp moving objects such as the handle of a door, or of a moving bus. Damage is exhibited as **sensory ataxia**. The symptoms in extreme cases are the inability to stand unsupported when the feet are spread apart and the patient is looking down at them. The patient will sway when the feet are together and eyes are closed (**Romberg's sign**). Also, the patient stamps the feet when walking to enhance remaining proprioceptive facility (the 'stamp and stick' gait).

Diseases that damage the dorsal columns include **multiple sclerosis**, which is an immune demyelinating disease of the nervous system. Here, there is specific damage to the cuneate fasciculus, causing loss of proprioception in hands and fingers, and an inability to identify shapes through touch alone (**astereognosis**). Deficiency of vitamin B_{12} (cyanocobalamin) leads to **subacute combined degeneration** of spinal cord, as well as to pernicious anemia. **Tabes dorsalis** is a late symptom of CNS syphilitic infection, which affects principally the lumbosacral columns and roots, and the patient exhibits sensory ataxia.

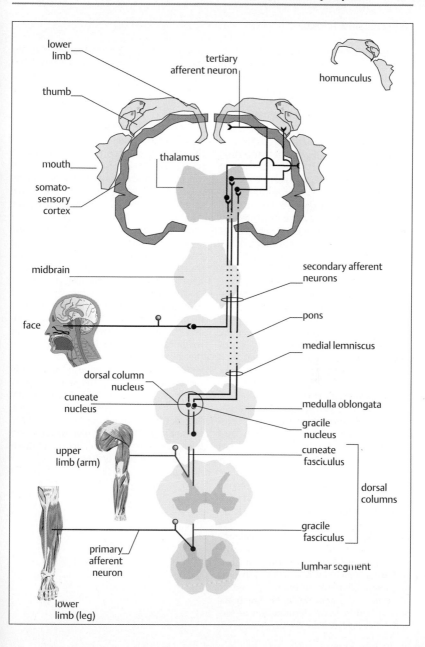

lower limb

thumb

tertiary afferent neuron

homunculus

thalamus

mouth

somato-sensory cortex

midbrain

secondary afferent neurons

face

pons

medial lemniscus

dorsal column nucleus

cuneate nucleus

medulla oblongata

gracile nucleus

upper limb (arm)

cuneate fasciculus

dorsal columns

primary afferent neuron

gracile fasciculus

lumbar segment

lower limb (leg)

Spinothalamic Pathway

The **spinothalamic pathway** lies in the ventral horn of the spinal cord, lateral and ventral to the gray matter. It is made up of second-order afferent sensory neurons that originate in Rexed's laminae I, III, IV, and V of the dorsal horn gray matter. These cross over to the contralateral side in the anterior commissure and run rostrally in two separate tracts, the **medial** (**anterior**) **spinothalamic tract** and the **lateral spinothalamic tract**. (Note that axons that transmit temperature and pain decussate within one spinal segment of their origin, whereas those transmitting pressure and touch may ascend through several spinal segments before decussation occurs.) The spinothalamic tract is also sometimes called the **anterolateral tract**. In the brain stem the two tracts merge to become the spinal lemniscus, which runs close to the medial lemniscus, and which picks up the trigeminal afferent fibers from the head (see p. 159). The tract terminates in the **thalamus** in the **ventral posterior nucleus** immediately caudal to the terminations of the medial lemniscus pathway. From there, third-order neurons project to the somatosensory cortex.

Functions of the spinothalamic pathway: As mentioned above, the spinothalamic tract carries conscious **pain and temperature** sensation. It also carries **crude perception** of **touch** and **pressure**. Spinothalamic neurons can be classified as (i) **low threshold units** which respond only to light touch of, e.g., skin; (ii) **wide dynamic range units** (**WDR**), which respond to nociceptive stimuli; (iii) **high threshold** (**HT**) **units**, which respond only to relatively high stimuli which activate nociceptive receptors; (iv) **thermosensitive units**, which respond only to warming or cooling of thermoreceptors in skin. In addition, there appears to be functional differentiation in the termination of second-order neurons in the thalamus. For example, more posterior terminations may carry sensation of non-localized immediate perception of pain, whereas those ending higher in the ventral posterior nucleus may mediate exact localization of the pain.

Information about the role of the spinothalamic tract comes largely from the surgical procedure of **cordotomy**, to relieve the pain in, e.g., terminally ill cancer patients. A needle is passed into the subarachnoid space and into the spinal column and up the anterolateral region. Progress is monitored using X-rays. A stimulating electrode inside the needle generates a small pulse, and in the right place should elicit pain on the contralateral side of the body. The pathway is then destroyed by an electrolytic lesion.

The spinothalamic tract can become damaged in the rare condition of **syringomyelia**, when the central canal distends and compresses adjacent pathways. The lesion or **syrinx** (a fusiform cyst) damages the decussating fibers of the tract in the ventral white commissure, commonly in the cervical region of the spinal column, resulting in selective loss of temperature and pain appreciation in the upper limbs. Proprioceptive sensation and light touch are not lost. The patient will inadvertently burn or injure hands and arms and dislocate joints without feeling pain.

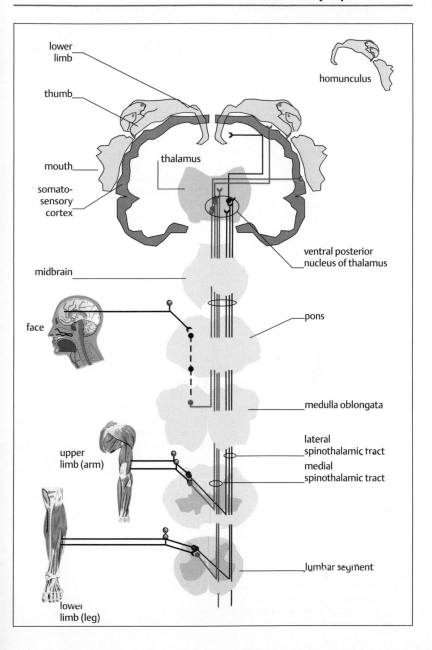

lower limb

homunculus

thumb

mouth

thalamus

somato-sensory cortex

ventral posterior nucleus of thalamus

midbrain

pons

face

medulla oblongata

upper limb (arm)

lateral spinothalamic tract

medial spinothalamic tract

lumbar segment

lower limb (leg)

Spinocerebellar Tracts

There are four fiber tracts that run up the spinal cord to the cerebellum. These are the **ventral spinocerebellar (SP) tract**, the **dorsal SP tract**, the **rostral SP tract**, and the **cuneocerebellar tract**. The spinocerebellar tracts serve the modality of **unconscious proprioception**.

The **dorsal and ventral SP tracts** run up the spinal cord near the dorsolateral and ventrolateral surfaces respectively. Both tracts consist of second-order neurons that receive their inputs in the gray matter near the base of the dorsal horn from terminations of 1A afferents from the muscle spindles, Golgi tendon organs, and certain touch receptors. From there, the second-order neurons run directly into the cerebellum where they terminate, mainly in the vermis.

The **dorsal** (posterior) **SP tract** originates in lamina VII in the **dorsal nucleus of Clarke** (nucleus dorsalis, thoracic nucleus). The primary 1A afferent fibers enter the cord and synapse either directly in the ventral horn with motoneurons to an agonist muscle or with interneurons to the antagonist muscle, thus completing the reflex arc. Also, the afferents send collaterals that travel up the cord to the dorsal nucleus, which extends from T1 to L1. Here, the afferents synapse with the second-order neurons of the dorsal spinocerebellar tract. In this way information from proprioceptors can be used for reflex muscle responses and also be relayed to the cerebellum. In addition, the dorsal nucleus receives inputs from skin. The dorsal spinocerebellar tract consists of the largest afferent fibers in the nervous system, being about 20 μm in diameter, and of high conductance velocity (120 m/sec). The tract rises ipsilaterally and enters the cerebellum through the inferior cerebellar peduncle.

The **ventral spinocerebellar tract** consists of second-order neurons that arise from a spinal border cell in lamina VII in the dorsal nucleus, decussate to the contralateral ventral cord, and ascend to the cerebellum, which they enter through the superior cerebellar peduncle. Some of the axons of this tract may then cross over to the other side of the cerebellum. The **rostral spinocerebellar tract** arises in the upper (cervical) portion of the cord and travels ipsilaterally to the cerebellum. The **cuneocerebellar tract** arises from the **accessory cuneate nucleus**, which lies outside and immediately above the cuneate nucleus (see p. 10). Primary afferent 1A fibers reach the accessory cuneate nucleus through the cuneate fasciculus and synapse with the second-order fibers of the cuneocerebellar tract. These fibers ascend to the cerebellum via the inferior cerebellar peduncle. Some other cell groups in the spinal cord, for example the central cervical nucleus (CCN), send projections to the cerebellum. CCN fibers send information mainly from receptors around the cervical joints.

Spinocerebellar pathways that travel uninterrupted by synapses (in the midbrain) to the cerebellum are termed **direct spinocerebellar tracts**, while those that may be interrupted by synapses are termed **indirect spinocerebellar tracts**. Most of the fibers of the spinocerebellar tracts terminate in the cerebellum ipsilaterally with the cord. The tracts terminate in the cerebellum in an orderly manner reflecting their somatotopic organization.

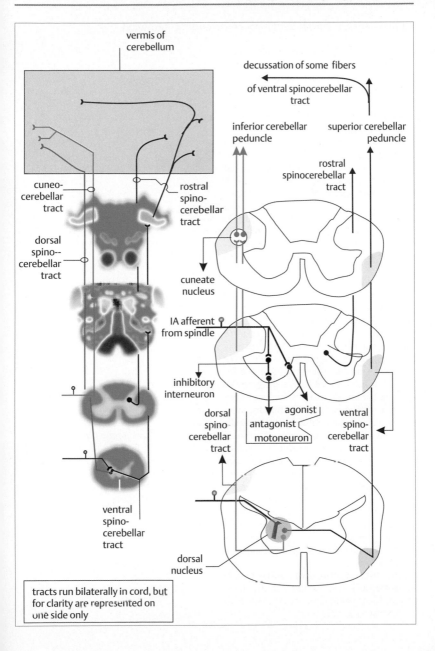

vermis of
cerebellum

decussation of some fibers
of ventral spinocerebellar
tract

inferior cerebellar
peduncle

superior cerebellar
peduncle

rostral
spinocerebellar
tract

cuneo-
cerebellar
tract

rostral
spino-
cerebellar
tract

cuneate
nucleus

dorsal
spino--
cerebellar
tract

IA afferent
from spindle

inhibitory
interneuron

dorsal
spino
cerebellar
tract

antagonist

agonist

motoneuron

ventral
spino-
cerebellar
tract

ventral
spino-
cerebellar
tract

dorsal
nucleus

tracts run bilaterally in cord, but
for clarity are represented on
one side only

Somatosensory Tracts: Summary of Ascending Pathways

There are a number of other minor **ascending somatosensory** tracts in addition to the major **dorsal column lemniscal**, **spinothalamic**, and **spinocerebellar** tracts. These carry information, indirectly, from peripheral cutaneous sensory receptors, sense organs such as eyes, or ears, or from proprioceptors, and arise in the spinal cord.

Indirect spinocerebellar tracts: The **spinotectal tract** (see also p. 2) is a small crossed tract, a supplementary **pain** pathway that is thought to arise in dorsal horn cells in the spinal cord and ascends closely associated with the lateral spinothalamic tract. It terminates in the **superior colliculus**, where its information is integrated with visual inputs to the colliculus. The tract is believed to carry pain afferents to the tectum, which is concerned with reflex head movements in response to pain. The **spino-olivary tract** is a small, crossed tract, which carries tactile information to the inferior olivary nucleus, a folded gray mass in the medulla oblongata. The inferior olivary nucleus integrates sensory information and projects this to the cerebellum via the inferior cerebellar peduncle. The tract may be involved in motor learning processes in the cerebellum, and modifies olivary discharges during motor movement when, for example, the organism encounters unexpected physical obstacles during movement in darkness. The **spinoreticular tract** is a phylogenetically ancient polysynaptic pathway that ascends bilaterally to the brain stem reticular formation, from where fibers ascend to the cerebellum via the inferior peduncles. The tract is believed to mediate arousal.

The **trigeminothalamic tract** carries somatosensory information from the head region. The trigeminal system is dealt with more fully on p. 222.

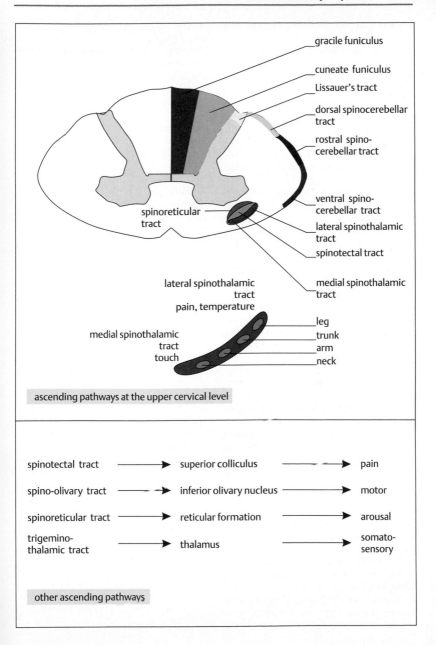

gracile funiculus

cuneate funiculus

Lissauer's tract

dorsal spinocerebellar tract

rostral spino-cerebellar tract

ventral spino-cerebellar tract

lateral spinothalamic tract

spinotectal tract

medial spinothalamic tract

spinoreticular tract

lateral spinothalamic tract
pain, temperature

medial spinothalamic tract
touch

leg
trunk
arm
neck

ascending pathways at the upper cervical level

spinotectal tract → superior colliculus → pain

spino-olivary tract → inferior olivary nucleus → motor

spinoreticular tract → reticular formation → arousal

trigemino-thalamic tract → thalamus → somato-sensory

other ascending pathways

Nociception I: Pain Pathways and Components

Pain can be defined as an unpleasant emotional and sensory experience, which may be associated with actual or potential tissue damage. There are thus two main components: the **motivational-affective** (emotional) component, and the **sensory-discriminative** component. Also, **nociception** and **pain** are not necessarily the same. **Nociception** is the awareness of the stimulation of nociceptors by a noxious stimulus. The information is relayed via primary afferents to the spinal cord and hence to the brain where the location, onset, intensity, and duration of the stimulus are appreciated. **Pain** is the subjective response of the individual to the nociceptive input to the brain, and it may be totally unrelated to the actual physical parameters of intensity and duration of the stimulus. The pain experienced may be determined by several emotional and cognitive factors, including anxiety, anticipation, past experience, and sociocultural influences. This is the motivational-affective component that overlies the sensory-discriminative (nociceptive) component.

Two types of input serve the sensory-discriminative component. We may experience a sharp, highly localized **pricking** or **first pain**, and a more prolonged, slower or **burning** (**second**) **pain**. Pricking pain is thought to be carried by Aδ fibers, and burning pain by C fibers. Both inputs terminate principally in **laminae I**, **II**, and **III** of the dorsal horn in the spinal cord, where most, if not all, of the nociceptive inputs from the periphery terminate. Other laminae, for example V and VIII, also appear to be involved in the control of pain transmission.

The **control of pain transmission and perception** is poorly understood, but we know that there are powerful descending pathways from the brain to the laminae that control the type and degree of nociceptive transmission up to the brain, where it is ultimately appreciated. Knowledge of these mechanisms is important for pharmacological and surgical control of pain in patients.

The brain areas known to be concerned in pain control are the **prefrontal cortex**, **the somatosensory cortex**, the periventricular nucleus in the **hypothalamus**, the **periaqueductal gray matter** in the midbrain (**PAG**), the nucleus raphe magnus in the **reticular formation** of the medulla, and the pars caudalis of the trigeminal nucleus (see also p. 222). It is known, for example, that stimulation of the PAG in conscious rats induces analgesia and abolishes surgical pain. Patients with chronic severe pain have been helped to some extent by stimulation of the PAG. The main pathway for pain control by the PAG appears to be to the raphe nucleus magnus and other nearby nuclei in the reticular formation. Important fibers descend from these nuclei down the spinal column in the dorsal part of the lateral funiculus. If these fibers are cut, then stimulation of the PAG no longer produces analgesia. The limbic system and neocortical regions appear to be involved in the emotional and cognitive responses to pain and the anticipation of pain, but very little is known of the pathways and mechanisms involved.

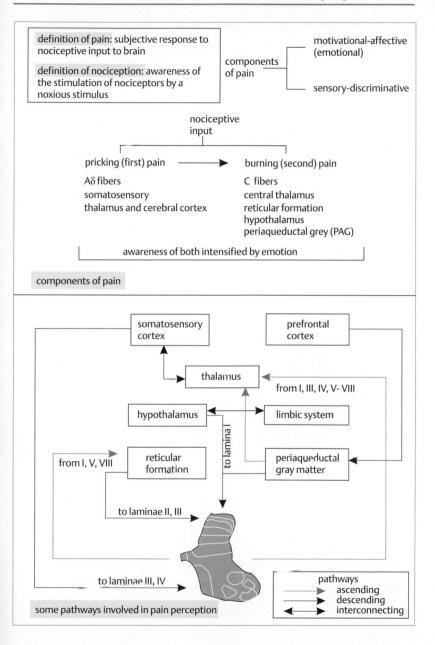

definition of pain: subjective response to nociceptive input to brain

definition of nociception: awareness of the stimulation of nociceptors by a noxious stimulus

components of pain
— motivational-affective (emotional)
— sensory-discriminative

nociceptive input

pricking (first) pain ⟶ burning (second) pain

Aδ fibers
somatosensory
thalamus and cerebral cortex

C fibers
central thalamus
reticular formation
hypothalamus
periaqueductal grey (PAG)

awareness of both intensified by emotion

components of pain

somatosensory cortex

prefrontal cortex

thalamus

from I, III, IV, V- VIII

hypothalamus

limbic system

to lamina I

from I, V, VIII

reticular formation

periaqueductal gray matter

to laminae II, III

to laminae III, IV

pathways
ascending
descending
interconnecting

some pathways involved in pain perception

Nociception II: Afferent Inputs to the Dorsal Horn and Ascending Pathways

Afferent nociceptive inputs to the dorsal horn are carried by the **Aδ** and **C** fibers. Aδ fibers terminate in laminae I and V, and C fibers in laminae I and II (**substantia gelatinosa**). Upon entering the cord, the fibers bifurcate or divide into collaterals, which may synapse with neurons in the dorsal horn, or ascend one or more segments in the Tract of Lissauer (see also p. 156) before entering the cord to synapse.

There are many **interneurons** linking the two layers, and these interneurons serve to modulate the release of neurotransmitters from the afferent terminals. In addition, descending fibers from the brain, and particularly from the nucleus **raphe** magnus, terminate in these layers, and these modulate the activity of the interneurons to control and limit the afferent input of nociception to the brain. In summary, there are three main types of pathways in the dorsal horn for transmission of nociceptive signals. (i) Nociceptive afferents from the periphery may synapse directly with neurons of the ascending anterolateral pathway. (ii) The afferents may synapse with excitatory interneurons, which relay nociceptive inputs to ascending fibers. (iii) Afferents may synapse with inhibitory inputs which inhibit or block altogether the transmission of the nociceptive impulse. Knowledge of these interconnections is useful when attempting to understand the clinical implications of pain, such as, for example, referred pain (see p. 174), and the effects of nerve damage on the transmission or lack of transmission of pain within the spinal cord. This knowledge has also given rise to theories of pain transmission to the brain, the best known being the **gating theory of pain**.

According to the gating theory of pain, there is a balance in the dorsal horn between the degree of stimulation of dorsal horn neurons by larger cutaneous affer-

ents, and stimulation by the smaller incoming nociceptive fibers. Thus, Aα+ afferents stimulate inhibitory interneurons in lamina IV, which inhibit afferents in I and II, which in turn inhibit the firing of the spinothalamic (anterolateral) fibers which carry nociceptive impulses up to the brain. For example, the application of mechanical pressure such as rubbing, or of heat to the skin (Aα), will decrease the conscious perception of an applied noxious stimulus such as a pinprick, to the skin. Conversely, if the painful input (Aδ, C) is strong enough, it will overcome the inhibitory influence of the interneurons activated by Aα afferents.

There are several ascending nociceptive tracts projecting from the laminae to the brain. The most prominent is the **spinothalamic (anterolateral) tract** (see also p. 160), originating from neurons in laminae I and V-VIII, and terminating in the thalamus. The **spinoreticular tract** (see p. 164) originates in laminae VII and VIII, and sends projection neurons that terminate either in the reticular formation or the thalamus. The **spinomesencephalic** tract originates in laminae I and V, and projects to the mesencephalic reticular formation, the lateral portion of the periaqueductal gray matter (PAG), and to other sites in the midbrain. Other neurons project from laminae III and IV in the **spinocervicothalamic** tract, while some run from III and IV to the gracile and cuneate nuclei.

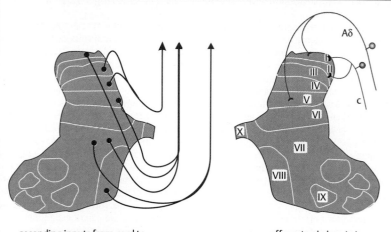

ascending inputs from cord to
contralateral thalamic nuclei

afferent pain inputs to
spinal cord

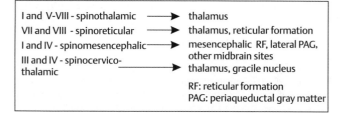

I and V–VIII – spinothalamic	→	thalamus
VII and VIII – spinoreticular	→	thalamus, reticular formation
I and IV – spinomesencephalic	→	mesencephalic RF, lateral PAG, other midbrain sites
III and IV – spinocervico-thalamic	→	thalamus, gracile nucleus

RF: reticular formation
PAG: periaqueductal gray matter

afferent nociceptive inputs to spinal cord and ascending pathways

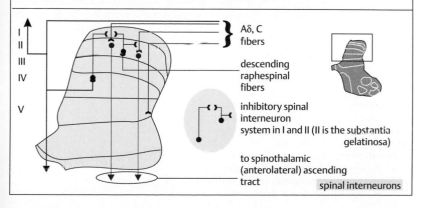

Aδ, C
fibers

descending
raphespinal
fibers

inhibitory spinal
interneuron
system in I and II (II is the substantia
gelatinosa)

to spinothalamic
(anterolateral) ascending
tract

spinal interneurons

Nociception III: Descending Brain Stem Pathways Affecting Transmission

The transmission of nociceptive impulses to the brain is controlled by the brain through modulatory circuits within it and through descending pathways that synapse with the various relay nuclei from the dorsal horn upwards. The main central components known to modulate nociceptive transmission through descending pathways include (i) the somatosensory cortex, (ii) the thalamus, (iii) the hypothalamus, (iv) the midbrain periaqueductal gray matter, (v) the **nucleus raphe magnus** in the medulla, and (vi) interconnections within the dorsal horn (see also p. 168).

An important efferent pathway is that from the **periventricular nucleus of the hypothalamus to the periaqueductal gray matter** (PAG). The pathway utilizes the endogenous opioid, **enkephalin**, as neurotransmitter. Enkephalins are small peptides that bind to the morphine receptor subtypes and are thought to be of major importance in the control of pain from the dorsal horn upwards. Fiber tracts descend from the PAG to the nucleus raphe magnus, where they form excitatory serotonergic synapses. The tracts also exert their excitatory action through interneurons, which have been shown to release one or more of a variety of putative neurotransmitters, including glutamate, neurotensin, and somatostatin. From the nucleus raphe magnus there is a descending pathway, the **raphespinal tract**, which projects to the dorsal horn, to laminae II and III. This synapses with enkephalinergic interneurons, which in turn act both pre- and postsynaptically to inhibit the transmission of nociceptive impulses to the brain through the spinothalamic and other tracts.

In addition, there are fiber tracts directly from the hypothalamus to the dorsal horn (hypothalamospinal tract), and from the PAG to the dorsal horn (see p. 166). It has been discovered that both cholecystokinin and substance P are released at terminals where PAG fiber tracts terminate in the dorsal horn, and may be neurotransmitters mediating the inhibitory action of PAG projection fibers on nociceptive transmission.

Knowledge of the existence of these descending pathways from the brain has prompted the use of electrical stimulation of areas, or stimulation-induced analgesia (SIA), in the hope that these will help to alleviate chronic pain, admittedly with highly variable success rates. Also, knowledge of the neurotransmitters involved has resulted in the use of exogenously applied synthetic opioids, applied either systematically, or locally to the spinal cord by epidural injection, in the hope that these will produce analgesia. The validity of the gating theory of pain (see p. 168) is supported by treatments in which the dorsal columns are stimulated by chronically implanted electrodes. This produces an antidromic firing of the column fibers resulting in the stimulation of inhibitory enkephalinergic interneurons in the dorsal horn, which in turn blocks nociceptive transmission. It is possible that techniques such as acupuncture also stimulate descending pathways and enkephalinergic interneurons to produce relief from pain.

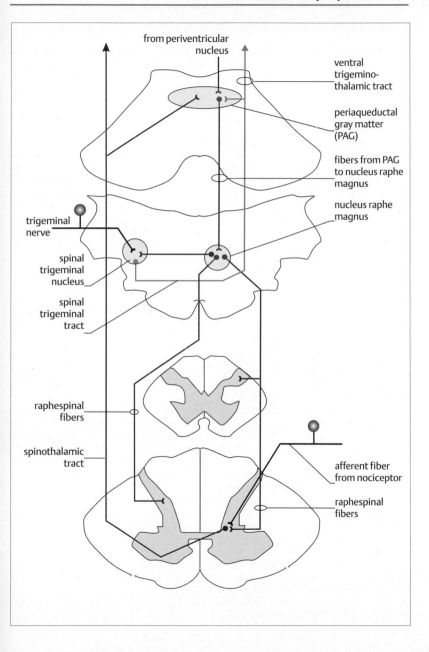

from periventricular
nucleus

ventral
trigemino-
thalamic tract

periaqueductal
gray matter
(PAG)

fibers from PAG
to nucleus raphe
magnus

nucleus raphe
magnus

trigeminal
nerve

spinal
trigeminal
nucleus

spinal
trigeminal
tract

raphespinal
fibers

spinothalamic
tract

afferent fiber
from nociceptor

raphespinal
fibers

Nociception IV: Visceral Afferents

Inputs, including nociceptive inputs from the external environment, are detected by cutaneous receptors and relayed to the brain via the spinal cord and the various ascending pathways. At the same time, the brain continuously receives sensory information from the internal environment from visceral receptors and the **visceral afferent pathways**.

Visceral receptors have been classified as one of two main types, **nociceptive** or physiological. The physiological receptors may be rapid or slowly adapting mechanoreceptors, baroreceptors, chemoreceptors, osmoreceptors, and thermal receptors. Nociceptors are free nerve endings that transmit stimuli that are ultimately perceived as, for example, visceral bloating, GIT cramp, appendicitis, or cardiac ischemia.

The afferent fibers that transmit visceral sensory information travel in the nerves of the sympathetic and, more commonly, of the parasympathetic system. Traditionally, these were thought to comprise only efferent fibers, but are now known to contain afferent fibers as well. For example, over 80% of the fibers in the vagus nerve (see p. 228) are afferent viscerosensory fibers. However, almost all the nociceptive input to the CNS is transmitted through sympathetic nerves.

Nociceptive visceral inputs to the CNS travel through the **splanchnic** and **cardiac** nerves. Fibers enter the sympathetic trunk and travel through the white ramus (see also p. 242) and join the spinal nerve. The cell bodies of origin of the sympathetic nociceptive afferents lie in the **dorsal root ganglia** from level T1 through L2. From there, the central afferents enter the CNS through the lateral portion of the dorsal root, and may ascend or descend in the dorsolateral (posterolateral) funiculus before they terminate in laminae I and V. Some of the fibers that terminate in I and V send projections to VII and VIII as well. The cells in laminae I and V that synapse with these inputs join the **contralateral spinothalamic (anterolateral) tract**, while those in laminae VII and VIII send projections bilaterally in the **spinoreticular** tracts.

Cells of the spinothalamic tracts that receive sympathetic viscerosensory nociceptive inputs in laminae I and V either cross in the ventral white commissure and ascend contralaterally, or ascend on the ipsilateral side. On both sides, the ascending fibers terminate in the **thalamus** in the **ventral posterolateral (dorsolateral) nuclei**, from where fibers ascend to the **parietal operculum** in the inferolateral part of the postcentral gyrus and to the insular cortex. In contrast to the exquisitely accurate nature of cutaneous nociceptive localization achieved by the cortex, that of visceral localization is relatively poor, due to low density of visceral nociceptors, and to the relatively large receptive fields.

Other ascending pathways, the **spinoreticular fibers**, arise in laminae VII and VIII (see also p. 164) and terminate in the reticular formation. From here, **reticuloreticular fibers** ascend to the periaqueductal gray where they terminate on cells, which project as the **reticulothalamic fibers** to the thalamus, while others terminate in the hypothalamus. The **reticulohypothalamic fibers** travel to the hypothalamus and have important functional implications. For example, increased heart rate can result from abnormal bowel distention.

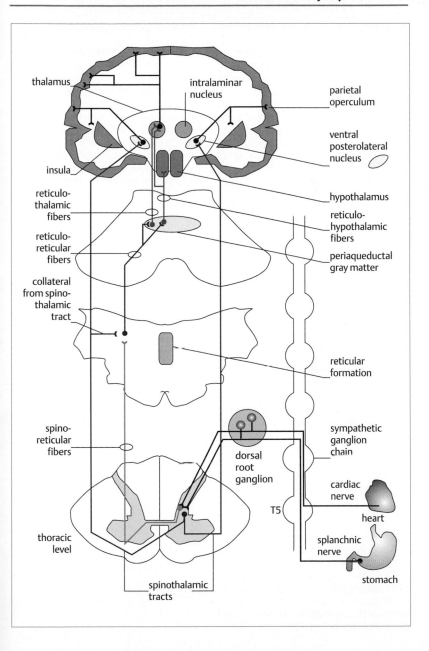

thalamus

intralaminar
nucleus

parietal
operculum

ventral
posterolateral
nucleus

insula

reticulo-
thalamic
fibers

hypothalamus

reticulo-
hypothalamic
fibers

reticulo-
reticular
fibers

periaqueductal
gray matter

collateral
from spino-
thalamic
tract

reticular
formation

spino-
reticular
fibers

sympathetic
ganglion
chain

dorsal
root
ganglion

cardiac
nerve

heart

T5

thoracic
level

splanchnic
nerve

stomach

spinothalamic
tracts

Nociception V: Referred Cardiac Pain

Referred pain is the sensation of pain in an area of the body distant from the site of origin of the original nociceptive receptor activation. Most commonly, it is the experience of cutaneous, muscle, or bone pain through activation of visceral nociceptor nerve endings. The phenomenon of referred pain occurs through the existence of common central points of convergence of nociceptive afferent inputs from the viscera and somatic structures.

Referred pain can be explained through knowledge of the spinothalamic tract. This is because the same second-order neuron receives inputs from the viscera (e.g. the heart) and the skin. Thus, when viscera are diseased (e.g. myocardial infarction), the brain may interpret the pain as coming from the left arm. Similarly, injury to the diaphragm may be perceived as a pain below the right shoulder blade. This phenomenon has useful diagnostic value. If a second-order neuron of the spinothalamic tract is being stimulated by nociceptive impulses from (say) heart, then touching the area of skin which sends afferent inputs to the neuron may also cause pain, even with a relatively light touch, because the second-order neuron has already been excited by the input from the heart nociceptor.

In the heart, for example, the condition known as angina is characterized by a constricting pain felt by the patient behind the sternum and often radiating down the left arm and sometimes up into the throat, and, rarely, down the right arm. Since cardiac disease is more commonly confined to the left side of the heart, this would explain the bias of referred cardiac pain to the left somatic structures.

The heart sends nociceptive afferents to the spinal cord through the cervical and thoracic cardiac nerves. These enter the sympathetic trunk and the cervical nerves join the **superior**, **middle**, and **inferior** **sympathetic ganglia**, while thoracic nerves enter the **thoracic ganglia** from **T1** through **T5**. Ultimately, these primary afferents terminate in the dorsal horn in laminae I and V. It is here that referred pain mechanisms originate, because the nerve cells in these laminae also receive nociceptive cutaneous afferents from the dermatomes (see p. 154) in the left arm and chest wall. Other second-order neurons in these laminae in other spinal segments may also be activated through the activation of collaterals running from segment to segment. Thus, the somatosensory cortex eventually receives nociceptive information from the heart, which it may interpret as having originated in the chest wall and upper limb. The same principle underlies referred pain from other visceral structures. The sites of referred pain from bladder, kidney, liver, and colon, for example, have been mapped to areas on the trunk.

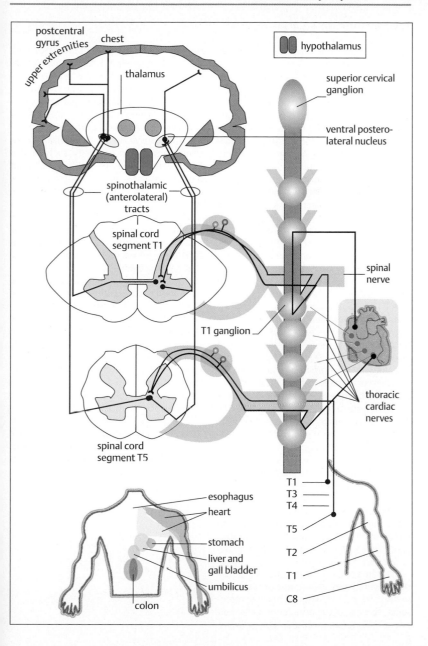

The Somatosensory Cortex

Ascending somatosensory projections are relayed, ultimately, to specific regions of the **cerebral cortex**, specifically to the parietal lobe, which lies behind the frontal lobe (see also p. 338), and which is bounded inferiorly by the temporal lobe and posteriorly by the occipital lobe. This region is the primary somatosensory cortex, also called area SI, or Brodmann's areas 1, 2, and 3 (see p. 336).

The somatosensory cortex has been mapped in relation to the inputs it receives from the ventral posterior nucleus of the thalamus. The cortex preserves the original topographical organization of skin with respect to the various modalities of sensation; the organization of the somatosensory cortex faithfully represents the contralateral area of skin. The somatosensory cortex thus is the final destination of afferent inputs carried by the medial lemniscus (proprioception and fine touch), trigeminothalamic (sensation from the head region), spinal lemniscus (coarse pressure and touch), and the spinothalamic tracts (temperature and pain).

There is a smaller somatosensory area, termed SII, found in primates, which is different from area SI in that it receives somatosensory inputs from both sides of the body, and in terms of some of the modalities it receives. Area SII is located on the medial surface of the parietal operculum, and receives a much larger nociceptive input from the thalamic nuclei than that received by area SI. During PET scans of the brain area SII is highlighted when the subject experiences painful peripheral stimuli. Areas SI and SII are known to coordinate activity in the process of tactile discrimination by the brain.

The area of cortex that subserves a particular cutaneous area is not proportional to the size of the body surface it represents; the size of the area reflects the density of cutaneous receptors. For example,

the lips, which are richly innervated with sensory receptors, are represented in the somatosensory cortex by a disproportionately high area. Similarly, the palmar surface of the hands, the digits, and particularly the thumb, the tongue, pharynx, and the face are well represented in the somatosensory cortex. Conversely, relatively large body surfaces such as the limbs, which are not richly innervated, have far smaller area of somatosensory cortex devoted to their afferent input information.

The arrangement of the topographical somatosensory cortical map has several interesting features, especially in clinical situations. For example, it should be noted that the representations of the digits and the face are close together. Patients who have undergone upper limb amputation report that they have experienced so-called 'phantom finger' sensations when touching their faces on the same side as the amputation. This phenomenon, which may be reported within two or so weeks of amputation, probably reflects the unmasking of overlapping, pre-existing areas served by neurons projecting from the thalamus to the cortex.

Damage to the somatosensory cortex is associated with partial seizures. So-called sensory seizures, which are sensations passing down the contralateral side of the body, are experienced.

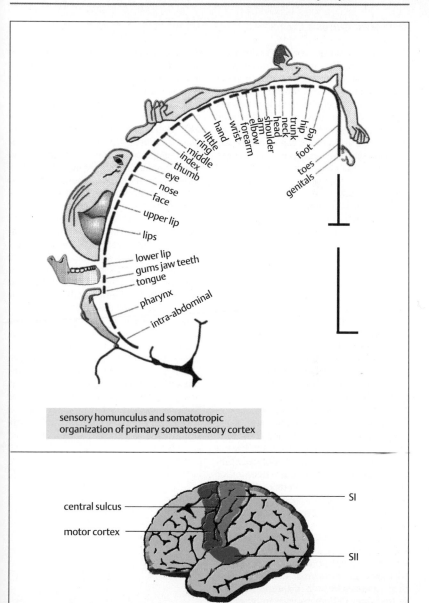

sensory homunculus and somatotropic
organization of primary somatosensory cortex

The Motor Cortex

The **primary motor cortex** (Brodmann's area 4; see p. 336) is somatotopically arranged as a **contralateral motor map** of the body. The representation of the head is found laterally, close by the lateral fissure, and the hands, limbs, and trunk lie more medially. These areas were mapped by stimulating areas of the motor cortex and observing the movements of the muscles. They were also elucidated as a result of the observation of the spread of seizures from distal sites such as fingers, up the arms and to the trunk, which reflected the spread of seizure activity in the motor cortex.

As with the somatosensory cortical map, the distribution of brain areas is disproportionate in size. Areas of the body that require greater precision of movement, such as the face, thumb, fingers, and hands, have a much larger area of motor cortex dedicated to their control than do the trunk or the limbs.

Adjacent to the primary motor area is the **premotor area** (Brodmann's area 6). Stimulation of neurons in this area also elicits motor movements in the body. These neurons project axons to the primary motor cortex, to subcortical areas, and through to the spinal cord. Two main premotor areas have been described. These are the **premotor cortex** (also referred to as **MII**), which lies on the lateral surface of the hemisphere, and the **supplementary motor cortex**, which has also been called the secondary motor cortex. The supplementary motor cortex lies on the superior and medial aspects of the hemisphere.

It is interesting that in all primates, the size of the primary motor cortex in relation to body weight is constant for all species, whereas the size of the supplementary motor cortex is disproportionately much larger in humans than in other primates. There is another difference between the primary and premotor areas, in that stimulation of primary motor units will elicit relatively precise, well-defined movements on the contralateral side of the body, while stimulation of premotor units generally elicits more complex movements. These movements are coordinated and generally involve contractions of muscles at more than one joint. When the supplementary motor areas are stimulated, these movements can also occur bilaterally. In addition to these differences between primary and premotor cortex, the premotor units require greater stimulus currents to generate impulses that will result in body movements. Premotor areas may occur elsewhere in the brain. For example, there are areas of the cingulate gyrus, which is a form of primitive cortex, whose function may be related to the role of motivation, i.e. emotional status, in the planning of motor movements.

Inputs to the motor cortex have been described (see p. 30), but it is worth summarizing here that the motor cortex receives its inputs from three main sources. These are (i) the peripheral body via the thalamic relay nuclei-somatosensory cortex system, from the premotor cortex, and from the sensory association areas of the cortex, (ii) from the cerebellum, and (iii) from the basal ganglia.

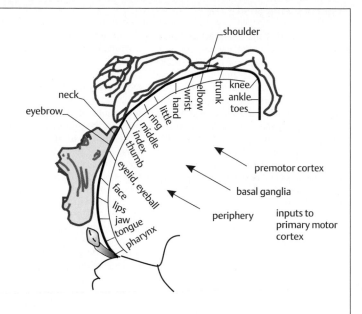

MI motor cortex, showing relative size of body representation

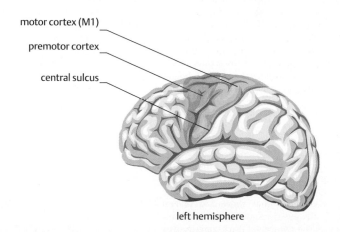

left hemisphere

motor and premotor areas

Origin of the Pyramidal Tract

The **pyramidal tract**, or **corticospinal tract** as it is also known, carries from the cerebral cortex the impulses that make possible the execution of precise voluntary movements. The tract is made up of axons that originate from cell bodies, or perikarya, or neurons in the cerebral cortex. It is the only pathway whose axons pass uninterrupted by any synapses from the cerebral cortex to their ultimate destinations in the spinal cord. It is called the pyramidal tract because of the shape of the pyramidal cell bodies or perikarya from which the axons originate. The term *pyramidal* is also used in connection with this tract to describe an area of the ventral surface of the medulla oblongata where the pyramidal tract crosses over (decussates) to the other side of the spinal cord (see p. 6). It has been estimated that there are around 1 million fibers in the pyramidal tract.

Many, perhaps most, of the axons of the pyramidal tract originate in the primary motor cortex, which is situated in the precentral gyrus (see p. 338). Many axons, however, arise outside the primary motor cortex; these areas include the area in front of the central sulcus, and in areas SI and SII (see p. 176). All the axons of the pyramidal tract originate from cell bodies lying in layer 5 of the cerebral cortex, and, contrary to some earlier reports, not all are the giant Betz cells.

The axons of the pyramidal tract leave the cortex and converge through the **corona radiata** of the cerebral white matter and pass into the posterior limb of the **internal capsule**. As they pass through, they retain the original somatotopic organization. Note that there are several other pathways through the internal capsule, and the pyramidal tract constitutes a minority of these fibers. For example, fibers descend from the cortex to the midbrain; fibers ascend from the thalamus to the cortex; the optic radiations to the occipital cortex pass through the internal capsule. Therefore injury to the internal capsule may result in both sensory and motor disturbance. The fibers pass into the midbrain or mesencephalon, where they spread out to mingle with various other tracts in the middle two-thirds of the crus cerebri (see p. 6), and from there, they pass down to the medulla, where, as mentioned above, decussation may occur. After decussation, the fiber bundles descend as the lateral corticospinal tract (see also p. 182), and the tract gradually lessens in thickness as fibers leave it on its way down to the lumbar spinal cord.

Not all of the fibers of the pyramidal tract are destined for the spinal cord. At the level of the midbrain, a bundle of fibers splits off to form the corticonuclear or corticobulbar tract, which will pass down to the nuclei of the cranial motor nerves (see p. 182). These fibers control muscles of the head, i.e. the face, pharynx, tongue, and the larynx. Some of the fibers of this tract will decussate, but others will innervate cranial nerves ipsilaterally.

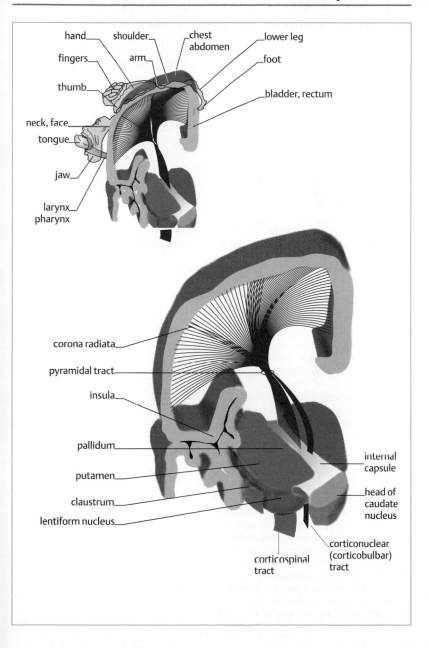

Descending Motor Tracts and Cranial Nerve Nuclei

The **pyramidal tracts** carry efferent information from the motor cortex down through the brain to the spinal cord, where they synapse with cells of motoneurons, which supply skeletal muscle. But not all of these tracts travel to the spinal cord.

There are two main divisions of the motor tracts which descend from the corona radiata and which emerge from the internal capsule. These two divisions are the **corticonuclear** (**corticobulbar**) **tracts** and the **corticospinal tracts** (see also p. 2). The corticospinal tracts in turn separate in the **uncrossed anterior corticospinal tracts**, and the **lateral, mainly crossed, corticospinal tracts**.

The fibers of the corticonuclear (corticobulbar) tract leave the pyramidal tract at the level of the mesencephalon (midbrain), and travel to the **cranial nerve nuclei**. Some of these fibers decussate, or cross to the contralateral side, while others remain ipsilateral, and travel to nuclei on the same side of the brain. The cranial nerve nuclei are involved in the control of facial and oral muscles (see also p. 222).

Cranial nucleus I is the olfactory nucleus receiving afferent inputs from the olfactory mucosa; II is the optic nerve midbrain nucleus receiving afferents from the retina; III is the oculomotor nerve and sends efferents to muscles of the eye; IV is the trochlear nucleus, which receives afferents from somatic proprioceptors, and sends efferents to the superior oblique muscle of the eye.

The nuclei from V through XII are organized in seven columns within the brain stem, according to their embryological origin. Nucleus V is the trigeminal, which sends efferents to the masticatory muscles of the mouth, and receives afferents from proprioceptors and cutaneous afferents from face and mouth. Nucleus VI is the abducens, which drives eye movements through the lateral rectus muscle; VII is the mixed sensory and motor nucleus, which innervates the lachrymal, salivary glands, and muscles of facial expression, and receives afferents from taste receptors of some mouth areas, as well as sensation from the external skin of the ear; VIII is the vestibulocochlear, which receives sensory afferents carrying information about balance, posture, hearing and head orientation in space; IX is the glossopharyngeal, a mixed nucleus, which drives swallowing and parotid gland secretion, and receives inputs from taste buds of part of the tongue, and from the carotid body; X is the vagus, a mixed nucleus, which innervates smooth muscle in heart, blood vessels, and many other types of smooth muscle and which receives several afferent inputs carrying visceral sensation; XII is the spinal accessory, a motor nucleus that drives the muscles of larynx and pharynx, and the sternocleidomastoid and trapezius muscles; XII is the origin of the hypoglossal nerve, which drives the muscles of the tongue.

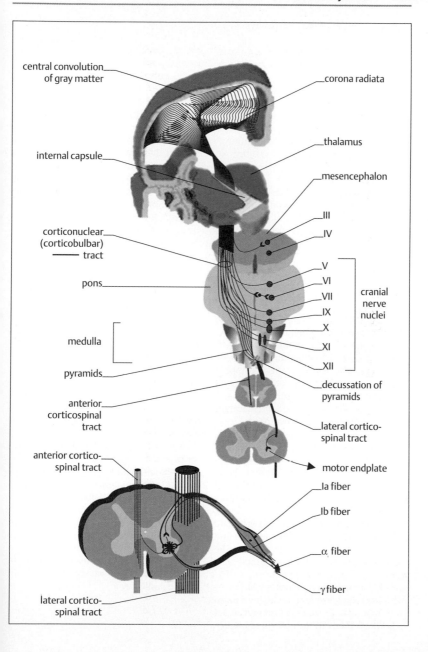

central convolution of gray matter

corona radiata

thalamus

internal capsule

mesencephalon

III

IV

corticonuclear (corticobulbar) tract

V

VI

VII

IX

X

XI

XII

cranial nerve nuclei

pons

medulla

pyramids

decussation of pyramids

anterior corticospinal tract

lateral cortico-spinal tract

motor endplate

anterior cortico-spinal tract

Ia fiber

Ib fiber

α fiber

γ fiber

lateral cortico-spinal tract

Extrapyramidal Motor Pathways

The **extrapyramidal pathways** are those motor pathways that do not pass through the pyramids of the medulla oblongata. They consist of central pathways that modulate CNS motor areas in **cerebral cortex**, **cerebellum**, the **brain stem**, and **spinal cord**. The primary function of the extrapyramidal system is the 'fine-tuning' of voluntary movement to render it amenable to higher levels of conscious control. The absence of such fine-tuning becomes obvious in conditions such as parkinsonism (see p. 370), when voluntary movement is hampered through the presence of uncontrollable tremor in the hands, for example.

Extrapyramidal fibers may originate in the frontal or parietal cortex, and travel to the cerebellum, or to other major extrapyramidal sites such as the **striatum**, the **substantia nigra**, **reticular formation**, **tegmental nuclei**, and the **red nucleus**. The **corticopontocerebellar tracts**, for example, connect the cerebral cortex with the contralateral cerebellum. Since the cerebellum also receives afferent inputs from the peripheral musculature, it is well placed to integrate this information and produce responses designed to maintain posture and purposeful movement.

From these central structures, second-, or third-order neurons, or both, project downwards through the spinal cord in various pathways, and at different levels give off branches that synapse with motoneurons or interneurons in the gray matter of the spinal cord.

The **reticulospinal pathways** originate in the reticular formation of the pons and medulla. The pathways from the pons lie medially in the cord as the ipsilateral pontine reticulospinal tract, while those that arise in the medulla travel as the lateral or medullary reticulospinal tract. These pathways modulate α- and γ-motoneuron activity, particularly in the control of breathing, and circulatory pressor and depressor activity.

The **rubrospinal tract** originates in the red nucleus in the midbrain tegmentum, decussates in the ventral tegmental decussation, and travels down the cord partly mingled with the lateral corticospinal tract. The pathway is excitatory to motoneurons that contract limb flexor muscles.

The **tectospinal tract** fibers arise in the superior colliculus of the midbrain and decussate in the dorsal tegmental decussation. The pathway descends the cord proximal to the ventral median fissure, and most fibers terminate in cervical segments. The tract is believed to carry motor responses to visual inputs received in the superior colliculus.

The **vestibulospinal tracts** originate in the **vestibular nuclei**, which receive inputs from the labyrinthine system of the ear via the cerebellum and the vestibular nerve. The **medial vestibular nucleus** gives rise to the ipsilateral medial longitudinal fasciculus, or medial vestibulospinal tract, while the lateral vestibular nucleus gives rise to the lateral vestibulospinal tract, which excites spinal motoneurons which contract extensor muscles involved in antigravity maintenance of posture.

It is important to note that both pyramidal and extrapyramidal descending influences ultimately meet at the motoneuron to modulate its activity. The clinical implications of damage to both extrapyramidal and pyramidal tracts are dealt with elsewhere (see pp. 42, 370), but it should be appreciated that damage to only the pyramidal system will result in flaccid paralysis, whereas damage to extrapyramidal pathways as well results in spastic paralysis.

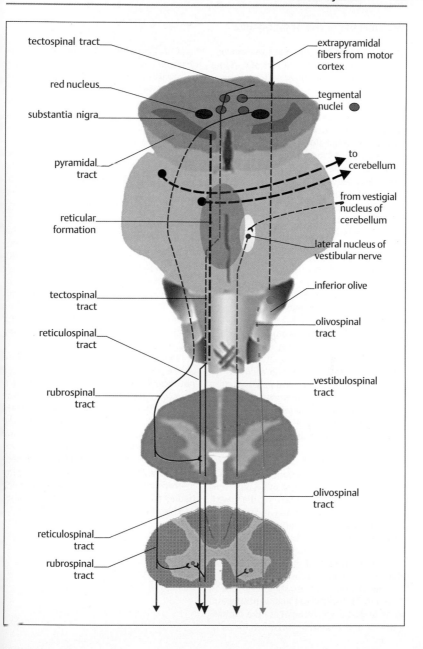

tectospinal tract

extrapyramidal fibers from motor cortex

red nucleus

tegmental nuclei

substantia nigra

pyramidal tract

to cerebellum

from vestigial nucleus of cerebellum

reticular formation

lateral nucleus of vestibular nerve

tectospinal tract

inferior olive

olivospinal tract

reticulospinal tract

vestibulospinal tract

rubrospinal tract

olivospinal tract

reticulospinal tract

rubrospinal tract

Components of the Basal Ganglia

The term **basal ganglia** refers to five sub-cortical nuclei situated bilaterally in the white matter of the cerebral hemispheres. The word *ganglia* is inappropriate, as these are not strictly ganglia, but nerve cell nuclei. These nuclei are the **caudate nucleus, putamen, subthalamic nucleus, substantia nigra**, and **the globus pallidus**. In more recent texts, the reader may find the **nucleus accumbens** and the **olfactory tubercle** included with the basal ganglia as associated nuclei. The globus pallidus and putamen are sometimes referred to as the lentiform nucleus. The caudate nucleus and the putamen are cytoarchitecturally similar structures with small neuronal cell bodies, and are referred to as the **striatum** or **neostriatum**. The name implies that these structures are phylogenetically newer than the globus pallidus, which is also called the **paleostriatum**, or **pallidum**. The globus pallidus is composed of **external** and **internal segments**. The cell bodies of the paleostriatum are larger than those of the neostriatum, and resemble those of motoneurons, to some extent. Together, the neostriatum and paleostriatum are called the **corpus striatum**.

The subthalamic nucleus lies ventral to the thalamus, at the junction of the thalamus and the midbrain. The **substantia nigra** (see also p. 23) lies in the midbrain, and consists of two distinct zones; there is a darkly staining dorsal zone, called the pars compacta, and a pale ventral zone called the pars reticulata, with neuronal cell bodies similar to those seen in the globus pallidus. *Substantia nigra* is a Latin term meaning *black substance*; in humans, the area appears black when stained because of dopaminergic cell bodies rich in neuromelanin.

The nuclei have in some texts been grouped as the **dorsal** and **ventral** basal ganglia. The **dorsal nuclei** are the caudate nucleus and putamen (together the neo-striatum), and the globus pallidus (paleo-striatum). Associated with these are the parabrachial pontine reticular formation, which contains the pedunculopontine tegmental nucleus, the subthalamic nucleus and the substantia nigra. The ventral nuclei are situated beneath the anterior commissure, and include the nucleus accumbens, basal nucleus of Meynert, the olfactory tubercle, and the substantia innominata. These nuclei are closely associated with the amygdala and the ventral tegmental area. In addition to these groupings, in some texts the basal ganglia have been divided into two functional units, namely (i) the striatal complex, consisting of caudate nucleus, putamen, nucleus accumbens, and olfactory tubercle and (ii) the pallidal complex, consisting of globus pallidus and the substantia innominata. The olfactory tubercle has been linked with the striatum because of cyto-architectural and functional similarities, but receives mainly olfactory inputs.

The striatal complex is characterized by the presence of **striosomes**, also called **patches**. These are areas within the striatum that stain negatively for the enzyme acetylcholinesterase (see p. 100), but stain positively for several neuropeptides, and for opioid receptors. The rest of the striatal complex, called the matrix, stains positively for acetylcholinesterase. Most neo-striatal neurons are called medium spiny neurons because of the medium-sized cell bodies and because there are many spines on their dendrites.

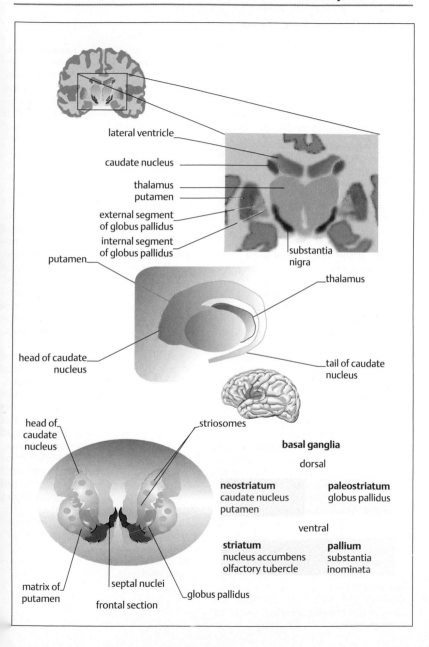

lateral ventricle

caudate nucleus

thalamus
putamen

external segment
of globus pallidus

internal segment
of globus pallidus

substantia
nigra

putamen

thalamus

head of caudate
nucleus

tail of caudate
nucleus

head of
caudate
nucleus

striosomes

basal ganglia

dorsal

neostriatum
caudate nucleus
putamen

paleostriatum
globus pallidus

ventral

striatum
nucleus accumbens
olfactory tubercle

pallium
substantia
inominata

matrix of
putamen

septal nuclei

globus pallidus

frontal section

Connections of the Basal Ganglia

The basal ganglia receive inputs from the **cerebral cortex**, send efferents to it, and inter-communicate extensively. Much of the information received from the cortex contains somatotopically-arranged data. In addition, there are thalamic connections. Most afferent projections to the basal ganglia terminate within the **neostriatum**. The three major contributors to the basal ganglia are the **cerebral cortex**, the intralaminar nuclei of the **thalamus**, and dopaminergic pathways from the midbrain. The dopaminergic striatum inputs from the mesencephalon (midbrain) are known to be involved in at least one motor disease. The destruction of this pathway is the cause of Parkinson's disease (see p. 370).

The basal ganglia send major efferent inputs to the cortex via the thalamus. The thalamus is sometimes referred to as a 'relay' station whose role is the passive transmission of information received from areas such as the basal ganglia, but evidence is growing that the thalamus integrates information received from different sources. The thalamic ventral lateral nucleus receives inputs from the reticular formation, and the ventral anterior nucleus receives cortical inputs, which may be integrated with those from the basal ganglia; the possible functional significance of these interactions is unclear, but may include a role in the control of, for example, the level of consciousness.

Inputs to the basal ganglia from the **thalamus** include the important afferents from the intralaminar nuclei of the thalamus to the neostriatum. This information is topographically organized; the fibers arise mainly in the thalamic corticomedian nucleus, which receives fiber bundles from the cerebral cortex, and the fibers to the basal ganglia from the thalamic corticomedian nucleus terminate in the **putamen**.

There appear to be separate basal ganglia parallel circuits; for example, there are two basic circuits, consisting of **direct** and **indirect** pathways. Generally speaking, the direct pathway facilitates the streaming of impulses through the **thalamus**, while the indirect pathway inhibits impulse passage through the thalamus; the pathways therefore provide a regulator of thalamus activation.

The **direct pathway**: excitatory corticofugal fibers project to the striatum, from where inhibitory fibers pass to the internal segment of the **globus pallidus** and the **pars reticulata**. From the internal segment and the pars reticulata, inhibitory fibers project to the thalamus, which sends excitatory fibers back to the cortex. Inhibitory pars reticulata and internal segment cells discharge spontaneously, unless inhibited, and therefore tonically inhibit thalamic discharge to the cortex. Therefore, discharge of the direct pathway causes thalamic disinhibition and cortical excitation.

The **indirect pathway**: inhibits thalamic discharge through an inhibitory striatopallidal pathway that projects to the external segment of the globus pallidus. The external segment cells fire spontaneously and send tonically inhibitory fibers to the **subthalamic nucleus**. The striatum, via the pallidum, thus disinhibits the subthalamic nucleus, which also receives an excitatory projection from the cortex. The net result is the inhibition of thalamocortical pathways.

At least five parallel circuits of information flow have been identified in the basal ganglia. These are the motor loop, limbic loop, dorsolateral prefrontal loop, lateral orbitofrontal loop, and oculomotor loop.

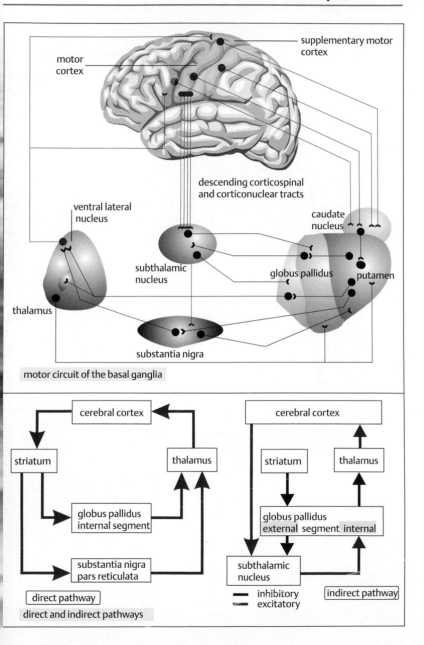

supplementary motor cortex

motor cortex

descending corticospinal and corticonuclear tracts

ventral lateral nucleus

caudate nucleus

subthalamic nucleus

globus pallidus

putamen

thalamus

substantia nigra

motor circuit of the basal ganglia

cerebral cortex

striatum

thalamus

globus pallidus internal segment

substantia nigra pars reticulata

direct pathway

cerebral cortex

striatum

thalamus

globus pallidus external segment internal

subthalamic nucleus

— inhibitory
— excitatory

indirect pathway

direct and indirect pathways

Basal Ganglia Neurotransmitters

The neurotransmitters of the basal ganglia have been studied extensively, in view of their importance in human disease. Very many neuroactive substances have been described in the basal ganglia, but the functional significance of most of them is still unknown. Nevertheless, the study of basal ganglia neurotransmitters and their neuronal distribution is helping to throw light on basal ganglia function in both health and disease.

The inputs to the striatum from the cerebral cortex appear to be all **excitatory glutamatergic** pathways. It is possibly a general rule that all corticofugal excitatory pathways are glutamatergic. Pathways from the striatum to other basal ganglia units, for example **striatonigral** and **striatopallidal** pathways are inhibitory, and are mediated by the neurotransmitter γ-aminobutyric acid (GABA). There is evidence that the peptide substance P may also be an inhibitory neurotransmitter in the striatonigral pathway. The pathway from the external to internal segments of the globus pallidus are also inhibitory, mediated by GABA. The cortex also sends excitatory glutamatergic fibers to the **subthalamic nucleus**, which in turn projects excitatory glutamatergic fibers to the internal segment of the **globus pallidus**.

The **thalamus** is an important component of the motor circuit of the basal ganglia and the **cerebral cortex**, and all excitatory interconnections between the thalamus and the cortex appear to be glutamatergic. The thalamus also sends excitatory glutamatergic fibers to the striatum.

The pattern of inhibitory and excitatory connections between the various components of the basal ganglia underlines the complex nature of motor control, but allows hypotheses about the relationship between them to be formulated. For example, if the cortex excites the striatum, this in turn would presumably excite inhibitory pathways from the striatum to the globus pallidus. Suppression of the globus pallidus would result in a decreased firing of globus pallidus inhibitory pathways to the thalamus, and the net result would be a stimulation of thalamo-cortical excitation of the cerebral cortex.

This pattern of electrical firing can be related to movements of the animal. When the animal is at rest, there is comparatively little electrical activity in the striatum, while there is considerable firing in the globus pallidus and the substantia nigra. Therefore, when the animal is resting, the thalamus is being actively inhibited by the globus pallidus. If, however, a decision is made to initiate a movement, the motor cortex and related cortical areas will activate striatal neurons, which results, ultimately, in the activation of excitatory thalamo-cortical pathways.

Dopamine is an extremely important neurotransmitter of the basal ganglia; its pathways originate in the **substantia nigra**, and project both to the **globus pallidus** and the **striatum**, as well as to sites in the midbrain reticular formation, and the superior colliculus. Loss of the nigro-striatal pathways results in parkinsonian symptoms (see p. 370), and this is a clue to dopamine and nigrostriatal roles in the control of muscle tone at rest, and in the initiation of movement. The role of dopamine in the basal ganglia is dealt with in more detail on p. 192.

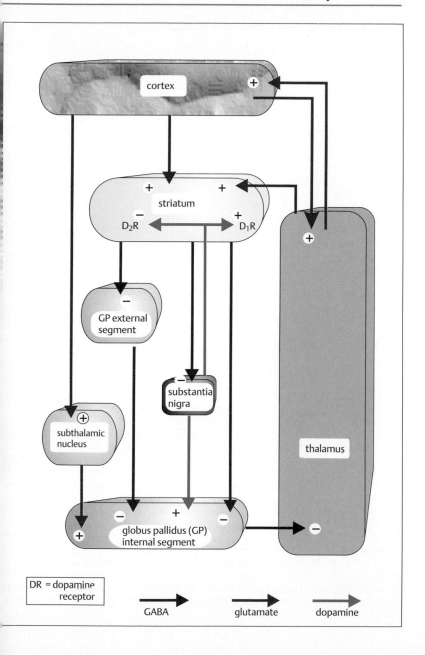

DR = dopamine receptor

GABA   glutamate   dopamine

Basal Ganglia Neurotransmitters and Receptors

The **dopaminergic nigrostriatal** pathway is the largest brain pathway using **dopamine** as neurotransmitter, and has been extensively studied not least because of its importance in degenerative brain disease. It has been found recently that there is an interaction between striatal dopaminergic inputs and those that use as neurotransmitter the nucleoside **adenosine**. In addition, hybridization studies have revealed the presence of subtypes of dopamine and adenosine receptors, situated both pre- and postsynaptically on presynaptic terminals and cell bodies respectively, in **striatum**, **globus pallidus**, and the **substantia nigra**. These findings underline the complexity of action of dopamine in the basal ganglia.

There is some evidence about the actions of dopamine in the striatum. Most of the cell bodies in the striatum are **GABA ergic**, and are projection neurons, and the next numerous are **cholinergic** interneurons. The GABAergic projection neurons to the globus pallidus also contain enkaphalins, while those projecting to the substantia nigra also contain substance P and dynorphin. In the striatum, GABAergic cell bodies that project to the substantia nigra contain on their surface mainly D_1 dopamine receptors, while those that project to the globus pallidus contain mainly D_2 receptors. Striatal cholinergic interneuron cell bodies appear to contain both D_1 and D_2 receptors. In addition, numerous presynaptic D_1 receptors have been found at striatonigral terminals. Similarly, D_2 receptors have been localized to striatopallidal terminals.

There is evidence that adenosine modulates dopamine release from nerve terminals in the striatum through A_1 receptors. Adenosine A_1 receptor mRNA has been found in striatal GABAergic projection neurons and acetylcholine interneurons. Similarly, A_1 receptors have been detected at nerve terminals in globus pallidus and substantia nigra. The evidence suggests that D_1, D_2, and A_1 receptor subtypes are not expressed in the globus pallidus or the substantia nigra but by the striatofugal nerves themselves. In addition, there are high concentrations of the adenosine A_{2A} receptor subtype in the striatum, and in the globus pallidus, where they are co-localized with presynaptic D_2 receptors.

The functional significance of these receptors is uncertain. There is evidence, however, that adenosine acts in the striatum to antagonize dopamine D_2 receptor-induced decreases in extracellular (i.e. released) GABA in the ipsilateral globus pallidus. GABA is an inhibitory neurotransmitter. There is perhaps a balance between dopamine and adenosine influences on pallidal GABAergic projection neurons which ultimately affects motor activity in the thalamus and the cortex.

The basal ganglia are part of the cortical-subcortical circuits that control the parallel processing of motor learning and performance. The overall output of the basal ganglia appears to be a tonic inhibitory one on motor activity. The pathways involved are both direct and indirect. The pathways may balance each other, being inhibitory and excitatory, respectively. It is possible that dopamine through D_2 receptors inhibits indirect pathways, and through D_1 receptors stimulates direct pathways. Adenosine may act as a counterbalance to the activating and inhibiting effects of dopamine. The evidence so far suggests that the receptor interactions are (A_1-D_1) and (A_{2A}-D_2). Clearly, the interactions are complex, and theories of the role of basal ganglia action need to take into account the integration of several projection and interneuronal pathways.

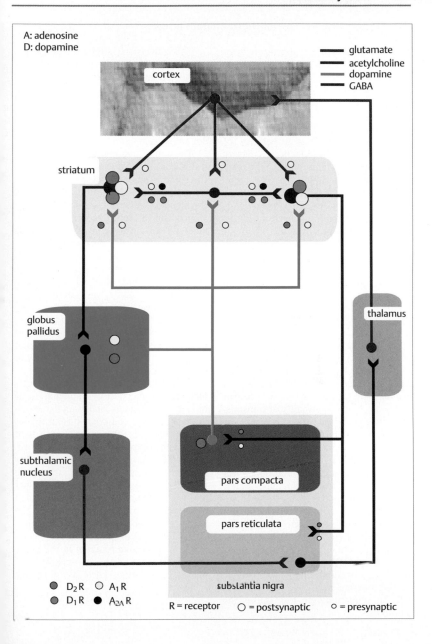

A: adenosine
D: dopamine

glutamate
acetylcholine
dopamine
GABA

cortex

striatum

globus
pallidus

thalamus

subthalamic
nucleus

pars compacta

pars reticulata

substantia nigra

● D₂ R ○ A₁ R
● D₁ R ● A₂ₐ R   R = receptor ○ = postsynaptic ○ = presynaptic

Basal Ganglia Disease: Loss of Nigrostriatal Pathway

Damage to the basal ganglia through injury, stroke, or degenerative diseases produces characteristic motor, cognitive, and emotional symptoms. Motor disturbances may present as hyper- or hypokinesias. Hypokinesias may be akinesias (failure to initiate movement) or bradykinesias (reduction in amplitude and velocity of movement). There is evidence that basal ganglia activity is greatest during the planning stage of a voluntary movement, which may explain the akinesia to some extent. Bradykinesia is caused by a disturbance of the equilibrium between direct and indirect motor pathways.

Parkinson's disease (see also p. 370) is a progressive loss of movement accompanied by affective disorders. The etiology of Parkinson's disease is unknown. Most patients do not exhibit symptoms until the fifth or sixth decade. Motor symptoms are akinesia, bradykinesia, oculomotor disturbance (e.g. absence of blinking), so-called cogwheel rigidity, and loss of postural reflexes. Patients exhibit both normal and shuffling gait, have flexed posture and a 'pill-rolling' tremor of frequency 3 to 6 per second. There is evidence that the cause of the tremor is an abnormality of transmission between the cerebral cortex and the motoneuron cell body.

The disease is caused by the progressive degeneration of the **dopaminergic nigrostriatal** pathway. Symptoms appear when the loss of striatal dopaminergic terminals reaches between 80-90%. At autopsy, the pars compacta lacks neuromelanin i.e. dopaminergic cell bodies. There is evidence of degeneration in other brain areas including the midbrain raphe nuclei, the nucleus ceruleus and the pars reticulata. Other aminergic (noradrenergic and serotonergic) pathways degenerate as well, but dopaminergic loss causes the symptoms.

This conclusion is supported by the discovery that MPTP (1-methyl-4-phenyl-1,2,3,6-tetrahydropyridine), a contaminant of illicitly prepared heroin, caused parkinsonian symptoms in 20-year-old users. At autopsy, the pars compacta of the substantia nigra was virtually devoid of dopaminergic neurons.

The aim of treatment is to replace the lost dopamine. This is attempted through the administration of a dopamine precursor, **L-dopa**, since dopamine will not cross the blood-brain barrier. L-dopa is particularly useful for counteracting the bradykinesia. The drug does not slow the course of the disease, and, disappointingly, its beneficial effects wane with time. Furthermore, the drug produces side effects. The hypothalamus and other brain areas have dopaminergic inputs, and patients experience nausea, loss of appetite, abnormal blood pressure control, mood changes, and sleep disturbance. Atropine-like drugs have also been used, which suggests that symptoms may be related to overactivity of striatal acetylcholine neurons.

A newer and still unconvincing treatment is the injection or implantation of human or autologous fetal brain tissue rich in dopaminergic cell bodies. Fetal tissues are not rejected. The results of treatment have been disappointing so far. Very recently, there have been reports that injection of a vector containing the human gene for glial cell line-derived neurotrophic factor (GDNF) into the rat mesencephalon protected dopaminergic neurons from the destructive effects of 6-hydroxydopamine.

Tardive dyskinesia is another disturbance of dopamine function in the brain, caused iatrogenically by administration of psychoactive drugs such as phenothiazines.

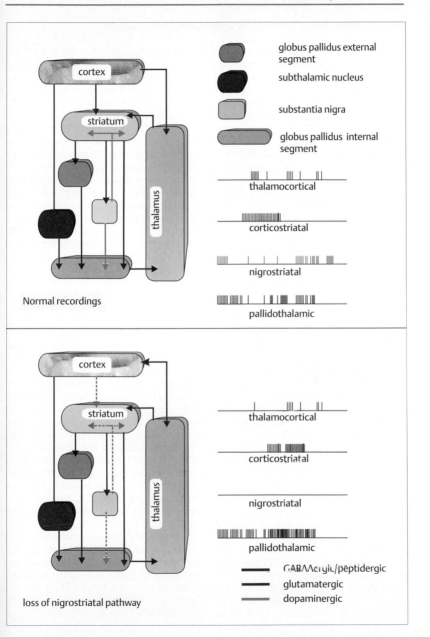

globus pallidus external segment

subthalamic nucleus

substantia nigra

globus pallidus internal segment

thalamocortical

corticostriatal

nigrostriatal

pallidothalamic

Normal recordings

thalamocortical

corticostriatal

nigrostriatal

pallidothalamic

loss of nigrostriatal pathway

GABAergic/peptidergic

glutamatergic

dopaminergic

Basal Ganglia Lesions in Striatum and Subthalamic Nucleus

Some previously unexplained disturbances of motor function, especially those involving hyperkinetic disturbances, have been found to be due to neurochemical lesions in the **striatum** or the **subthalamic nucleus**. In principle, the hyperkinesias may be explained (perhaps oversimplified) as an abnormally high flow of impulses through the thalamocortical pathway due to a disturbance of the normal balance between (direct pathway) excitation and (indirect pathway) inhibition of pallidothalamic pathways (see p. 188).

The hyperkinetic disturbances present as **dyskinesias**, and the three most common are **athetoid** movements, **ballismus**, and **choreiform** movements. Athetoid movements are uncontrollable writhing motions of distal limbs; ballismus is the involuntary (ballistic) jerking of a lower or upper limb; choreiform movements are involuntary dance-like jerkings of the limbs, or movements of the facial muscles.

Huntington's disease, also called Huntington's chorea (*chorea*: Greek for dance), is an autosomal dominant genetic disease that stems from a mutation on the short arm of **chromosome 4**. Clearly, anyone who inherits the mutation will develop Huntington's disease, which can be screened for before parturition.

The disease often presents during the fourth decade of life, with behavioral symptoms, including nervous irritability, depression, absent-mindedness, manipulative difficulties, and sudden falling down. With time, choreiform movements become more frequent, and the patient cannot control the jerky, rapid movements of limbs and face. At the same time, the mood changes become more frequent and intense, and cognitive powers begin to diminish. The patient becomes bedridden, and in advanced stages dementia sets in. Patients usually die within 15 years of onset of overt symptoms. There is no effective treatment for the disease.

The etiology is unknown, but at autopsy the striatum is virtually completely lost. There is a massive depletion of GABAergic neurons. It has been reported that, in early stages, striatal loss is limited to inputs to the external segment of the globus pallidus, while in later life the projections to the internal segment are affected as well. The cause of cell loss is unknown, although it has been hypothesized that cells are destroyed by glutamate excitotoxicity. Glutamate may not be eliminated fast enough in these patients, and remains bound to N-methyl-D-aspartate (NMDA) receptors for an abnormally long time. This would create damagingly high intracellular levels of calcium ions.

Recent reports link Huntington's and some other neurological disorders to the formation of abnormally long chains of glutamine, (polyglutamines), which somehow destroy neurons. Polyglutamines result from the presence in genes of abnormally large numbers (more than 40) of CAG repeats. CAG codes for glutamine. Abnormal CAG repeat numbers are associated with several diseases, including Huntington's, spinocerebellar ataxias 1 and 3, and X-linked spinobulbar muscular dystrophy (Kennedy's disease). Polyglutamines bind to an enzyme, glyceraldehyde-3-phosphate dehydrogenase (GAPDH), and the complex could contribute to neuronal loss. GAPDH is involved in glucose metabolism, and brain scans suggest that glucose metabolism is impaired well before signs of neuronal loss.

Another hypothesis states that the symptoms may be caused (at least in part) through disinhibition of excitatory dopaminergic projections to the striatum. It has been observed that L-dopa exacerbates the choreiform movements in Huntingdon's disease.

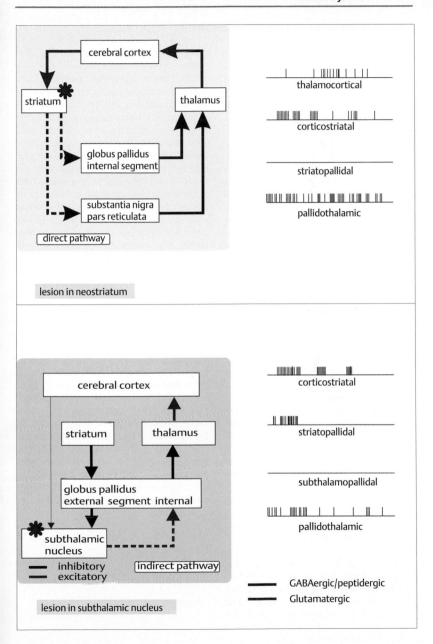

Functional Organization of the Cerebellum

The **cerebellum** is an important member of the central motor control system. As with the basal ganglia, the cerebellum forms part of extensive motor loops concerned with the initiation and coordination of movement. The cerebellum appears to be an integrating center for afferent sensory and other inputs. There are about 40 times the numbers of afferent inputs than there are efferent outputs from the cerebellum. The cerebellum receives afferents from ascending spinal tracts, the cerebral cortex, the eye, and from the vestibular apparatus.

Functionally, the cerebellum can usefully be considered as three separate compartments or modules, each consisting of an area of cerebellar cortex together with its associated deep-lying white matter and nuclei. These are the **vestibulocerebellum**, **spinocerebellum** and **the pontocerebellum**. The vestibulocerebellum consists of the flocculonodular node together with the adjacent areas of the **vermis** (vermian lobule 9).

The **vestibulocerebellar cortex** receives afferents from the vestibular nucleus and the ipsilateral vestibular ganglion. This module is called the archicerebellum (see also p. 18), since it is phylogenetically the oldest part of the cerebellum. The vestibulocerebellar outflow is concerned chiefly with the orientation of the head and body in space, and with certain eye movements.

The **spinocerebellar module** consists of the intermediate and adjacent vermian zone. The module receives its inputs from ascending **spinocerebella**r and **cuneocerebellar tracts**. Fibers that enter the vermian zone project collaterals to the fastigial nucleus. Those that enter the intermediate zone send collaterals to the globose and emboliform nuclei. The spinocerebellar outputs are concerned with the control of axial and limb musculature.

The **pontocerebellar module** (also called the cerebrocerebellar or neocerebellar module) is the largest zone, and consists of the lateral area. This module receives most of its inputs as crossed afferents from the basal pontine nuclei through the **middle cerebellar peduncle**. A major pathway exists from the cerebral cortex to the ipsilateral pontine nucleus and incoming afferents project collaterals to the dentate nucleus. Another important afferent pathway is the **olivocerebellar** pathway from the principal **inferior olivary nucleus**. The **pontocerebellum**, which is phylogenetically the newest module, is important in the planning and timing of movements of the hand and forearm. It sends corticonuclear projections to the dentate nucleus, which in turn projects to the cerebral cortex. The dentate nucleus, also, is the source of cerebellar efferent fibers to the cerebral cortex.

The inputs to the cerebellum are **topographically organized**; the same area of the body may be represented in more than one area of the cerebellum. This has been called **fractured somatotopy**. This phenomenon may be due, at least in part, to the fact that the cerebellum receives inputs from several different sources. Sensory information may be fed directly to the cortex, or may arrive after being processed in, for example, the cerebral cortex, and be sent to another cerebellar cortical area.

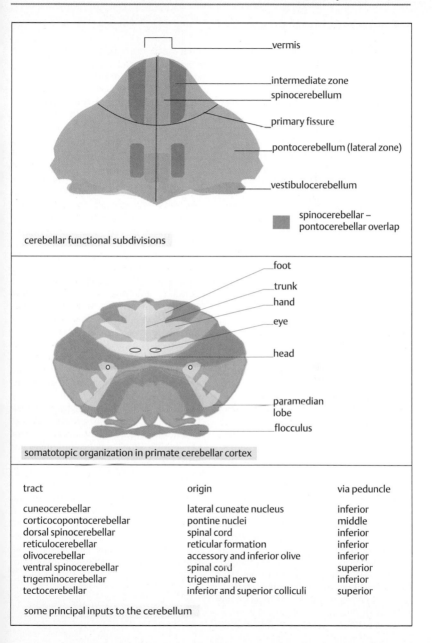

cerebellar functional subdivisions

- vermis
- intermediate zone
- spinocerebellum
- primary fissure
- pontocerebellum (lateral zone)
- vestibulocerebellum

spinocerebellar – pontocerebellar overlap

somatotopic organization in primate cerebellar cortex

- foot
- trunk
- hand
- eye
- head
- paramedian lobe
- flocculus

tract	origin	via peduncle
cuneocerebellar	lateral cuneate nucleus	inferior
corticocopontocerebellar	pontine nuclei	middle
dorsal spinocerebellar	spinal cord	inferior
reticulocerebellar	reticular formation	inferior
olivocerebellar	accessory and inferior olive	inferior
ventral spinocerebellar	spinal cord	superior
trigeminocerebellar	trigeminal nerve	inferior
tectocerebellar	inferior and superior colliculi	superior

some principal inputs to the cerebellum

The Vestibulocerebellar Module

The **vestibulocerebellum** (archicerebellum) is phylogenetically the oldest cerebellar module. The **flocculonodular** and adjacent **vermian cerebellar cortex** receive information about the orientation of the head and body in space from the vestibular ganglion, and receive other inputs from the contralateral accessory **olivary nuclei** (see p. 12). The vestibulocerebellum also receives inputs concerning eye movements from the basal pons.

The vestibulocerebellum sends cerebellar **corticovestibular** efferents from the **flocculonodular lobe** to the **vestibular nuclei**. It also sends cerebellar **corticonuclear** fibers to the **fastigial nucleus**, which in turn projects excitatory fibers to the vestibular nuclei. The cerebellar afferents are GABAergic inhibitory fibers. The **fastigial body** also projects bilateral excitatory fibers to the vestibular nuclei and to nuclei in the midbrain **reticular formation**. From the vestibular nuclei fibers descend as the medial and lateral **vestibulospinal tracts**. The vestibular nuclei project bilaterally to the cranial nerves, namely III, IV, and VI, in tracts that ascend in the medial longitudinal fasciculus.

In addition to the flocculonodular lobe, the vermis also sends efferents to the vestibular nuclei, and receives afferents from them. The **lateral vermian** zones receive ipsilateral secondary vestibular afferents, and send reciprocal efferents to these nuclei. The vermis projects also to the contralateral **ventral lateral thalamus**, and from there to the trunk areas of the **motor cortex**. Both the flocculonodular node and the lateral vermian zones project efferents to the ipsilateral fastigial nuclei. The fastigial nucleus and the vestibulocerebellar module therefore work together to exert their functional effects. The vestibulocerebellum receives information about head movements from the semicircular canals, and about its spatial orientation from the vestibular system.

Through the descending **medial** and **lateral vestibulospinal tracts**, the vestibulocerebellar module controls postural equilibrium, balance, and the judgement of limb movements. This is achieved through synaptic contact with ventral horn motoneurons, which innervate axial and proximal limb muscles. These functions are revealed after injury to midline structures, for example the fastigial nucleus, or to the flocculonodular node. Symptoms range from tremor to complete inability to maintain posture.

Damage to the flocculonodular node produces equilibrium loss. The patient cannot stand steadily (**astasia**), and cannot maintain equilibrium while walking (**abasia**). The gait when walking is unsteady and reminiscent of alcohol toxicity (truncal or axial ataxia; flocculonodular syndrome). The ataxia results from the inability of the muscles to act in coordination. The patient tends to fall over to the side, or backwards, or forwards when ambulating. When standing, patients may stand with feet wider apart than normal; this is to compensate for a loss of balance. In addition to these symptoms, the patient may exhibit axial and head tremors (titubation). Eye movement abnormalities may be seen, including nystagmus, a rapid, uncoordinated movement of the eyes.

The interruption of pathways to and from the flocculonodular node results in characteristic abolition of certain reflexes. For example, patients whose flocculonodular nodes and part of the uvula have been damaged no longer suffer from motion sickness.

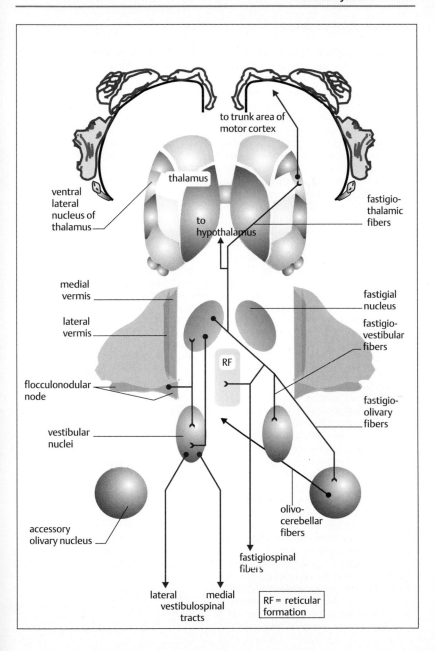

The Spinocerebellar Module

The **spinocerebellum** (paleocerebellum) is so called because the vermian and intermediate zones receive important inputs from the **ventral** and **dorsal spinocerebellar tracts**. Through these inputs, the cerebellum monitors body position and movement. These zones also receive afferents from the upper extremities via the cuneocerebellar tract. The cerebellum also receives inputs from the contralateral **accessory olivary nuclei**. The cerebellum integrates this information and projects it to the **cerebral cortex** via the **thalamus**. The impulses that travel up to the cerebellar cortex in the ascending spinocerebellar tract are arranged in topographical order. The parts of the body are faithfully relayed in topographical order to the ipsilateral cerebellar cortex.

The spinocerebellum exerts control over axial musculature through the efferent outputs from the vermian cortex and the **fastigial nuclei**. It controls limb movements through outputs to the **globose** and **emboliform nuclei**. Afferent information coming from the cerebellar cortex into the emboliform and globose nuclei is arranged in topographical order. Note that the paravermian cortical areas project to both nuclei, while the vermian cortex projects to the fastigial nuclei. From the fastigial nuclei, outputs cross to the contralateral vestibular and accessory olivary nuclei, and into the midbrain **reticular formation**. The fastigial nucleus also projects contralaterally to send fastigiospinal fibers down through the spinal cord, where they terminate in the medial ventral horn. The information sent from the cerebellar cortex to the ipsilateral fastigial nucleus is arranged in topographical order. Fibers from the anterior part of the vermian cerebellar cortex enter the fastigial nucleus at its top or rostral end, while those from the posterior vermian cerebellar cortex enter the fastigial nucleus at its caudal end.

The **emboliform** and **globose** nuclei (also called **anterior** and **posterior interposed nuclei**, respectively) send efferent projections via the superior cerebellar peduncle to the contralateral side of the brain.

Some fibers, the cerebellorubral fibers, ascend and terminate in the **red nucleus**, while others ascend further to the **ventral lateral nucleus** of the thalamus. The system consisting of the red nucleus, together with its descending rubrospinal fibers and the primary motor cortex, with its descending corticospinal fibers, together control contralateral spinal ventral horn motoneurons that drive the distal limbs.

Other emboliform and globose nuclear efferents project caudally and descend to the midbrain reticular formation (cerebelloreticular fibers), while others project to the contralateral olivary nuclei. The reticular formation and the accessory olivary nuclei in turn project reciprocally back to the emboliform and globose nuclei.

In summary, the role of the spinocerebellum is the maintenance of body posture as an **antigravity regulatory system**. The spinocerebellum controls the level of muscular tension or tone required to maintain posture while standing or moving.

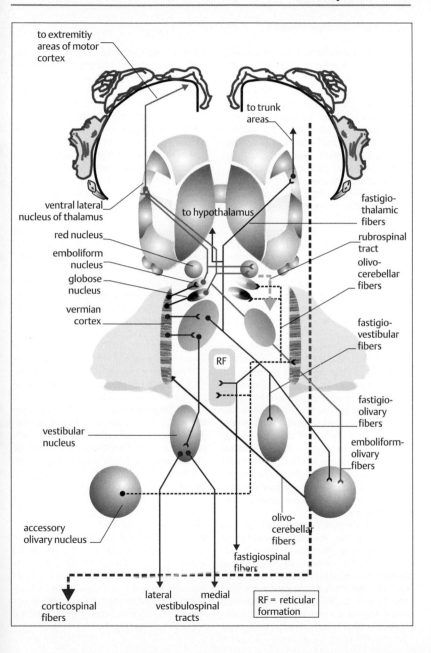

to extremitiy areas of motor cortex

to trunk areas

ventral lateral nucleus of thalamus

to hypothalamus

fastigio-thalamic fibers

red nucleus

emboliform nucleus

globose nucleus

vermian cortex

rubrospinal tract

olivo-cerebellar fibers

fastigio-vestibular fibers

RF

fastigio-olivary fibers

vestibular nucleus

emboliform-olivary fibers

accessory olivary nucleus

olivo-cerebellar fibers

fastigiospinal fibers

corticospinal fibers

lateral vestibulospinal tracts

medial

RF = reticular formation

The Pontocerebellar Module

The **pontocerebellum (neocerebellum, cerebrocerebellum)** is involved in the planning and control of timing of precise movements that require dexterity of the extremities, particularly of the hand, arm, and forearm. The system comprises, mainly, the **cerebral cortex**, the **pontine nuclei**, the **principal inferior olivary nucleus**, the **dentate nucleus**, and the **lateral cerebellar cortex**.

The lateral cerebellar cortex receives major inputs from the contralateral basal pontine nuclei through the middle cerebellar peduncle. The pontine nuclei receive inputs from the ipsilateral cerebral cortex, which explains why the pontocerebellum is also called the cerebrocerebellum. The lateral cerebellar cortex also receives inputs from the contralateral principal inferior olivary nucleus, which sends collaterals to the dentate nucleus. The information in these fibers is organized topographically.

The major outputs of the pontocerebellum are corticonuclear fibers from the lateral zone of the cerebellar cortex to the dentate nucleus, and dentatofugal efferents through the decussation of the superior cerebellar peduncles. Fibers pass rostrally to the contralateral **red nucleus** (dentatorubral fibers) and to the **thalamus** (dentatothalamic fibers), to the **ventral lateral nucleus**, and to the centromedian and intralaminar nuclei. From the ventral lateral nucleus, fibers project extensively to many regions of the cerebral **pre-motor and motor cortex.**

Descending dentatofugal fibers project caudally to the contralateral principal olivary nucleus (dentato-olivary fibers) and, to a lesser extent, to contralateral **pontine** and **reticular formation** nuclei. From the olivary nucleus, reciprocal outputs project to the contralateral lateral zone of the pontocerebellar cortex (**olivo-cerebellar** fibers), and also to the dentate nucleus (**olivodentate fibers**). Similarly, there are outputs from pontine nuclei to the contralateral pontocerebellum. There are also major descending projections from the motor cortex to the ipsilateral pons (**corticopontine** fibers).

The functional correlates of all these connections are not clear; there is, however, evidence that the dentato-ventral lateral nucleus-motor cortex connection drives the initiation of movement in response to a visual stimulus. It has also been shown that outputs from the pontocerebellum to the motor cortex are involved in the planning and execution of the timing and duration of muscle agonist-antagonist timing of excitation and inhibition.

Injury to the pontocerebellar module can result in severe disruption of movement. The ipsilateral side is affected because pontocerebellar efferents project to the contralateral motor cortex, which in turn projects caudally in corticospinal fibers that decussate in the pyramids. Injury is more serious if both cerebellar cortex and dentate nucleus are injured. These lesions result in a partial or complete loss of coordinated movement, termed **dyssynergia** or **decomposition of movement**. Patients may exhibit ataxia, or unsteady gait, hypotonia, which is a loss of muscle tone, and may tend to fall on the lesioned side. **Tremor** often accompanies the lesions, and is most noticeable during movement (intention tremor). (Note that in Parkinson's disease the tremor is more noticeable when the patient is not moving.) Tremor is also evident when the patient stretches out an arm i.e. works against gravity (static tremor). A diagnostic symptom is impaired check or **rebound**, when the patient cannot operate normal agonist-antagonist function. Other symptoms include **dysarthria** (slurred speech), and **nystagmus**.

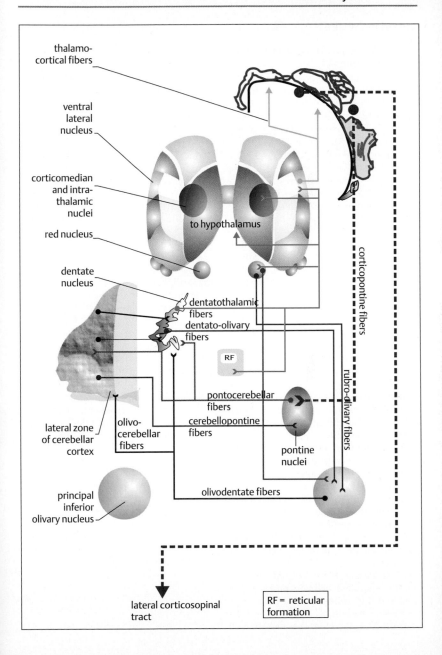

Control of Posture

Posture is body position, which is designed to maintain support against the force of gravity. Put another way, it is the arrangement of vertical position relative to the body supports in contact with the ground. In humans, the support area when standing is covered by the feet, a relatively small area, and the center of gravity is high. Therefore relatively little tilt will destabilize the vertical position. The body is equipped with mechanisms that sense changes in the orientation of the body and of the support area, and with mechanisms that respond to alter posture so as to maintain stability.

Two sources of information monitor changes in body position and ground support: the **head** and the **feet**. The feet have **pressure receptors**, which monitor changes in pressure distribution points; the head has special senses, the **vestibular** and **visual** systems, which monitor motion and position of the body relative to the external environment. The head also possesses a **brain** which integrates information from the feet and the other two systems, and which can instruct the musculature to respond appropriately. Posture maintenance is therefore an excellent paradigm of the integration of the somatosensory and motor systems.

The vestibular system informs the brain about the **velocity** of body movement relative to the semicircular canals, and about the static body position relative to the direction of gravity from the point of view of the semicircular canals. The semicircular canals respond extremely fast to body changes, and are able virtually to warn in advance of an impending upset to body balance.

An important aim is to keep the head upright regardless of body position, the **head righting reflex**. This in turn keeps the **eyes** in the optimal orientation; if the head tilts, for example, the eyeballs will rotate reflexly in an attempt to retain their optimal position for sensing body orientation. Visual responses, like those of the vestibular system may be **static** or **dynamic**. Static responses are those to nonmoving objects such as a tree or the horizon. Dynamic responses are those to moving objects such as trains or revolving doors. The visual responses are slower than those of the vestibular system.

To maintain posture, the brain also needs to know the position of the head relative to the body. This is provided by the **neck reflexes**, which are mediated by joint proprioceptors, mainly around the vertebrae. This does not mean that the head always has to be kept upright; posture can be maintained whatever the position of the head relative to the body.

From the scheme provided opposite, it is clear that the orientation of the body in space is sensed by three independent mechanisms. Swimmers, for example, are kept informed of their orientation under water, even with closed eyes and no pressure on their feet, purely through the responses of the vestibular system. And even if the eyes are kept open while the body revolves rapidly, the person will nevertheless still fall to the ground due to the violent disturbances in the semicircular canals.

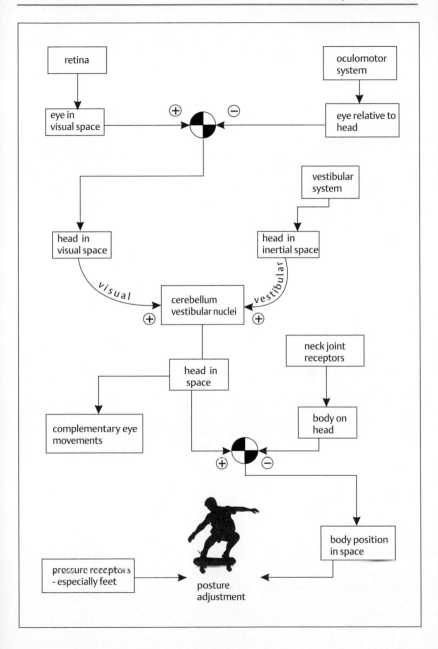

The Reticular Formation

The term **brain stem** is used here to define the anatomically visible brain areas referred to as the medulla, pons, and mesencephalon. In some texts (not this one) it also encompasses the diencephalon. The brain stem is not a functional unit, and can be thought of as two distinct parts: (i) the **reticular formation**, which appears to exert a form of control over the spinal cord and over (ii) the **cranial nerve nuclei**. The term 'reticular formation' is derived from the microscopic appearance of the region as a dense, almost impenetrable network of seemingly randomly scattered nerve cells. Doubtless the term will eventually be displaced by more precise and appropriate terminology as the secrets of the reticular formation are unraveled, and its regional differences in structure and function are better defined.

The reticular formation is a poorly understood, complex network of neurons extending centrally in the stem from the medulla along the length of the brain to the top of the mesencephalon, where it merges with many thalamic nuclei. It occupies much of the space not taken by the tracts and cranial nerve nuclei. It is a phylogenetically ancient part of the brain whose functions include (for want of a better term) the processing of sensory inputs

Historically, very little was known about the reticular formation until the electrophysiological experiments of Moruzzi and Magoun, who showed in the 1940s and 1950s that it was required for maintenance of wakefulness and alertness. The Spanish microscopist, Cajal, had already shown that the reticular formation had some form of topographical organization according to cell size and connections. Later studies revealed the extensive interconnections between the reticular formation and the cerebral cortex, thalamus, limbic system, hypothalamus, cranial nerve nuclei and other brain stem nuclei, and with the spinal cord. A large number of different neurotransmitters have been found in the reticular formation, including the catecholamines, indolamines, enkaphalins, and other peptides, which is suggestive of the vast number of different inputs and interneuronal connections of the reticular formation.

It is believed that the reticular formation is largely an integrative center. It is involved in the regulation of respiration, cardiovascular function, muscle tone, the level of consciousness, and the appropriate motor response to sensory stimuli. The reticular formation is therefore 'aware' of every sensory input received by the body at a given moment in time and receives a huge number of ascending and descending inputs to achieve this state of awareness.

Structurally, the reticular formation has now been subdivided into three main columns of nerve cells. The medially situated, unpaired **raphe nuclei**, or median column, lies in the midline brain stem tegmentum. Immediately lateral to the midline are the paired **medial** and **lateral** columns. A frequently occurring anatomical feature of the neurons of the reticular formation is the presence of several collateral processes that run parallel to the long axis of the brain stem. There are also extensive connections between reticular formation cells and the ascending tracts, suggestive of the integrative activity of the reticular formation.

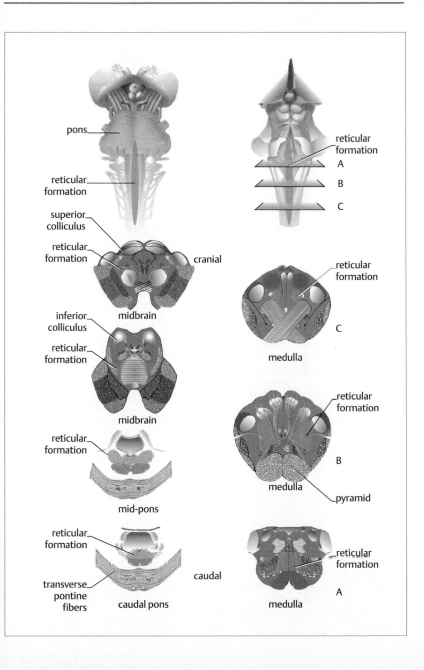

pons

reticular formation

superior colliculus

reticular formation

cranial

midbrain

inferior colliculus

reticular formation

midbrain

reticular formation

mid-pons

reticular formation

transverse pontine fibers

caudal

caudal pons

reticular formation

A

B

C

reticular formation

C

medulla

reticular formation

B

medulla

pyramid

reticular formation

A

medulla

Afferent Connections to the Reticular Formation

The reticular formation receives much afferent input, both from the spinal cord and from other parts of the brain. The **lateral column** of the reticular formation is an important reception area for incoming sensory and other afferent inputs; inputs from collaterals arising from ascending spinal sensory tracts and from **spinoreticular** tracts are especially prominent. The lateral column is made up of nuclei consisting chiefly of small cells, including the parvicellular nucleus in the medulla and pons and the parabrachial nucleus in the pons and midbrain.

Ascending **spinoreticular** fibers travel in the ventral portion of the lateral funiculus with spinothalamic fibers (see p. 160), but they diverge in the caudal **medulla**. The fibers of the spinoreticular tracts terminate in the lateral column of the reticular formation, but give off long collaterals that travel further up to the thalamus. Sensory inputs to the lateral column are relayed to the **medial column** and the **raphe nuclei**. For example, the parvicellular nucleus relays inputs from the ascending auditory, trigeminothalamic, and spinothalamic pathways to the medial column and raphe nucleus. Functionally, these ascending pathway systems modulate sensory inputs to maintain alertness. In addition, the reticular formation may receive information about **nociceptive** and **thermoceptive** signals through collaterals given off by the spinothalamic tracts. The reticular formation also receives information about visual signals through inputs from the superior colliculus.

The reticular formation receives several other sensory inputs in addition to those from the ascending spinal tracts. For example, the lateral column receives visceral inputs in collaterals from ascending fibers of the **tractus solitarius** (solitary tract), which originates in the nucleus of the tractus solitarius, which in turn receives inputs from the vagus and other sensory nerves. The lateral column receives auditory inputs from the vestibular nuclei.

The reticular formation receives descending inputs from the cerebral cortex through corticoreticular fibers that originate principally in cortical regions giving rise to the pyramidal tract. These fibers terminate mainly in areas of the reticular formation that project caudally to the spinal cord; this system is the corticoreticulospinal pathway, which is involved in the control both of automatic and voluntary motor activity. The reticular formation also receives inputs from the **cerebellum**. These originate principally in the fastigial nucleus, and the pathway is important in the mediation of cerebellar control over the activity of both α and γ spinal motoneurons.

The **periaqueductal gray** matter (PAG) surrounds the cerebral aqueduct. Many of its larger neurons form complex connections with the midbrain reticular formation. The PAG also has powerful reciprocal connections with the frontal cortex, hypothalamus, and with the 5-HT (serotonergic) neurons of the medulla. Together with the reticular formation, the PAG plays an important part in the integration of nociceptive, autonomic, and limbic activities.

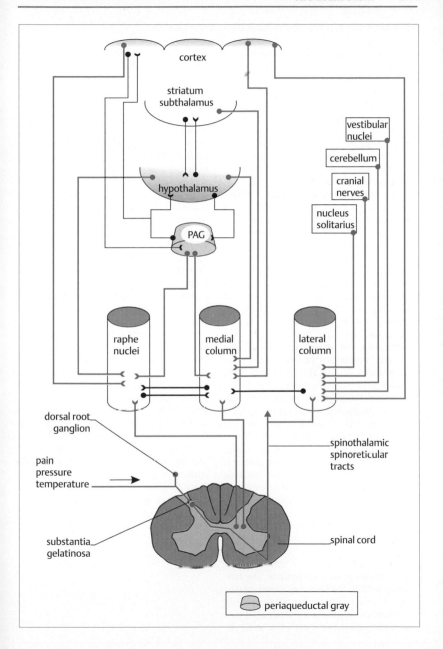

cortex

striatum
subthalamus

vestibular
nuclei

cerebellum

cranial
nerves

nucleus
solitarius

hypothalamus

PAG

raphe
nuclei

medial
column

lateral
column

dorsal root
ganglion

spinothalamic
spinoreticular
tracts

pain
pressure
temperature

substantia
gelatinosa

spinal cord

periaqueductal gray

Efferent Connections of the Reticular Formation

The **raphe nuclei** and **medial column** are the principal sources of efferent projections from the reticular formation to other brain areas. The **medial column** contains large cell bodies in the gigantocellular, ventral reticular, and pontine reticular nuclei. These cells put out long ascending and descending axons with many collaterals that interconnect ascending and descending neurons. Many of these collaterals also travel to the cranial nerves.

Descending **reticulospinal fibers** travel either crossed or uncrossed in the ventral portion of the lateral funiculus and also in the ventral funiculus. These fibers give off collaterals on their way down the spinal cord, and usually terminate on spinal interneurons, which synapse in turn with ventral horn motoneurons. The reticulospinal neurons may be excitatory or inhibitory, and one reticular formation neuron is thus able to influence more than one motoneuron at different spinal levels. Functionally, the reticulospinal tracts are involved in voluntary movements of proximal muscles, and in the control of **body posture** related to the orientation of the body and head with respect to environmental signals. There are at least two areas of the reticular formation involved in the control of skeletal muscle tone. There is a medullary region which when stimulated inhibits the stretch reflex. There is also a more rostral region in the midbrain with opposite effects, in that stimulation of this region increases the activity of the γ motoneurons. The effects of stimulation are diffuse, which underlines the complex nature of the reticular formation efferents involved.

The reticular formation sends important efferents to the **cerebellum**. The reticulotegmental nucleus lies close to the pontine nuclei, and receives afferents from the superior colliculus. The nucleus in turn sends projections to cerebellar cells in-

volved in eye movements. The lateral reticular nucleus lies laterally to the inferior olive in the medulla. It receives inputs from the spinal cord and from the vestibular nuclei and its cerebellar projections may carry information concerning head movements. The paramedian reticular nucleus lies medially in the medulla; the function of its cerebellar projection is unknown.

The reticular formation profoundly affects the state of **consciousness** (see p. 214). There is evidence that this is achieved through mainly cholinergic projections from the mesencephalic reticular formation to the intralaminar **thalamic** nuclei, which project in turn to the **cerebral cortex**. In addition, there are direct projections from the **raphe nucleus** and the nucleus locus ceruleus to the cerebral cortex, which mediate wakefulness and attention.

The reticular formation receives respiratory afferents whose signals originate in the walls of blood vessels and in the lungs. It therefore monitors **respiration**. Similarly, **cardiovascular** activity is monitored by the reticular formation. The efferent projections from the reticular formation whereby it alters respiratory and cardiovascular tone are complex and very poorly understood. The reticular formation is known, however, to send reticulospinal fibers that synapse in sympathetic ganglia and in the dorsal motor nucleus of the vagus.

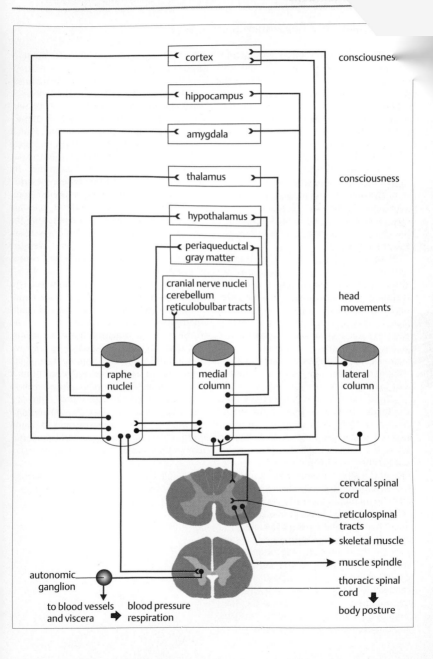

reticular formation is required for normal attention, wakefulness, and normal wake-sleep patterns. If the brain stem is sectioned or damaged at the mesencephalic level, the experimental animal or patient falls unconscious. This happens even if the major ascending sensory tracts, i.e. the medial lemniscus, spinothalamic tract, and the auditory and visual inputs are still intact. Furthermore, the animal cannot be aroused by any sensory input. It is likely that the direct **reticulocortical** pathways and the reticulothalamic pathways, which terminate in the intralaminar thalamic nuclei, are essential for arousal and consciousness.

Many of the activational fibers from the reticular formation to the **thalamus** are **cholinergic**. The projections from the **intralaminar thalamic nuclei** to the **cerebral cortex** are extensive and widespread. It is believed that the reticular formation exerts a tonic control over cerebrocortical activity, which maintains the animal in a state of consciousness, with variable states of attention, depending on the frequency and intensity of sensory inputs.

There are also direct projections from the **locus ceruleus** and the **raphe nuclei** to the cerebral cortex. Those from the raphe nucleus are mainly **serotonergic**, while those from the locus ceruleus are **noradrenergic**. The serotonergic cell bodies of the raphe nucleus extend from the mesencephalon caudally through the pons into the medulla, while the noradrenergic cell bodies of the locus ceruleus are confined mainly to the **pons**. The serotonergic neurons of the midbrain ramify extensively in the brain stem, and extend to the cerebral cortex and to the **cerebellum**, while those in the medulla extend caudally to the spinal cord. At least 90% of the noradrenergic cell bodies of the brain stem are confined to the locus ceruleus, and project not only to the cerebral cortex,

but also to the cerebellum and caudally into the **spinal cord**.

The reticular activating system serves not only to maintain consciousness, but also to highlight attention to certain sensory inputs. This is achieved mainly through its inputs to the thalamus, which in turn activate certain cerebrocortical areas to focus attention on a particular sensory stimulus. This is exemplified by the sudden arousal from a near-soporific state by an alarming sensory input. The reticular activating system directs not only cognitive processes to the source of the stimulus, but alerts the motor systems, which direct the head, gaze, and even the postural orientation of the body towards the stimulus.

The reticular activating system is also a regulator of the degree of activation allowed to reach the cerebral cortex. The diffuse direct reticulocortical inputs and those from the thalamus are in some way gated so that the cortex does not receive too intense a level of stimulation, which could result in inappropriate emotional and cognitive responses to stimuli. This is partly achieved through inputs from the reticular formation to the thalamic reticular nucleus, which monitors and gates the output from the thalamic intralaminar nuclei to the cerebral cortex.

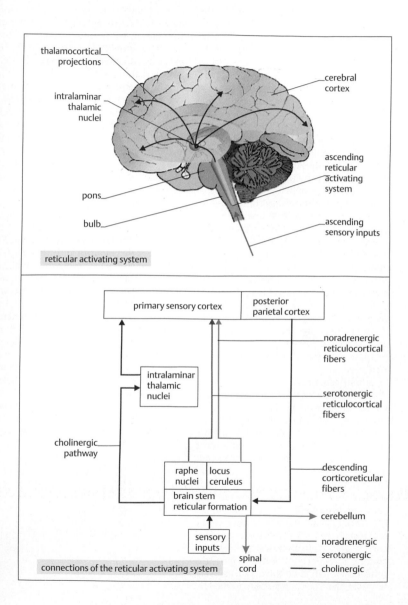

thalamocortical projections

intralaminar thalamic nuclei

cerebral cortex

ascending reticular activating system

pons

bulb

ascending sensory inputs

reticular activating system

primary sensory cortex

posterior parietal cortex

noradrenergic reticulocortical fibers

intralaminar thalamic nuclei

serotonergic reticulocortical fibers

cholinergic pathway

raphe nuclei | locus ceruleus

brain stem reticular formation

descending corticoreticular fibers

cerebellum

sensory inputs

spinal cord

noradrenergic
serotonergic
cholinergic

connections of the reticular activating system

Sleep and The Reticular Formation

The **reticular formation** plays a role in the rhythmical cycle of **sleep** and wakefulness. Evidence for its role can be obtained by using the **electroencephalogram**, or **EEG**, which is a surface recording of electrical patterns. Further evidence is obtained from experimental evidence based on lesioning of selected areas in the reticular formation.

The EEG obtained during sleep suggests that the brain passes through several stages of sleep. Wakefulness is characterized by high frequency, low voltage activity. During the early phases of sleep, after about 90 minutes, high frequency, low voltage activity is observed, accompanied by movements of the eyeball and dreaming. This is the so-called **rapid eye movement** (REM) sleep phase. With time during sleep, the EEG becomes progressively more low frequency, high voltage in character (so-called **slow-wave sleep**) until eventually the order is back to REM sleep. This sequence may be repeated about five or six times during each physiological sleep period. During the sleep period, intervals between REM episodes decrease, and the length of REM periods increases.

Stimulating the reticular formation can alter the pattern of EEG activity in **conscious** animals. The EEG shows high frequency, low voltage activity. If the ascending reticular formation efferents are interrupted through a lesion or a section of the mesencephalon, the animal loses consciousness, and stimulation of the reticular formation no longer produces any change in the EEG. The ascending reticular pathways which effect the changes in the EEG do not involve the participation of any of the major sensory inputs to the **cerebral cortex**, since they can be lesioned without altering the effects of stimulation of the reticular formation on the EEG. It is likely, however, that the changes seen in the EEG after stimulation of the reticular formation involve the reticulothalamic pathway; stimulation of the intralaminar thalamic nuclei produces similar changes to the EEG as those seen after stimulation of the reticular formation.

The reticular formation is important also in the factors that cause the animal to fall asleep. If the reticular formation is lesioned in the **mid-pons**, the animal is no longer able to fall asleep. Furthermore, if a hypnotic drug such as a barbiturate is applied selectively to the pontine-mesencephalon area, the animal becomes anesthetized and loses consciousness. The EEG pattern becomes synchronized for slow wave sleep. If, however, the drug is then restricted to the **caudal** area of the pons, the animal wakes up and the EEG pattern is **desynchronized**. This suggests that the rostral pontine-mesencephalic reticular formation activates and arouses from sleep, while the caudal pons reticular formation is sleep inducing.

The identity of the specific reticular formation nuclei involved in sleep is not known with certainty. There is evidence that the serotonergic raphe nuclei are involved, since the intracerebral injection of 5-HT induces sleep in cats. Nevertheless, lesioning of the raphe nucleus does not permanently abolish sleep. It is now known that the raphe nuclei are partly responsible for the inhibition of REM sleep.

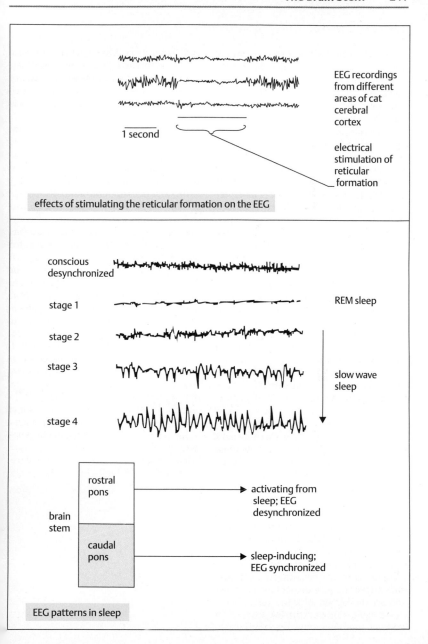

EEG recordings from different areas of cat cerebral cortex

1 second

electrical stimulation of reticular formation

effects of stimulating the reticular formation on the EEG

conscious desynchronized

stage 1 — REM sleep

stage 2

stage 3 — slow wave sleep

stage 4

brain stem
- rostral pons → activating from sleep; EEG desynchronized
- caudal pons → sleep-inducing; EEG synchronized

EEG patterns in sleep

The Cranial Nerves

There are twelve bilateral pairs of **cranial nerves**, which are identified by Roman numerals in rostrocaudal order of their attachment to the brain. The first two, the **olfactory** and **optic** nerves, are attached directly to the forebrain, while the others are attached to the brain stem. Cranial nerves may be **sensory** or **motor**, and may serve more than one function.

There are various types of nerves, classified in terms of their function. **Branchial efferents** (**BE**) innervate muscles that are derived phylogenetically from the branchial or gill arches of fish. They mediate chewing (**V**), facial expressions (**VII**), swallowing (**IX** and **X**), vocalization (**X**), and head turning (**XI**). **Somatic efferent** (**SE**) nerves innervate the skeletal muscles derived from the somites. They mediate eye movements (**III**, **IV**, and **VI**) and tongue movements (**XII**). **Visceral efferents** (**VE**) are preganglionic cranioparasympathetic fibers that innervate smooth muscles of the inner eye (**III**), the lacrimal and salivary glands (**VII**, **IX**), and bowel, heart, and lung muscles that mediate secretions and movement (**XI**).

Somatic afferent (**SA**) fibers carry sensory inputs from the mucous membranes and skin of the head to the CNS (**V**). There are also afferent fibers in nerves **VII** and **IX**, which terminate in the trigeminal nuclei. **Visceral afferents** (**VA**) carry sensory inputs from the blood vessels, GIT, heart, and lungs (**IX** and **X**). Taste (gustatory) inputs are carried by fibers in **VII**, **IX**, and **X**. **Special sensory** (**SSE**) fibers carry messages about olfactory inputs (**I**), vision (**II**), and balance or equilibrium (**VII**).

The cranial nerves are associated with certain **ganglia**. The ganglia associated with **afferent** inputs do not have synapses, and are analogous with the spinal dorsal root ganglia. Ganglia with synapses lie on **efferent** autonomic motor routes. The ganglia serving efferent pathways are classically designated part of either the sympathetic or parasympathetic nervous systems. The **sympathetic ganglia** form a chain of three in the neck area, and consist of the inferior, middle, and superior cervical ganglia, whose postganglionic fibers form a sympathetic carotid plexus. The cranial **parasympathetic ganglia** of the autonomic nervous system are the ciliary (**III**), pterygopalatine and submandibular (**VII**), otic (**IX**), and intramural (**X**). Ganglia **III**, **VII**, and **IX** are associated with fibers of the trigeminal nerve (**V**), some of which may actually pass through these ganglia.

Although the olfactory peduncle is designated as cranial nerve **I**, the true olfactory cranial nerves are relatively short fiber tracts that connect the olfactory mucosa of the nose with the olfactory bulb. The optic nerve, which is designated cranial nerve **II**, has its distal origins in the ganglion cells of the retina (see p. 274), and courses through the optic papilla to the orbit of the eye. After the nerve passes through the optic chiasm at the base of the brain, it becomes known as the optic tract. The afferent cranial nerves that carry inputs to the head terminate in **cranial nerve nuclei**. Efferent cranial nerves also arise in brain stem cranial nerve nuclei.

number	name	description	associated ganglion and type
I	olfactory	SSE	
II	optic	SSE	
III	oculomotor	SE, VE	ciliary - parasympathetic
IV	trochlear	SE	
V	trigeminal	SA, BE	semilunar (SA)
VI	abducens	SE	
VII	facial	BE, SA, VA, VE	geniculate, Pt., submand. (VA)
VIII	vestibulocochlear	SSE	spiral, vestibular (SSE)
IX	glossopharyngeal	BE, SA, VA, VE	otic (VE); inferior, superior (SA, VA)
X	vagus	BE, SA, VA, VE	intramural, inferior, superior (SA, VA)
XI	accessory	BE	
XII	hypoglossal	SE	

BE: branchial efferent; SA: somatic afferent; SE: somatic efferent;
SSE: special sensory; VA: visceral afferent; VE: visceral efferent; Pt: pterygopalatine;
submand: submandibular

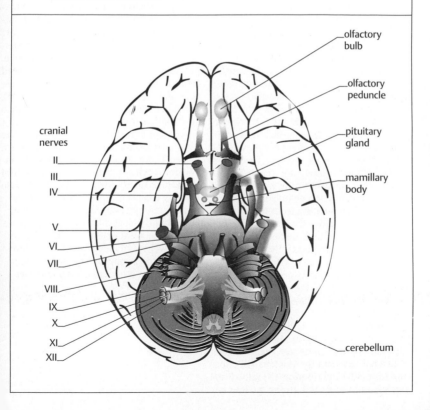

The Cranial Nerve Nuclei

During embryonic development, there is a vertical column in the brain stem from which the different nerve fiber types are derived. As the fetus develops, the column splits into different columns, which migrate away from it. In the mature nervous system, **afferent** cranial nuclei tend to lie more **laterally** in the brain stem, while **efferent** nuclei lie **medially**.

The most medially placed of the somatic efferent nuclei are termed **general somatic efferent nuclei**, and lie caudally to rostrally in the order oculomotor (**III**), **abducens** (**VI**), **hypoglossal** (**XII**), and **accessory** (**XI**). These nuclei innervate muscles that are derived from the embryonic somites; these muscles are termed **myotome** muscles. The **oculomotor** nucleus lies in the ventral apex of the periaqueductal gray matter at superior collicular level. Its efferent nerve fibers constitute the oculomotor nerve, and innervate the extraocular muscles with the exception of the superior oblique, and the levator palpebrae superioris. The **trochlear nucleus** lies at the level of the inferior colliculus, and its efferents supply the superior oblique muscle of the eye. The hypoglossal efferents innervate the extrinsic and intrinsic muscles of the tongue.

The somatic efferent nuclei that have migrated more laterally from the midline of the brain stem are the **motor trigeminal nucleus** (**V**), **facial nucleus** (**VII**), and the **nucleus ambiguus** (**IX**). They are termed **special somatic efferent nuclei**. They innervate muscles derived from the branchial arches. These are striated muscles of the pharynx, and the masticatory and facial muscles.

Lateral to the special somatic efferent nuclei are the **parasympathetic visceral efferent nuclei**. These are the **Edinger-Westphal oculomotor nucleus** (**III**), the **superior** (**VII**) and **inferior** (**IX**) **salivatory nuclei**, and the **dorsal motor nucleus of the vagus** (**X**). The **visceral afferents** terminate in one nucleus, the nucleus of the **tractus solitarius**. The Edinger-Westphal nucleus is the most rostrally placed, and lies in the periaqueductal gray matter near the oculomotor nucleus. Its efferents terminate in the ciliary ganglion, from where postganglionic efferents travel to the ciliary muscles and sphincter pupillae of the eye. The dorsal motor nucleus of the vagus is the largest of the parasympathetic preganglionic nuclei, and lies beneath the floor of the fourth ventricle. Its efferents travel to many different visceral abdominal and thoracic targets. The superior and inferior salivatory nuclei lie in the tegmentum of the pons. The superior salivatory nucleus projects efferents in the facial nerve, and these supply the pterygopalatine and submandibular ganglia. The postganglionic efferents travel to the mucous membranes of the mouth and nose and the lacrimal glands, and the submandibular efferents to the sublingual and submandibular glands.

The **somatic afferent nuclei** are the most laterally placed of the cranial nerve nuclei. These are the **trigeminal nucleus** (**V**), the **cochlear nuclei** (**VIII**), and the **vestibular nuclei**(**VIII**). The term **special sensory** has been used to describe the olfactory and optic nerves, because of their origins in the specialized sensory organs, namely the nasal epithelium and the eye, respectively, and because of their forebrain origins, as opposed to the brain stem origins of the other cranial nerve nuclei.

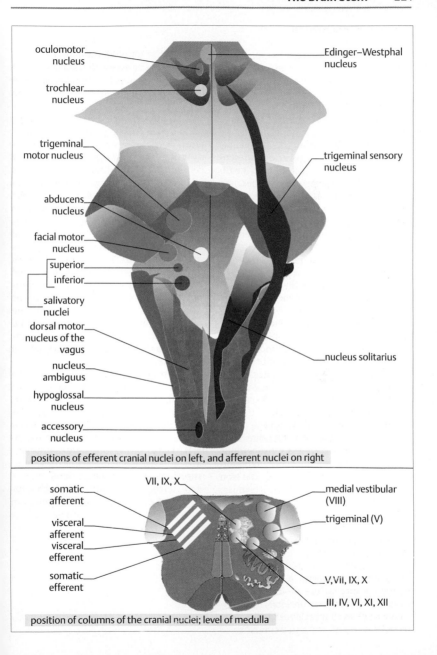

oculomotor nucleus

Edinger–Westphal nucleus

trochlear nucleus

trigeminal motor nucleus

trigeminal sensory nucleus

abducens nucleus

facial motor nucleus

superior

inferior

salivatory nuclei

dorsal motor nucleus of the vagus

nucleus ambiguus

nucleus solitarius

hypoglossal nucleus

accessory nucleus

positions of efferent cranial nuclei on left, and afferent nuclei on right

VII, IX, X

somatic afferent

medial vestibular (VIII)

visceral afferent

trigeminal (V)

visceral efferent

somatic efferent

V, VII, IX, X

III, IV, VI, XI, XII

position of columns of the cranial nuclei; level of medulla

Trigeminal Innervation

The **trigeminal nerve** is primarily **sensory**, and covers a large area of the skin of the **face**, **dura mater**, **major intracranial blood vessels**, the **teeth**, and the **oronasal mucosa**. The nerve also supplies the **masticatory muscles** with both sensory afferents and motor efferents. The three main divisions of the trigeminal sensory nuclei are the **principal**, **mesencephalic**, and **spinal** nuclei. The **trigeminal sensory** (gasserian) **ganglion** lies near the apex of the petrous temporal bone and gives rise to three main sensory divisions: **ophthalmic**, **maxillary**, and **mandibular**. The motor root lies medial to the sensory root. The **motor nucleus** lies in the lateral pontine tegmentum and supplies the masticatory muscles and the tensor tympani and tensor veli palatini muscles. The **supratrigeminal nucleus**, which is a pattern generator for mastication rhythms, lies at its upper end. Both motor nuclei receive corticonuclear fibers, which mediate voluntary control over muscle movements. Where the trigeminal exits from the brain stem, it is close to two vessels, namely the superior petrosal vein and the superior cerebellar artery. Compression of the nerve root by these vessels causes the pain known as **trigeminal neuralgia**.

The **ophthalmic** division enters the orbit of the eye, and carries sensory inputs from the upper eyelid, cornea, supratentorial dura, globe, the mucosa of the frontal, ethmoidal, and sphenoidal sinuses, and from areas of the scalp and face. The **mandibular** division is mixed, containing motor and sensory fibers. It exits the cranium through the foramen ovale, and innervates the gingiva and lower teeth, and the skin of the lower face, extending into the temporal area. A branch of the nerve, the **lingual nerve**, innervates the tongue. The **maxillary** division travels forward in a groove on the floor of the middle cranial fossa, and exits the cranial cavity through the foramen rotundum. It innervates the lower eyelid, the upper teeth and gingiva, the hard palate, the skin above the mouth, and the posterior region of the nasal cavity.

The **motor nucleus** of the trigeminal nerve lies in the lateral tegmentum of the pons, situated ventromedially to the principal sensory trigeminal nucleus. It consists of large multipolar neurons, which are lower motoneurons for skeletal muscles that are involved in reflexes mediated by the trigeminal nerve. These motoneurons are controlled in turn by upper motoneurons projecting from the facial area of the precentral gyrus and other cortical motor areas. There are also smaller interneurons in the nucleus, and inputs from the reticular formation. The motor nucleus is innervated also by several diffuse inputs from the limbic system, and these, together with inputs from the reticular formation, enable the production of appropriate facial expressions as part of an emotional response.

The **principal trigeminal nucleus** projects **afferents** in the contralateral medial lemniscus to the ventral posterior nucleus of the **thalamus**. These carry both mechanical and tactile information. Other fibers travel ipsilaterally to the thalamus, and the afferents constitute the ventral and dorsal trigeminothalamic tracts, respectively. The **spinal nucleus** projects pain, temperature, and some touch information to the contralateral thalamus.

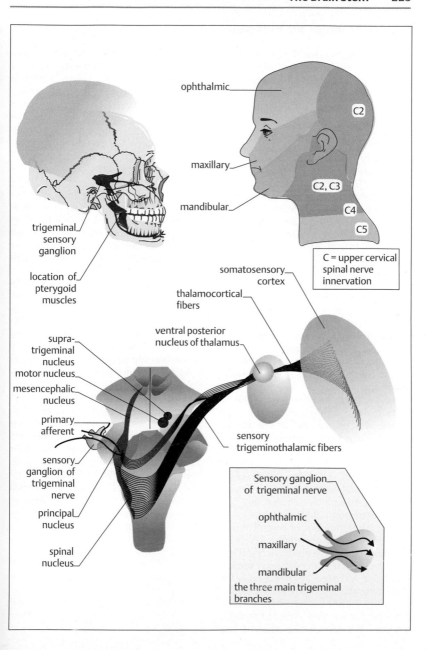

Trigeminal Function and Pathology

The **trigeminal nerve** is the principal **sensory nerve of the head**, and also innervates the **masticatory muscles**. The sensory fibers carry modalities of temperature, touch, pain, pressure, and proprioceptive information from the temporomandibular joint and the muscles of mastication.

Sensory inputs converge on to different central sensory nuclei. Pressure and touch terminate in the principal nucleus, pain and temperature in the **spinal nucleus**, and proprioceptive afferents in the mesencephalic nucleus. These are the only primary afferent fibers whose cell bodies lie in the CNS. In addition to the afferent projections to the thalamus, the trigeminal nuclei project to the cerebellum, and also establish reflex arcs with brain stem reticular formation nuclei. The trigeminal system mediates several head **reflexes**, and **mastication**.

Mastication (chewing) is complex, involving both voluntary and reflex actions that require the coordinated activity of central nuclear groups, which supply motor nerves to the cheeks, tongue, mandible, and hyoid bone. Mastication appears to be controlled in the **premotor cortex**, directly in front of the cortical areas on which the homuncular face is represented. In the brain stem, mastication is controlled by the **supratrigeminal motor nucleus**, which projects directly to the **trigeminal motor nucleus** and also to ipsilateral trigeminocerebellar and contralateral trigeminothalamic nuclei.

The trigeminal nuclei control several reflexes. The **jaw-opening** reflex is initiated by stretch afferents, particularly in the anterior part of the **masseter muscle**, which are activated by dental occlusion. These provoke a supratrigeminal nuclear response, which inhibits closure motoneurons and activates jaw-opening motoneurons. The **jaw-closing** reflex is triggered by contact of food with the oral mucosa. The **jaw jerk** or **masseter** reflex is a monosynaptic tendon reflex, which is evoked when the chin is tapped with a downward stroke, which elicits a twitch of the jaw-closing muscles, including the masseter. Lesions in or near the motor nucleus, for example in **pseudobulbar palsy**, which is caused usually by thrombotic episodes in the brain stem, produces an abnormally brisk reflex response. The trigeminal is involved, together with the facial nerve, in the blink or **corneal reflex**, the **sucking reflex**, which is elicited by touching mechanoreceptor nerve endings in the lips of the neonate, and the **sneeze reflex**, produced by exciting touch receptors in the nasal mucosa.

Trigeminal neuralgia is the term given to the occurrence of intense pain, often in patients over 60 years, within one or more of the peripheral territorial divisions of the trigeminal system. The diagnosis involves the localization of the pain using a **trigeminal sensory map**; this is useful in differentiating the pain from that involving, for example, the facial nerve. **Infection of sensory nerve roots** by herpes zoster causes painful shingles-like symptoms. In winter, inflammatory conditions cause nociceptive activity in afferents from the mucosa of the middle ear, larynx, pharynx, and pharyngotympanic tube. **Dental** pain is ascribed to nociceptive activity in trigeminal afferents, and **frontal headache** may be due to activation of trigeminal afferents activated by lesions distorting cerebral arteries.

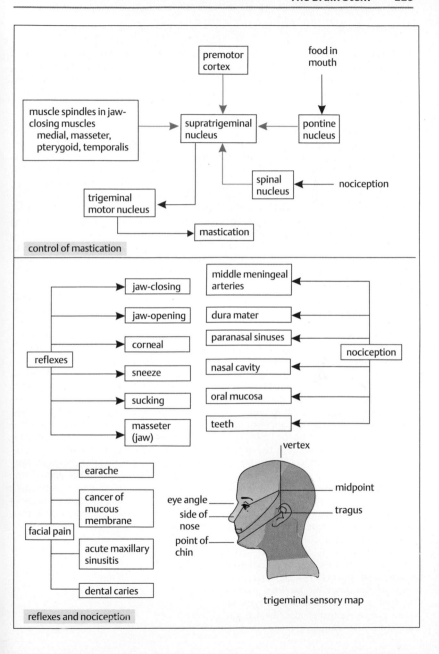

control of mastication

reflexes and nociception

trigeminal sensory map

The Facial Nerve

The **facial** (**VII**) **nerve** contains **motor**, **parasympathetic**, and **sensory fibers**. It supplies several **facial muscles**, including those involving facial expression. It also supplies the posterior digastric, stapedius, and stylohyoid muscles. The nerve has two roots: the nervus intermedius, which contains the parasympathetic and sensory fibers, and the facial nerve proper, which contains the motor fibers.

The **motor nucleus** of the facial nerve lies in the pons and receives fibers from the facial region of the contralateral motor cortex and from the ipsilateral cortex. The latter innervate motor nucleus cells that supply muscles of the upper face. This bilateral supply enables the paired muscular actions of blinking, tight eye closure, and voluntary wrinkling of the forehead. Contrast this with the **unilateral** voluntary control of mouth muscles. The fibers leaving the motor nucleus initially loop over the **abducens nucleus** beneath the floor of the fourth ventricle, after which they leave the brain stem in the facial nerve motor root, which passes through the **stylomastoid foramen**. The division of the motor nucleus into **supranuclear**, **nuclear**, and **infranuclear** nuclei is useful in diagnosis of facial nerve lesions. The supranuclear supply receives inputs from the limbic system via the nucleus accumbens, which makes the facial muscles responsive to emotional changes.

The nervus intermedius contains parasympathetic and sensory fibers. The parasympathetic root projects from the **superior salivatory nucleus**, and forms the motor component of the chorda tympani and greater petrosal nerves. The latter nerve synapses in the **pterygopalatine ganglion** with postganglionic fibers that innervate the **nasal** and **lacrimal glands**. The motor fibers of the chorda tympani synapse with postganglionic fibers in the **submandibular ganglion**; these fibers innervate the salivary sublingual and submandibular glands. The nervus intermedius has a sensory root in the **geniculate ganglion**, whose unipolar cell bodies receive inputs from the taste buds from the tongue and palate.

The facial nerve motor nucleus receives several afferent inputs from brain stem regions, which enable it to mediate reflexes, including the **corneal reflex**, which is the reflex closing of the eye in response to touching the cornea; this depends on inputs to the nucleus from the trigeminal sensory nucleus. Reflex eye closure in response to visual inputs depends on inputs from the superior colliculus. **Auditory inputs** from the olivary nucleus to the facial motor nucleus mediate reflex eye closure.

Lesions of the facial nerve are the most frequent cause of loss of facial reflexes and facial paralysis. **Supranuclear lesions** are usually caused by interruption of corticofugal fibers through a vascular stroke. The result is lower face motor weakness, which does not affect the upper face since this is bilaterally supplied. **Nuclear lesions** may be caused by thrombosis of a pontine branch of the basilar artery, resulting in complete paralysis of the abducens, or facial nerve, or both, and crossed hemiplegia. **Infranuclear lesions** include viral infection of the nerve, which swells and is compressed in a bony canal between the stylomastoid foramen and the geniculate ganglion. This results in the unilateral **Bell's palsy**, in which the patient cannot close the eye, retract the lip, or raise the eyebrow.

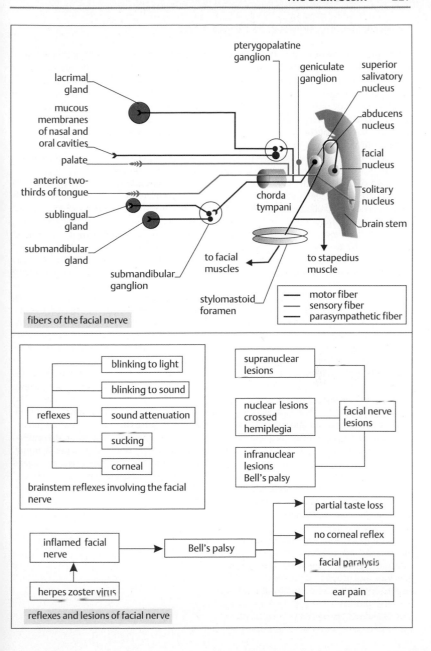

pterygopalatine ganglion

geniculate ganglion

superior salivatory nucleus

lacrimal gland

mucous membranes of nasal and oral cavities

abducens nucleus

facial nucleus

palate

anterior two-thirds of tongue

chorda tympani

solitary nucleus

sublingual gland

brain stem

submandibular gland

submandibular ganglion

to facial muscles

to stapedius muscle

stylomastoid foramen

— motor fiber
— sensory fiber
— parasympathetic fiber

fibers of the facial nerve

blinking to light

blinking to sound

reflexes — sound attenuation

sucking

corneal

brainstem reflexes involving the facial nerve

supranuclear lesions

nuclear lesions crossed hemiplegia

facial nerve lesions

infranuclear lesions Bell's palsy

inflamed facial nerve → Bell's palsy

partial taste loss

no corneal reflex

facial paralysis

ear pain

herpes zoster virus

reflexes and lesions of facial nerve

The Accessory, Hypoglossal, and Vagus Nerves

The **vagus**, **accessory**, and **hypoglossal** nerves are X, XI, and XII, respectively. The vagus is the main parasympathetic nerve, having very extensive motor and sensory components (see also p. 240: the autonomic nervous system). The **accessory nerve** is purely **motor**, and consists of **cranial** and **spinal** divisions. The cranial part has a linear set of rootlets that project bilaterally from the medulla, and lie just caudal to the vagal roots. The spinal part projects from the five most rostral segments of the spinal cord. The **hypoglossal** nerve is also a purely motor nerve, which supplies the extrinsic and intrinsic muscles of the **tongue**.

The **motor efferents** of the vagus originate in the **nucleus ambiguus** of the medulla, and innervate the muscles of the **larynx**, **pharynx**, soft palate, and the upper esophagus. Therefore, damage to the nucleus ambiguus affects speech and swallowing. Note that the caudal vagal efferents leave the brain stem in the cranial roots of the accessory nerve, but join the other vagal fibers at the **jugular foramen**. The **parasympathetic efferents** originate in the **dorsal motor nucleus of the vagus**, which lies beneath the floor of the fourth ventricle in the medulla. They innervate large parts of the cardiovascular, GIT, and respiratory systems. Sensory afferents of the vagus join the brain stem just caudal to the glossopharyngeal nerve, and carry inputs from the abdominal and thoracic viscera, from baroreceptors in the aortic arch, and chemoreceptors in the aortic bodies. They also carry general sensory inputs from part of the concha of the external ear, the tympanic membrane, external auditory meatus, the larynx, pharynx, and esophagus. Vagus visceral afferents outnumber efferents by at least 4:1 (see also p. 172).

Cranial accessory fibers become incorporated into the vagus at the **jugular fora-men**. The efferent cranial accessory division consists of visceral efferents from the nucleus ambiguus. These are the motor fibers of the vagus, which supply the larynx, pharynx, and upper third of the esophagus. The spinal fibers originate also in the nucleus ambiguus and travel with the vagus. They innervate the trapezius and sternomastoid muscles, which move head and shoulders.

The **hypoglossal** nerve originates in the **hypoglossal nucleus**, and travels through the medulla, emerging from the brain stem as a group of rootlets between the pyramid and the olive. The efferents mediate movement and shape of the **tongue**. The hypoglossal nucleus receives afferent inputs from the contralateral **motor cortex**, which are involved in voluntary tongue movements during speech. It also receives afferents from the trigeminal sensory nucleus and from the solitary nucleus (nucleus solitarius). These afferents are part of the reflex control of swallowing, chewing, and sucking.

If the hypoglossal nucleus nerve is lesioned unilaterally, this results in **tongue paralysis** on the **ipsilateral side**. The tongue atrophies and becomes distorted, mainly because the mucous membranes of the tongue are too large to be accommodated by the reduced tongue volume. Paresis of the tongue, which means muscular weakness, results.

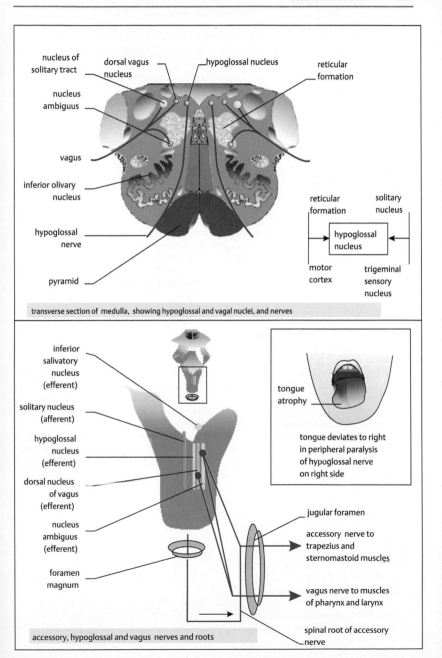

transverse section of medulla, showing hypoglossal and vagal nuclei, and nerves

accessory, hypoglossal and vagus nerves and roots

The Glossopharyngeal Nerve

The **glossopharyngeal nerve** (**IX**) is mainly sensory in function, but does have some preganglionic parasympathetic and motor fibers. On route to the brain stem, the nerve leaves the mucous membrane of the oropharynx and runs between the middle and superior constrictor muscles. Where the nerve enters the brain at the base of the skull, it joins the **vagus**, spinal accessory, and the sympathetic internal carotid branch of the superior cervical ganglion. The glossopharyngeal runs together with the vagus through the anterior compartment of the jugular foramen. The posterior compartment of the foramen accommodates the bulb of the internal jugular vein. In the foramen the glossopharyngeal has small inferior and superior ganglia which contain sensory unipolar neurons. It carries at least five afferent inputs to the brain stem, which it enters through a linearly arranged set of rootlets, which lie lateral to the olive in the rostral part of the medulla. The afferents terminate in the **trigeminal sensory nucleus**.

The glossopharyngeal nerve innervates the **taste buds** and receptors for general sensation of the pharynx and posterior third of the **tongue**; the nerve also innervates **carotid body** chemoreceptors, **carotid sinus** baroreceptors, the eustachian tube, and the middle ear. The gustatory afferents from the taste buds terminate centrally in the **gustatory nucleus**. The oropharynx is the largest peripheral sensory field of the nerve. The oropharynx is accessible to clinical investigation of the integrity of the glossopharyngeal. This is tested through the **gag reflex**, which is elicited by stroking the wall of the oropharynx. The patient swallows reflexly (and usually experiences nausea). In the brain stem, the reflex is mediated through connections between the **nucleus ambiguus** and the hypoglossal nucleus. Branches of the glossopharyngeal that serve modalities of touch in the oropharynx synapse in the brain stem in the **commissural nucleus**.

The **carotid branch** of the glossopharyngeal contains two sets of afferents. One set runs centrally from the **baroreceptor** stretch receptors in the wall of the **carotid sinus** at the beginning of the internal carotid artery. These receptors respond to changes in the systolic pressure. These afferents synapse centrally in the medial portion of the solitary nucleus. Another set of afferents run centrally from the glomus cells of the **carotid body**. The nerve endings of these afferents are chemoreceptors, which respond to O_2 and CO_2 partial pressure changes in the blood. Their afferents terminate centrally in the **dorsal respiratory nucleus**.

Just before it leaves the jugular foramen, the nerve gives off the **tympanic branch**, which spreads or ramifies over the tympanic membrane; this branch is often a source of referred pain to the ear. In the brain stem, the tympanic branch terminates in the spinal nucleus of the trigeminal nerve, which receives temperature and nociceptive inputs from the neck and head. The **motor** component of the glossopharyngeal originates in the rostral part of the medullary nucleus ambiguus, and innervates the **stylopharyngeus muscle**, which takes part in swallowing. A parasympathetic motor nerve runs from the inferior salivatory nucleus to the otic ganglion; the postganglionic nerve innervates the **salivary parotid gland**.

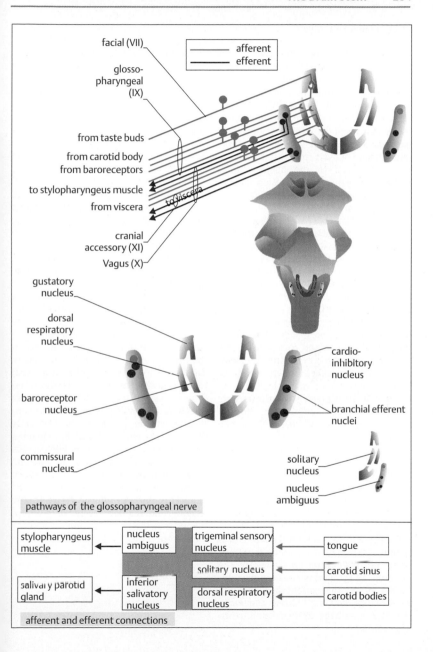

facial (VII)

glosso-pharyngeal (IX)

afferent
efferent

from taste buds

from carotid body
from baroreceptors

to stylopharyngeus muscle

from viscera

to viscera

cranial accessory (XI)

Vagus (X)

gustatory nucleus

dorsal respiratory nucleus

cardio-inhibitory nucleus

baroreceptor nucleus

branchial efferent nuclei

commissural nucleus

solitary nucleus

nucleus ambiguus

pathways of the glossopharyngeal nerve

stylopharyngeus muscle	←	nucleus ambiguus	trigeminal sensory nucleus	←	tongue
			solitary nucleus	←	carotid sinus
salivary parotid gland	←	inferior salivatory nucleus	dorsal respiratory nucleus	←	carotid bodies

afferent and efferent connections

Cranial Nerve Paralysis

Interruption of the **corticonuclear** supply to the brain stem nuclei (**supranuclear**), or damage to the nuclei (**nuclear**), causes paralysis of the muscles they innervate, and decreases or deletes their other **cranial** and **visceral** actions. Interruption is often the result of cerebral or brain stem **vascular strokes** that damage the pyramidal tract. Paralysis may result if structures peripheral to the nuclei (**infranuclear**) are damaged. The lesion may be caused by injury, by cardiovascular accident, or **tumor** growth.

Supranuclear lesions to nerves **IX**, **X**, and **XI** may be **unilateral** or **bilateral**. A muscle or organ that is bilaterally supplied is less vulnerable than one that receives a unilateral supply, and if the supply decussates, i.e. is crossed, then the contralateral muscle or organ will be affected. The **hypoglossal** nerve (**XII**), for example, innervates the extrinsic and intrinsic striated tongue muscle fibers. The descending fibers from the motor cortex decussate and terminate in the contralateral nucleus. The nuclei are paired in the medulla. Therefore unilateral supranuclear damage, for example **hemiplegic stroke**, interrupts outflow to the contralateral tongue muscles. (**Hemiplegia** is paralysis on one side of the body.) The patient can still swallow and talk because the nucleus ambiguus has a bilateral supranuclear supply. **Bilateral** supranuclear lesions may occur in patients who develop arteriosclerosis of the vertebrobasilar arterial system, with resultant brain stem thrombosis and bilateral damage to the supranuclear supply to the hypoglossal nuclei and **nucleus ambiguus**. This may also affect the facial nerve and **trigeminal** motor nuclei. The spectrum of symptoms is called **pseudobulbar palsy**; the patient has difficulty chewing, swallowing, talking, and walking, due to damage to descending corticospinal fibers.

Nuclear lesions in cranial nuclei of nerves **X**, **XI**, and **XII** result in **progressive bulbar palsy**. Damage to the nucleus ambiguus and hypoglossal nucleus demonstrates symptoms similar to those seen in pseudobulbar palsy; speech (phonation) and swallowing are difficult due to damage to the hypoglossal and cranial accessory nuclei, while damage to the facial and mandibular nuclei hamper articulation of the jaw and chewing.

Infranuclear lesions of nerves **IX**, **X**, **XI**, and **XII** are most commonly the result of a **tumor** that grows and spreads at the base of the skull. The tumor may be **primary**, in the nasopharynx, or **metastatic**, in the lymph nodes of the upper cervical chain. The primary tumor responsible for the metastasis may be within the larynx, pharynx, or tongue, or contained within an air sinus. It is usually possible to palpate a mass behind the ramus of the mandible. The symptoms of the tumor are pain and (i) **headache**, through inflammation of the meningeal branch of the vagus, (ii) difficulty with **swallowing** (dysphagia) due to pharyngomotor fiber paralysis, (iii) **hoarse** voice, through laryngomotor fiber paralysis, and (iv) **earache**, due to inflammation of the tympanic and auricular branches of nerves IX and X. Unilateral earache, without signs of middle ear disease, is often symptomatic of pharynx cancer. A lesion of the **spinal accessory nerve** may result in paralysis of the **trapezius muscle**, which atrophies. The clavicle and scapula are no longer supported and the shoulder drops. The neck contour becomes 'scalloped'.

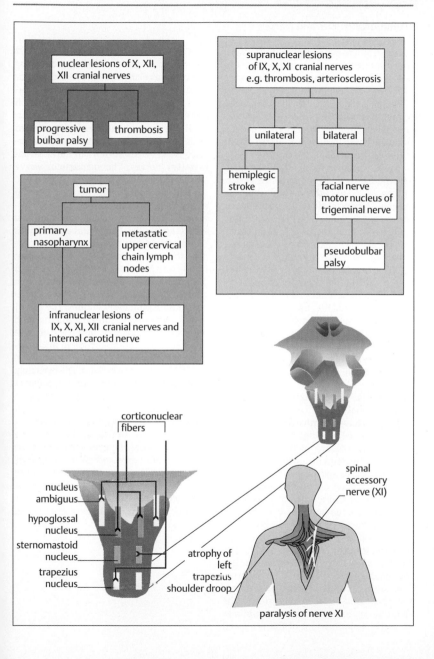

nuclear lesions of X, XII, XII cranial nerves

progressive bulbar palsy

thrombosis

tumor

primary nasopharynx

metastatic upper cervical chain lymph nodes

infranuclear lesions of IX, X, XI, XII cranial nerves and internal carotid nerve

supranuclear lesions of IX, X, XI cranial nerves e.g. thrombosis, arteriosclerosis

unilateral

bilateral

hemiplegic stroke

facial nerve motor nucleus of trigeminal nerve

pseudobulbar palsy

corticonuclear fibers

spinal accessory nerve (XI)

nucleus ambiguus

hypoglossal nucleus

sternomastoid nucleus

trapezius nucleus

atrophy of left trapezius shoulder droop

paralysis of nerve XI

Oculomotor Nuclei and Nerves

The main aim of **eye movement** is to focus external objects on to the fovea of the eye (see p. 236), and to keep the focus on the fovea. The eye has to be stabilized even when the head moves. Each eye has six **extraocular muscles**, and each eye has five movements, which are governed by three bilateral groups of **brain stem oculomotor nuclei**.

The extraocular muscles are the **inferior**, **medial**, **lateral**, and **superior rectus** muscles, and the **inferior** and **superior oblique**. The muscles enable the eye to **rotate** freely around its center in three planes: horizontal, vertical, and torsional. Horizontal movement takes place about the transverse (**z-**) **axis**, and the eye moves from side to side. When looking to the left, the left eye rotates laterally (**adduction**), and the right eye rotates medially (**abduction**). When looking up (**elevation**) or down (**depression**), the eye rotates around the **x-axis**. The eye can also rotate the cornea about the **y-axis** toward (**intorsion**) or away (**extorsion**) from the nose. Torsional rotations enable the gaze always to be stabilized perpendicular to the horizontal axis. All the extraocular muscles have some torsional action.

The **extraocular muscles** are aligned straight (**rectus**) or **oblique**, relative to the alignment of the eye in the socket. The four **rectus muscles** originate on the apex of the eye orbit, and insert on the sclera, which is the outer coat of the eyeball, situated anterior to the equator of the eye. The **lateral rectus** pulls the cornea laterally, while the **medial rectus** pulls it medially. The **superior rectus** pulls the eye upward, the **inferior** pulls it downward. The **superior oblique** muscle originates posteriorly in the orbit, is hooked onto a loop of connective tissue (**trochlea**), and travels posterolaterally to insert posterior to the equatorial plane. The **inferior oblique** originates at the bottom of the orbit and

runs posterolaterally and inserts behind the equatorial plane. All the extraocular muscles are relatively thin and richly supplied with muscle spindles, whose function may be integrated with information from the vestibular system and the retina.

The extraocular muscles are innervated with **somatic** efferent fibers by the **abducens** (**VI**), **oculomotor** (**III**), and **trochlear** (**IV**) nerves. The oculomotor nerve also carries autonomic parasympathetic visceral (intrinsic) efferent fibers to the ciliary ganglion, which supplies postganglionic fibers to the ciliary muscles and sphincter pupillae. The **abducens** supplies the lateral rectus and the **trochlear** supplies the superior oblique. The **oculomotor** nucleus lies near the Edinger-Westphal nucleus, which supplies the autonomic efferents. The two nuclei are sometimes called the oculomotor complex. The oculomotor nerve supplies inferior, medial, and superior rectus and inferior oblique muscles. The oculomotor nerve also supplies the **levator palpebrae superioris**, which lifts the upper eyelid. The eyes may move identically (**conjugate** movements). But the eyes can move in opposite directions (**disconjugate** movements) when converging or diverging to focus on moving objects and keep them focused onto each fovea. The eyes converge when objects move closer, and diverge when objects move away. This is controlled by the **vergence** system. The lens of the eye must also **accommodate** for moving objects through contractions of the ciliary muscle.

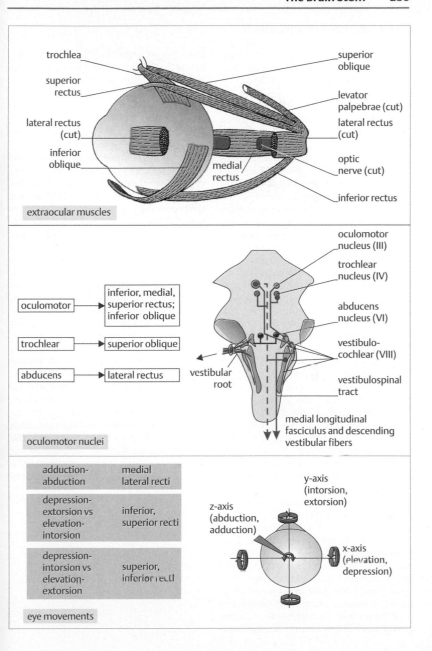

extraocular muscles

trochlea

superior rectus

lateral rectus (cut)

inferior oblique

medial rectus

superior oblique

levator palpebrae (cut)

lateral rectus (cut)

optic nerve (cut)

inferior rectus

oculomotor nuclei

oculomotor	→	inferior, medial, superior rectus; inferior oblique
trochlear	→	superior oblique
abducens	→	lateral rectus

oculomotor nucleus (III)

trochlear nucleus (IV)

abducens nucleus (VI)

vestibulo-cochlear (VIII)

vestibulospinal tract

vestibular root

medial longitudinal fasciculus and descending vestibular fibers

eye movements

adduction-abduction	medial lateral recti
depression-extorsion vs elevation-intorsion	inferior, superior recti
depression-intorsion vs elevation-extorsion	superior, inferior recti

y-axis (intorsion, extorsion)

z-axis (abduction, adduction)

x-axis (elevation, depression)

Control of Extraocular Muscles

The **extraocular muscles** and their nerves determine the **velocity** of movement and **position** of the eyes. They have to stabilize the gaze and keep the object in focus, regardless of head movement, or movement of the object. This is achieved through the versatility of eye movements and through several reflexes.

Gaze is stabilized through five systems that are controlled by the abducens, oculomotor, and vestibular nuclei in the brain stem. The **optokinetic** reflex keeps the object in focus during head rotation, and the **vestibulo-ocular** reflex does this during brief head movements. Both reflexes, which are very old in phylogenetic terms, keep the object on the fovea during head movement. Three **eye movements** that keep the object in focus are **saccadic**, **pursuit**, and **vergence**. All except vergence are **conjugate**; both eyes move in the same direction to the same degree.

The **vestibulo-ocular** system depends on impulses to the brain stem from the **semicircular canals**, which sense the speed of head rotation. As the head rotates in one direction, the eyes move in the other to keep the objects in focus; if they did not, **retinal slip** would occur. Without this reflex, we could not focus unless the head was stationary. During horizontal head movements, for example, if the head moves left, this fires hair cells in the left semicircular canal and inhibits firing in the right canal. In the midbrain, the impulses are integrated so that the ipsilateral medial rectus and contralateral lateral rectus muscles contract, thus pulling the eyes to the right. At the same time, the ipsilateral lateral rectus and contralateral medial rectus are inhibited. Disease of the labyrinth upsets the reflex, and results in **nystagmus**, which is jerky eye movements, unrelated to focusing. Different eye movements may be controlled and integrated by different centers in the brain stem. For example, horizontal eye movements are controlled by a group of cells in the pontine reticular formation, the so-called **PPRF**, which lies near the abducens nerve and projects fibers to it. A unilateral lesion to the PPRF reduces or completely blocks conjugate horizontal eye movements to the side of the lesion.

Optokinetic movements are the result of the integration of apparent movements of a stationary external visual field relative to movement of the head. The reflex drives the eyes in the opposite direction to that in which the head moves, and therefore complements the vestibulo-ocular reflex. It is the reflex that gives the impression that you are moving backwards, even when stationary, when something next to you moves forward. **Saccadic** movement is the fast movement of the eyes to keep an object in focus, especially when we shift gaze fast from one object to another. **Smooth pursuit** is used to keep tracking a moving object, and the vestibulo-ocular reflex is inhibited during smooth pursuit. During all these conjugate movements, complementary muscles are coordinated by the brain stem through the integration of ipsilateral and contralateral impulses using the decussating medial longitudinal fasciculi. Clearly, interruption of the fasciculi would paralyze focusing in the medial direction. **Vergence**, which is a non-conjugate system, has been discussed earlier (see p. 234).

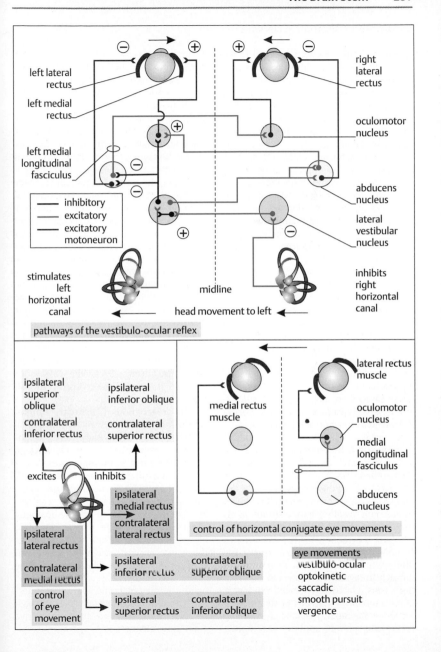

left lateral rectus

left medial rectus

left medial longitudinal fasciculus

right lateral rectus

oculomotor nucleus

abducens nucleus

lateral vestibular nucleus

inhibitory
excitatory
excitatory motoneuron

stimulates left horizontal canal

midline

inhibits right horizontal canal

head movement to left

pathways of the vestibulo-ocular reflex

ipsilateral superior oblique

ipsilateral inferior oblique

contralateral inferior rectus

contralateral superior rectus

excites   inhibits

ipsilateral medial rectus

contralateral lateral rectus

ipsilateral lateral rectus

contralateral medial rectus

ipsilateral inferior rectus

contralateral superior oblique

control of eye movement

ipsilateral superior rectus

contralateral inferior oblique

lateral rectus muscle

medial rectus muscle

oculomotor nucleus

medial longitudinal fasciculus

abducens nucleus

control of horizontal conjugate eye movements

eye movements
vestibulo-ocular
optokinetic
saccadic
smooth pursuit
vergence

Layout of the Autonomic Nervous System

The **autonomic nervous system** (**ANS**) carries all efferent impulses from the central nervous system, except for motor innervation of skeletal muscle. The ANS is mainly outside voluntary control and regulates (i) the heart beat, (ii) contraction of smooth muscle, (iii) all exocrine and some endocrine organs, and (iv) some of intermediary metabolism. Afferent sensory fibers run in the same nerve bundles that carry efferents, but only the efferents will be considered here. The ANS is anatomically and functionally divided into two main divisions, the **parasympathetic** and **sympathetic** divisions. Structurally, both divisions have **preganglionic** and **postganglionic** fibers. In both divisions, the neurotransmitter released from the preganglionic presynaptic nerve terminal is **acetylcholine** (**ACh**), which acts on postsynaptic, ganglionic **nicotinic receptors**. These are so called because nicotine can act as an agonist at the receptor sites. The neurotransmitter released from the postganglionic parasympathetic nerve terminal is also ACh, which acts on postsynaptic **muscarinic** receptors. The neurotransmitter released from postganglionic sympathetic nerve terminals is **norepinephrine** (**NA**), which acts on α and β receptors.

In several tissues, such as visceral smooth muscle in bladder and gut, the two divisions are present and appear to oppose each other. In others, such as sweat glands and most of the blood vessels, only the sympathetic division is present. In salivary glands both divisions have a stimulant effect on secretion.

There is evidence that the two systems do not operate independently in the periphery, but modulate each other's activity through **presynaptic reciprocal innervation**. Thus, electrically evoked release of ACh from parasympathetic postganglionic nerves in the small intestine is inhibited by the concomitant application of epinephrine or norepinephrine. Furthermore, when the parasympathetic nerve terminals release ACh, there is concomitant release of endogenous norepinephrine from neighboring sympathetic nerve terminals, and ACh release is inhibited. Conversely, norepinephrine release from sympathetic nerve terminals is modulated by the activity of parasympathetic nerves. There is much anatomical evidence that sympathetic noradrenergic and parasympathetic cholinergic nerve terminals lie closely together in the myenteric plexus. There appear to be presynaptic catecholaminergic terminals on those of the cholinergic nerve terminal, and, conversely, there are presynaptic parasympathetic, cholinergic nerve terminals on those of the sympathetic postganglionic nerves that terminate on the myenteric plexus. Similarly, in the heart, there is a reciprocal presynaptic modulation of neurotransmitter release between parasympathetic and sympathetic nerve terminals. This form of reciprocal inhibition, where the release of one neurotransmitter affects the release of another, is termed **heterotropic inhibition**.

The preganglionic fibers of the **sympathetic** division of the ANS leave the spinal cord in a spinal nerve and enter the paravertebral sympathetic ganglion through the **white rami communicantes**. These are called 'white' because they are myelinated. The preganglionic fibers that innervate structures in the head and thorax synapse in the ganglia of the sympathetic chain with cell bodies of postganglionic fibers. The postganglionic fibers return to the spinal nerve through the **gray rami communicantes**, so-called because the fibers are unmyelinated. On the other hand, the preganglionic fibers that innervate the abdominal and pelvic viscera pass through the chain to their respective abdominal plexuses.

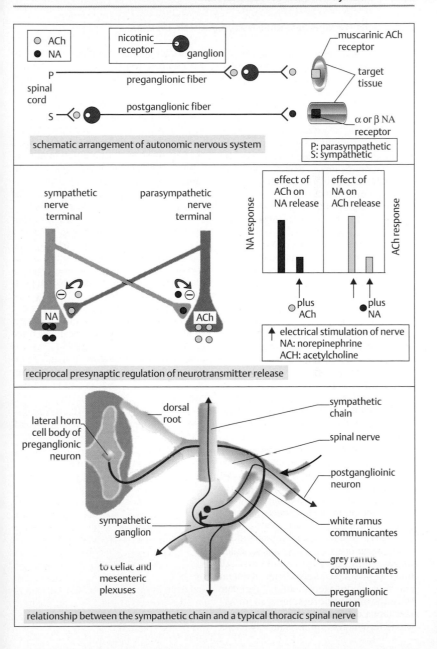

ACh
NA

nicotinic receptor
ganglion

muscarinic ACh receptor

target tissue

P
spinal cord

preganglionic fiber

S

postganglionic fiber

α or β NA receptor

schematic arrangement of autonomic nervous system

P: parasympathetic
S: sympathetic

sympathetic nerve terminal

parasympathetic nerve terminal

NA

ACh

effect of ACh on NA release

effect of NA on ACh release

NA response

ACh response

plus ACh

plus NA

electrical stimulation of nerve
NA: norepinephrine
ACH: acetylcholine

reciprocal presynaptic regulation of neurotransmitter release

dorsal root

sympathetic chain

lateral horn cell body of preganglionic neuron

spinal nerve

postganglioinic neuron

white ramus communicantes

sympathetic ganglion

grey ramus communicantes

to celiac and mesenteric plexuses

preganglionic neuron

relationship between the sympathetic chain and a typical thoracic spinal nerve

Autonomic Nervous System: Parasympathetic Division

The **parasympathetic** division of the autonomic nervous system (PNS) consists of preganglionic fibers that originate in three main areas of the central nervous system. These are the midbrain or tectum, the medulla, and the sacral outflow. The outflows emerge from two main regions, (i) the brain stem **cranial** outflow, and (ii) the **sacral** outflow. Preganglionic fibers are generally much longer than the postganglionic fibers and often the ganglia lie on the organ innervated.

The **midbrain** nuclei are the Edinger-Westphal nucleus of the third cranial nerve. The **medullary** nuclei subserve the seventh, ninth, and tenth cranial nerves. The seventh (**facial**) cranial nerve is the chorda tympani, which innervates the salivary sublingual and submaxillary glands. It also forms the greater superficial petrosal nerve. The **glossopharyngeal** is the ninth cranial nerve. Its parasympathetic components innervate the otic ganglion. The **vagus**, the tenth cranial nerve, arises in the medulla, and its preganglionic fibers generally synapse in ganglia embedded in target organs in the thorax and abdomen.

The **sacral** outflow arises from cell bodies in the second, third, and fourth segments of the sacral spinal cord. Their preganglionic fibers form the nervi erigentes, or pelvic nerves. The sacral outflow innervates the large intestine, the bladder, and reproductive organs.

The neurotransmitter released by the postganglionic presynaptic nerve terminal is ACh, which acts on postsynaptic **muscarinic receptors** on the membrane of the target organ or tissue. These are so called because muscarine, an alkaloid derived from a poisonous mushroom, *Amanita muscaria*, is an agonist at the receptor sites. The muscarinic receptor is an important target for drugs (see p. 246). ACh released from nerve terminals mainly exerts constrictor effects on smooth muscle. ACh will contract smooth muscle of the eye and gut. It is important to be aware that several tissues, especially the smooth muscle of the bronchial tree and the blood vessels, are poorly innervated by the parasympathetic nervous system (if at all) but still respond to exogenously applied ACh. This is because these muscles are rich in ACh receptors, although the physiological significance of their presence is unknown.

Clinical problems associated with the parasympathetic division of the ANS usually arise as a result of side effects or toxicity produced by chemical agents that act as either as agonists or antagonists at the muscarinic receptor. Excessive use of the muscarinic agonist pilocarpine, for example, results in decreased blood pressure, bronchoconstriction, GIT discomfort, and excessive sweating (although the last effect is due to stimulation of *sympathetic* cholinergic muscarinic receptors, see p. 242). Muscarinic antagonists, on the other hand, may produce urinary retention, mydriasis, tachycardia, and hypertension.

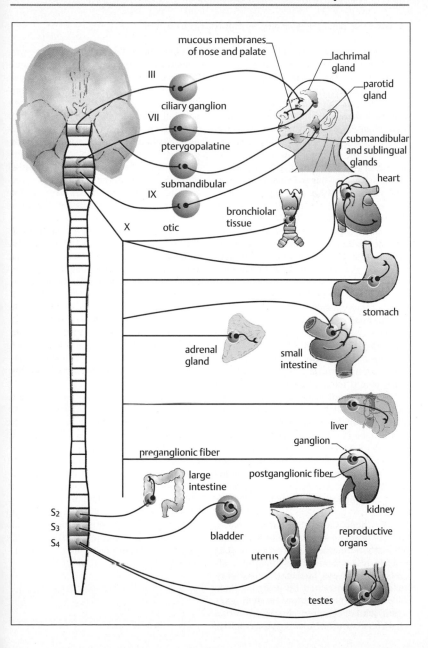

Autonomic Nervous System: Sympathetic Division

The **sympathetic** preganglionic neuron cell bodies are situated in the thoracic and upper two or three lumbar segments of the spinal cord. The cell bodies lie in the lateral horn of the spinal gray matter. The (usually) short **preganglionic fibers** leave the spinal cord in the ventral nerve root, and join the spinal nerve. These fibers synapse with the postganglionic fibers, either in one of the sympathetic ganglia, which lie in a **bilateral** longitudinal, paravertebral chain on either side of the spinal column, or in one of the plexuses, which surround the main branches of the abdominal aorta. These plexuses are the **coeliac, superior mesenteric**, and **inferior mesenteric** ganglia, and are unpaired. These ganglia are also termed prevertebral ganglia.

An exception to this general arrangement of the sympathetic division is that of the **adrenal medulla**. The adrenal gland lies above the kidney, and is structurally two separate organs. The outer shell of the adrenal gland is concerned with production of the steroid hormones, while the inner core is the adrenal medulla, a modified sympathetic ganglion. Thus, preganglionic cholinergic fibers run to the adrenal medulla, where they synapse with postganglionic cell bodies, which are in effect hormone-secreting cells. These cells respond to the arrival of impulses down the preganglionic fibers, by secreting the catecholamine hormones **epinephrine** and **norepinephrine** into the bloodstream.

The sympathetic division innervates most of the organs innervated by the parasympathetic division, and generally (but not always) opposes parasympathetic effects. Thus, the **eye, lacrimal**, and **salivary glands** are innervated by postganglionic fibers from the **superior cervical ganglion**, while fibers from the paravertebral chain innervate the **heart, larynx, trachea**, and **bronchi**. Fibers from the coeliac ganglion innervate the **oesophagus, stomach**, and **small intestine**, and some interconnect the **coeliac ganglion** and the **superior mesenteric ganglion**, which innervates the **large intestine**. The **inferior mesenteric ganglion** innervates the **kidney, bladder**, and the **reproductive organs**. In addition, several postganglionic fibers leave the **paravertebral chain of ganglia** and run to the blood vessels, erector pili, which are the muscles responsible for piloerection (hair raising), and the sweat glands.

The preganglionic fibers, like those of the parasympathetic division, release the **neurotransmitter, ACh**, which binds to nicotinic receptors on ganglionic postsynaptic cell bodies of postganglionic fibers. But the postganglionic fibers of the sympathetic division differ from those of the parasympathetic division since they release as their neurotransmitter the catecholamine norepinephrine, which binds to α or β receptors on the presynaptic noradrenergic nerve terminal, or on the postsynaptic membrane of the target organ. An exception to this general rule is the presence in the sympathetic division of postganglionic fibers, which innervate the sweat glands. These are cholinergic, and release ACh, which acts on muscarinic receptors on the membranes of the sweat glands. Stimulation of the sympathetic division of the ANS results in increased heart rate and force of contraction, raised blood pressure, and mobilization of glucose, and this division is therefore the focus of much attention in the treatment of diseases such as essential hypertension, and cardiac disorders.

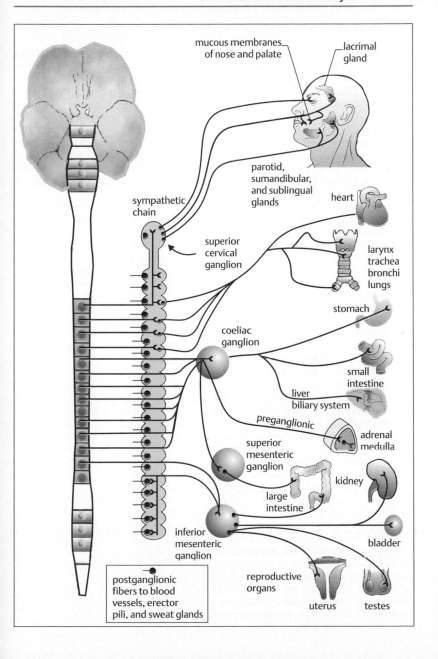

mucous membranes of nose and palate

lacrimal gland

parotid, sumandibular, and sublingual glands

sympathetic chain

superior cervical ganglion

heart

larynx trachea bronchi lungs

stomach

coeliac ganglion

small intestine

liver biliary system

preganglionic

adrenal medulla

superior mesenteric ganglion

kidney

large intestine

inferior mesenteric ganglion

bladder

reproductive organs

uterus

testes

postganglionic fibers to blood vessels, erector pili, and sweat glands

Autonomic Nervous System: Effects

Most organs receive dual **parasympathetic** and **sympathetic** innervation. Generally, these two divisions antagonize each other, although this is not always so. In some cases, for example the spleen and arterioles, the tissues receive only sympathetic fibers. The two systems, in opposing each other, actually work together to maintain a balance of organ and tissue function.

The anatomical arrangements of the two divisions highlight a general feature of their difference in function. In the sympathetic division, one thoracic or lumbar preganglionic nerve may ramify and synapse, ultimately, with the cell bodies of many postganglionic nerve fibers in the chain of ganglia. Thus, activation of the sympathetic nervous system through, for example anger, fear, excitement, or stress will have wide-ranging effects, affecting many different tissues, and prepare the body for the flight-or-fight response. **Heart rate** is speeded up, **blood pressure** rises, and **blood flow** is redirected to increase the perfusion of skeletal muscle. **Blood glucose** is raised, the **pupil dilates**, and **piloerection** occurs. There is generalized **constriction** of **skin** and **visceral blood vessels** to minimize blood loss through injury, and **sphincters constrict**.

Activation of the parasympathetic nervous system, on the other hand, results in a far more localized response, which reflects the more limited nature of the preganglionic and postganglionic parasympathetic innervation. Thus, for example, the craniosacral outflow consists mainly of single pre- and postganglionic synapses, resulting in a more limited, localized response. The overall effects of parasympathetic activity are associated with the conservation of energy and the maintenance of organ function during periods of less activity. These effects include a **slowing** of the **heart rate**, **lowering of blood pres-**sure, the activation of **digestive and gut activity**, **increased secretory activity from exocrine glands**, the **opening of sphincters**, **contraction of bladder smooth muscle**, **constriction of the pupil** of the eye, and **contraction of the ciliary muscle**. During sexual intercourse, the sympathetic and parasympathetic divisions do not oppose but complement each other, since **erection** is a **parasympathetic** activity, while **ejaculation** is **sympathetically** controlled.

The parasympathetic division is essential for life, whereas the sympathetic division is not. Before the introduction of drugs for the treatment of life-threatening hypertension, the only treatment was bilateral sympathectomy, which was the removal of the sympathetic, paravertebral chains of ganglia.

organ	sympathetic division		parasympathetic division (receptors all muscarinic; M)
	receptor	effect	
heart sinoatrial node	β₁	rate ↑	rate ↓
atrioventricular node	β₁	automaticity ↑	conduction velocity ↓ AV block
atrial muscle	β₁	force ↑	force ↓
ventricular muscle	β₁	automaticity ↑ force ↑	no effect
blood vessels arterioles brain skin viscera	α	constriction	no effect
coronary	α	constriction	
erectile tissue	α	constriction	dilatation
salivary glands	α	secretion ↓	secretion ↑
skeletal muscle	β₂	dilatation	no effect
	α	constriction	
veins	β₂	dilatation	no effect
viscera bronchi glands smooth muscle	β₂	no effect dilatation	secretion ↑ constriction
GI tract glands smooth muscle sphincters	α₂, β₂ α₂, β₂	no effect motility ↓ constriction	secretion ↑ motility ↑ dilatation
uterus non-pregnant pregnant	α β₂ α	relaxation contraction	response varies
male sex organs	α	ejaculation	erection
eye ciliary muscle pupil	β α	some relaxation dilatation	contraction constriction
lacrimal glands salivary glands	α β	no effect secretion ↑	secretion ↑ secretion ↑
liver	α β₂	gluconeogenesis glycogenolysis	no effect
kidney	β₂	renin secretion	no effect
skin pilomotor effect sweating	α M	piloerection ↑ sweating ↑	no effect no effect

Autonomic Nervous System: Agonists and Antagonists

Agonists activate the **receptors** with which they interact, while **antagonists** block the binding of the agonist to the receptor. Both agonists and antagonists of the **ACh** receptor, especially the **muscarinic** receptor, and of the **catecholaminergic** receptors, have several important therapeutic implications, many of which have been developed.

Muscarinic agonists include **ACh**, **muscarine**, **carbachol**, **methacholine**, and **pilocarpine**. Their effects are those of stimulation of the parasympathetic division of the ANS. **Oxotremorine** is a powerful muscarinic agonist acting mainly on receptors of the CNS. It is useful experimentally, but not therapeutically. Muscarinic agonists slow the heart and decrease cardiac output. They cause a fall in blood pressure through a direct effect on muscarinic receptors, which are present on smooth vascular muscle, even though there is no parasympathetic innervation. They contract GIT smooth muscle, resulting in cramps, and they stimulate exocrine secretions. The pupil is constricted, and the ciliary muscle contracts, thus accommodating for near vision. The main use of muscarinic agonists is in treatment of **glaucoma**, which is increased intraocular pressure. Because of their side effects, they have little if any systemic use.

Muscarinic antagonists are more important therapeutically. They are sometimes called **parasympatholytic**, since they reduce or abolish parasympathetic effects. The two best known are the naturally occurring **atropine** and **hyoscine**. **Homatropine** is a synthetic analogue of atropine. **Pirenzepine**, another synthetic analogue, acts mainly at M_1 receptors. Muscarinic antagonists block parasympathetic effects, inhibiting exocrine secretions, dilating the pupil (mydriasis), and relaxing biliary, bronchial, and urinary tract smooth muscle. Atropine excites the CNS, while hyoscine causes sedation. Paradoxically, atropine slows the heart (bradycardia), through a central action, although higher doses act directly on the heart to cause tachycardia. Muscarinic antagonists are used for surgical premedication, and short-acting agents such as **tropicamide** are used to dilate the pupil during ophthalmic examination. Hyoscine is used to prevent and treat motion sickness.

Epinephrine and **norepinephrine** are endogenous **sympathetic receptor agonists**, but are highly unstable, and a number of stable synthetic analogues have been developed. **Isoprotenerol** was developed to treat asthma through stimulation of β_2 receptors, but it also stimulates β_1 receptors, causing dysrhythmias. **Salbutamol** is more specific for β_2 receptors. **Phenylephrine** is an α receptor agonist used to treat nasal congestion by constricting nasal blood vessels. Epinephrine is used to treat anaphylactic shock during a type I hypersensitivity reaction. Stimulation of presynaptic α_2 receptors by the selective α_2 agonist **clonidine**, a treatment for essential hypertension, inhibits norepinephrine release from nerve terminals.

Sympathetic receptor antagonists have wide use in the treatment of cardiovascular disease. **Prazosin** and **indoramin**, selective antagonists at postsynaptic α_1 receptors, are useful in hypertension, and cause vasodilatation without tachycardia, since they do not inhibit α_2 receptors. Blockers of β receptors are also useful in hypertension, and in cardiac disorders such as angina pectoris and certain cardiac dysrhythmias. **Propranolol** blocks β_1 and β_2 **receptors**, and is therefore unsuitable in asthma, since it blocks bronchiolar dilatation mediated by β_2 receptors. Selective β_1 antagonists such as **atenolol** and **practolol** are more useful in cardiac disease.

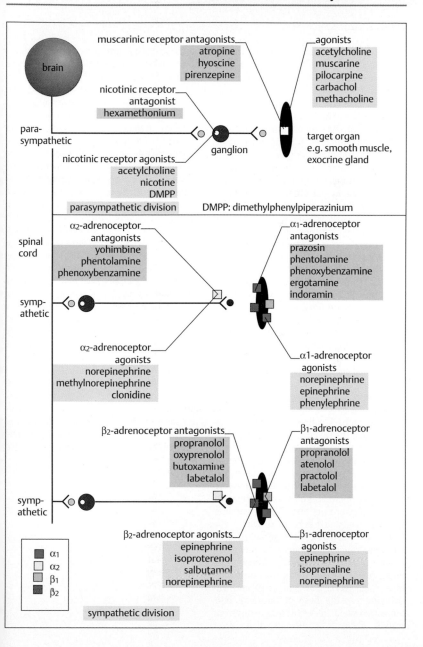

The Gustatory System

The **gustatory (taste) system** makes possible the phenomenon of **flavor perception**. Modalities of taste are sensed by **taste buds** in the oropharyngeal mucosa, which detects chemicals that are dissolved in the saliva. The information is transmitted by afferent conduction to the CNS, where the modality is recognized. Taste buds are modified oral mucosa cells, which transduce the chemical modality into an electrical impulse; this impulse travels through first-order neurons along one of more of the **cranial nerves VII, IX, and X** to the **solitary nucleus**. From there, second-order neurons project to the **thalamus** or **pons** depending on the species. Third-order neurons project to **diencephalic** areas involved in appetite control, food intake, and fluid and ion balance. From the thalamus, fibers project to the orbitofrontal and **insular cortex**.

Taste buds are complex structures that are situated on the tongue and distributed throughout the oropharyngeal mucosa. It is generally accepted that different **modalities** of taste are unequally distributed on the tongue and other oral mucosal surfaces. **Sour** taste is usually depicted as being on the sides of the tongue, while **bitter** is at the back. **Salt** and **sweet** are concentrated at the tip of the tongue. The taste bud consists of different cell types arranged concentrically, somewhat like the petals of a flower. **Light**, **dark**, and **intermediate cells** can be distinguished, based on the density of granules within them. At the apex, where the taste bud opens into the oral cavity, it has a **pore**, where the epithelial microvilli are situated. The different cell types appear to recognize different taste modalities. These are: sweet (e.g. **sucrose**), bitter (e.g. **quinine**), sour (e.g. **HCl**), and salt (e.g. **sodium chloride**). At the **base** of the taste bud, there are several nerve endings of different cranial nerves. Taste buds, like other epithelial cells, are constantly being renewed; this turnover is halted if the nerve endings are destroyed. The interaction between taste bud and nerve cell for both taste recognition and turnover appear to depend on the expression of a neural cell adhesion molecule (NCAM), and possibly a number of other surface antigens.

There is evidence that the detection of **sour** (i.e. acid or H^+) taste is mediated by the blockage on the **apical membrane** of **voltage-dependent** K^+ channels by H^+ ions. Na^+ ions move passively into the cell through channels, which can be blocked by **amiloride** (better known as a K^+-sparing diuretic) A **Na^+/K^+ ATPase pump** on the **basolateral membrane** of the cell pumps Na^+ back out of the cell. The detection of **sweet** taste may involve the activation of **adenylate cyclase**, and the generation of intracellular **cyclic AMP**, which closes voltage-dependent **K^+channels** on the basolateral membrane of the taste bud cell. In both cases, the net result is the influx of Ca^{2+} ions into the cell. Salty taste appears mediated by a Na^+ channel.

The neural representation of taste is not understood, but it appears that different cranial nerves may serve different proportions of the various taste modalities. The brain is programmed to react to taste not only with feeding behavior, but also with protective reactions.

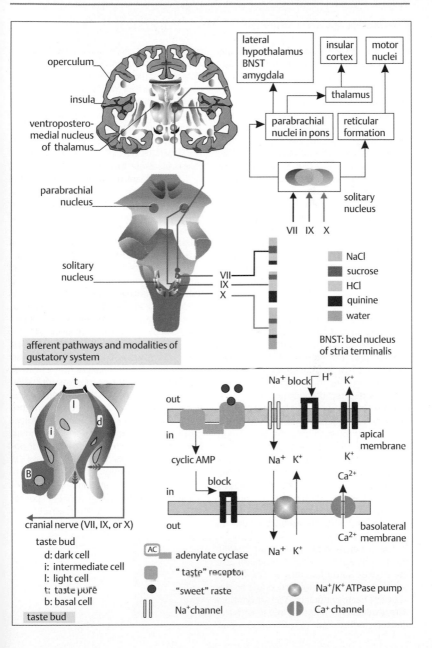

lateral hypothalamus
BNST
amygdala

insular cortex

motor nuclei

operculum

insula

ventroposteromedial nucleus of thalamus

thalamus

parabrachial nuclei in pons

reticular formation

parabrachial nucleus

solitary nucleus

solitary nucleus

VII IX X

VII
IX
X

NaCl
sucrose
HCl
quinine
water

afferent pathways and modalities of gustatory system

BNST: bed nucleus of stria terminalis

t

l

i

d

B

out

in

Na⁺ block   H⁺   K⁺

cyclic AMP

Na⁺   K⁺

apical membrane

K⁺

in

block

Ca²⁺

out

Na⁺   K⁺

basolateral membrane

Ca²⁺

cranial nerve (VII, IX, or X)

taste bud
d: dark cell
i: intermediate cell
l: light cell
t: taste pore
b: basal cell

AC   adenylate cyclase

"taste" receptor

"sweet" taste

Na⁺ channel

Na⁺/K⁺ ATPase pump

Ca⁺ channel

taste bud

The Olfactory System Pathways

The sense of smell is mediated by the **olfactory system**. This is the detection of airborne chemicals by specialized receptors in the olfactory mucosa. Animals that rely heavily on olfaction for survival and reproduction are termed **macrosmatic**, while humans, who do not, are **microsmatic**. Nevertheless, humans are able to detect many different airborne chemicals at low concentrations. Olfaction and taste work together to achieve the sensation referred to as **taste**; if for any reason olfaction is impaired, the patient complains that food cannot be properly tasted. In contrast to the taste system, which distinguishes relatively few modalities of sour, sweet, bitter, and salt, the olfactory system can distinguish very many different **odorants**, which contribute to the subtle modality of smell.

The olfactory system is completely neural, since the **receptors** are modified neurons that transduce and transmit olfactory inputs to the brain via the **olfactory bulb**, the **lateral olfactory tract**, and from there to the **olfactory cortex**. The olfactory system is unique among the senses, in that receptors project directly to cortex; the other senses relay through the thalamus. The **olfactory bulb** is part of the forebrain, situated on its ventral surface in the **olfactory sulcus**, and attached to it by the **olfactory tract**. The olfactory tract consists mainly of fibers of the **anterior olfactory nucleus**, the **lateral olfactory tract**, and the anterior limb of the anterior commissure. This tract carries many centrifugal fibers from the brain to the olfactory bulb.

The **lateral olfactory tract** (LOT), which transmits olfactory inputs to the brain, gives off collaterals to the limbic system, to the olfactory cortex, and to the anterior olfactory nucleus. The anterior olfactory nucleus projects mainly to both the olfactory bulbs and to its contralateral partner. The axons of the LOT travel caudally as the lateral olfactory stria; these synapse in the **piriform cortex**, a major component of the olfactory cortex, and the **olfactory tubercle**. The LOT projects further caudally to the **anterior cortical amygdaloid nucleus**, the lateral **entorhinal cortex** and the **periamygdaloid cortex**, which is part of the piriform cortex that overlies the amygdala.

The main areas of the olfactory cortex are the anterior cortical amygdaloid nucleus, anterior olfactory nucleus, lateral entorhinal cortex, periamygdaloid nucleus, piriform cortex, and olfactory tubercle. All these areas have reciprocal **intrinsic** connections. The main intrinsic connections stem from the anterior olfactory nucleus, lateral entorhinal cortex, and piriform cortex. The olfactory cortex is phylogenetically identified as paleocortex, because most of it contains three cell layers, while neocortex has six layers of cells.

The olfactory cortex projects to several other **extrinsic** areas. These are the olfactory bulb, which receives fibers from all areas of the olfactory cortex except the olfactory tubercle; to the **hippocampus** from the lateral entorhinal cortex, and to the lateral hypothalamus, mainly from the piriform cortex and anterior olfactory nucleus. The connections to the hippocampus mediate olfactory contribution to memory and learning. The connections to the hypothalamus mediate feeding behavior and perhaps emotional responses such as food-evoked rage responses.

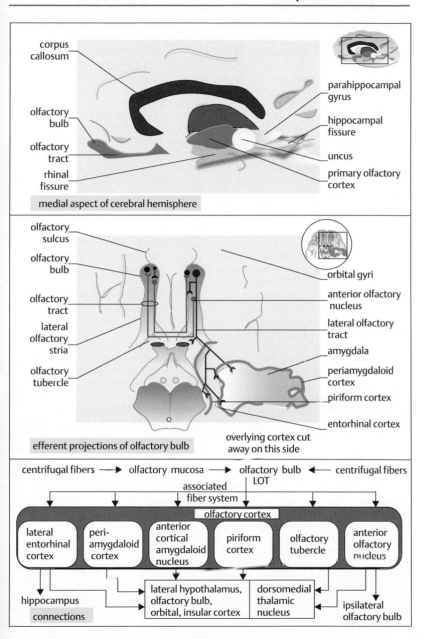

corpus callosum

parahippocampal gyrus

hippocampal fissure

olfactory bulb

olfactory tract

uncus

rhinal fissure

primary olfactory cortex

medial aspect of cerebral hemisphere

olfactory sulcus

olfactory bulb

orbital gyri

anterior olfactory nucleus

olfactory tract

lateral olfactory tract

lateral olfactory stria

amygdala

periamygdaloid cortex

olfactory tubercle

piriform cortex

entorhinal cortex

efferent projections of olfactory bulb

overlying cortex cut away on this side

centrifugal fibers → olfactory mucosa → olfactory bulb ← centrifugal fibers

LOT

associated fiber system

olfactory cortex

| lateral entorhinal cortex | peri-amygdaloid cortex | anterior cortical amygdaloid nucleus | piriform cortex | olfactory tubercle | anterior olfactory nucleus |

hippocampus

lateral hypothalamus, olfactory bulb, orbital, insular cortex

dorsomedial thalamic nucleus

ipsilateral olfactory bulb

connections

Olfactory System Organization

The principal sensory components of the **olfactory system** are the nasal **olfactory epithelium**, the **olfactory mucosa**, the **olfactory bulb**, and the **olfactory tract**. Each of these is highly organized and specialized. The olfactory bulb lies on the ventral surface of the forebrain above the **nasal olfactory epithelium** and mucosa, and is separated from it by the cribriform layer.

The **olfactory receptors** lie in the **olfactory mucosa**, which overlies the olfactory epithelium. The receptors occur on **cilia** on specialized **neurons**. The neuron is bipolar, and at the opposite end is an unmyelinated **axon**. The axons group together in **olfactory fila**, which become the **olfactory nerve**. The fila pass through the **cribriform plate** (the roof of the ethmoid bone, which contributes to the nasal cavity and orbits) and end in the olfactory bulb. The olfactory receptor neurons are unique in that, unlike other mammalian neurons, they are being continuously replaced. The olfactory epithelium also contains **basal** stem cells and **supporting** (sustentacular) cells. The olfactory receptor neurons are differentiated from the basal stem cells.

Olfactory stimuli (odorant molecules) enter the nasal cavity and pass through the nasal mucus into the **olfactory epithelium** bound to low-molecular weight, water-soluble proteins. After dissociating from the proteins, the odorants bind to G-protein-coupled receptors on the cilia of the neuron. The reaction is transduced into a rise in intracellular cyclic AMP, which opens gated cation channels. This causes a gradual depolarization, called a generator potential, which is transmitted across the neuron to the cell body. When a threshold potential is reached, the neutron fires off an action potential that travels along the axon to the olfactory bulb. There is evidence that the IP_3 (inositol 1,4,5-triphosphate) system is also involved.

The **olfactory bulb** appears as five well-defined **layers** or laminae of fibers and cell bodies, in microscopic section. The most superficial layer is the olfactory epithelium, whose neural receptor cell axons terminate in the olfactory **glomeruli**. In the glomeruli, the axons branch and synapse on apical dendrites of **tufted** and **mitral** cells. These are the efferent neurons of the olfactory bulb. **Periglomerular** cells branch extensively within glomeruli, and their axons may communicate with up to five glomeruli. Many thousands of cell inputs converge on to a single glomerulus, and all the inputs appear to be excitatory. The glomerulus also receives afferent inputs via centrifugal pathways; these include fibers from the ipsilateral anterior olfactory nucleus and the diagonal band of Broca. There are also serotonergic afferents from the midbrain raphe nuclei and noradrenergic afferents from the locus ceruleus.

The external plexiform layer contains GABAergic synaptic connections between apical dendrites of **granular cells** and basal dendrites of **tufted** and **mitral cells**, together with the cell bodies of tufted cells. Mitral and tufted cells feed back onto granular cells with excitatory glutamatergic dendrites. The **mitral layer** contains mitral cell bodies, and the **granule cell layer** contains the cell bodies of the granular cells, the interneurons of the olfactory bulb. This layer also receives inputs from the raphe nuclei, locus ceruleus and the diagonal band.

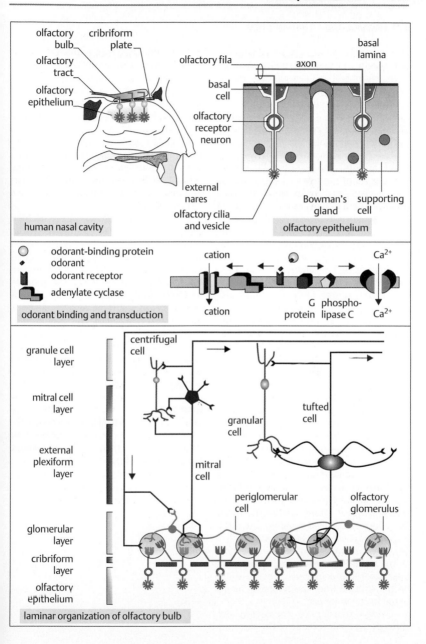

olfactory bulb
cribriform plate
olfactory tract
olfactory epithelium

olfactory fila
basal lamina
axon
basal cell
olfactory receptor neuron

external nares
olfactory cilia and vesicle

Bowman's gland
supporting cell

human nasal cavity

olfactory epithelium

○ odorant-binding protein
◆ odorant
▮ odorant receptor
adenylate cyclase

cation

cation

Ca²⁺

G protein   phospho-lipase C

Ca²⁺

odorant binding and transduction

granule cell layer

mitral cell layer

external plexiform layer

glomerular layer

cribriform layer

olfactory epithelium

centrifugal cell

granular cell

tufted cell

mitral cell

periglomerular cell

olfactory glomerulus

laminar organization of olfactory bulb

The Cochlea and Organ of Corti

The **auditory system**, in common with the other senses, consists of two main divisions: peripheral and central. The peripheral components are the **ear** and the nerves, which carry impulses to and from the ear. The central components are the CNS pathways and centers, which process auditory information.

The ear is conveniently divided into **outer**, **middle**, and **inner** ears. The outer ear consists of the external ear or **pinna**, and the ear canal, or **external auditory meatus**. The functions of the pinna are to direct sounds into the ear canal and to localize sounds. The size and shape of the pinna dictate the range of wavelengths detected. For example, sounds of very long wavelength, i.e. low frequency, that exceed the dimensions of the pinna will not be detected. Only sounds of frequency of 5 kHz or above are picked up by the pinna.

The middle ear consists of the eardrum or **tympanic membrane** and the **ossicles**, three bones called the **malleus**, **incus**, and **stapes**. These are also called, respectively, the hammer, anvil, and stirrup. The middle ear acts to conserve the energy of the sound waves that strike the tympanic membrane, which is transmitted to the cochlear fluid; it serves as an **impedance matching device**. It drastically reduces the surface area from the tympanic membrane to the stapes. The **force** applied to the tympanic membrane is equal to the **total surface area** of the membrane times the **pressure**. By reducing surface area to that of the footplate of the stapes, which lies opposite the **oval window**, the same force is applied to it by the stapes. The pressure amplification is about 25:1. Without this impedance matching system, less than 0.1% of sound wave energy would be transmitted from the tympanic membrane to the inner ear.

Energy transfer is conserved also through the conical shape of the eardrum, and through the lever arm action of the movement of the ossicles. Two muscles drive the ossicles, namely the stapedius and the tensor tympani. The stapedius is innervated by motoneurons in cranial nerve VII, from the facial nucleus. The tensor tympani is innervated by motoneurons in nerve V, from the motor nucleus of the trigeminal nerve. These muscles protect the ear from excessively loud sounds. When they contract, they cause the **ossicular chain** to stiffen; this decreases sound transmission.

The inner ear consists of the **cochlea**, the **vestibule**, and the **semicircular canals**. The cochlea is a spiral, snail-shaped organ that forms part of the bony labyrinth of the ear. The cochlea contains the organ of hearing, the so-called **organ of Corti**, which transduces the physical movement of sound waves into electrical impulses. It is a tightly coiled fluid-filled tube, whose base is closest to the stapes. The tube is partitioned lengthwise by a long **basilar membrane**, which widens progressively towards the apex. In cross-section, the cochlea is seen to have three compartments, the **scala tympani**, **scala media**, and **scala vestibuli**. At the apical end is the **helicotrema**, which allows the fluid pressure wave to travel into the scala tympani, from which it escapes through the **round window**.

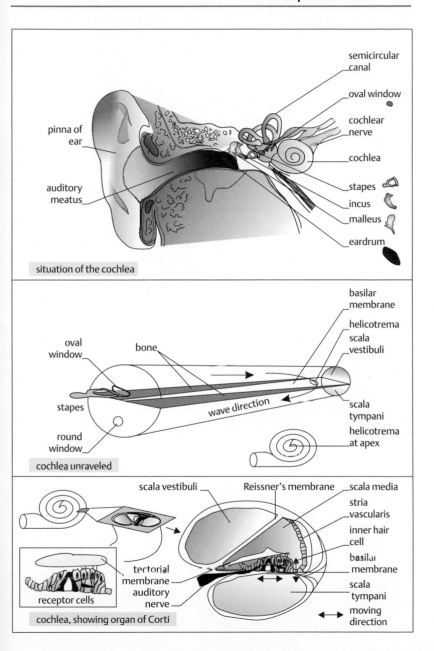

situation of the cochlea

cochlea unraveled

cochlea, showing organ of Corti

The Nature of Sound

Sound is caused by changes in pressure in a medium such as air. For example, the initial vibration of a loudspeaker diaphragm sets up a cone of rapidly moving air molecules. This moving boundary compresses the air immediately in front of it. If the loudspeaker continues to vibrate, the pressure differences will continue to move away from the original source of the air disturbance at a rate dependent on the elastic properties and density of the medium in which the pressure wave is traveling. In air, the speed of movement is about $340 \, \text{msec}^{-1}$, and around four times that speed in water. The pressure changes are appreciated by the auditory system as sound.

The application of regular pulses to a loudspeaker, or the oscillations caused by the vibrations of a tuning fork, will result in the simplest form of sound wave, caused by regular **sinusoidal** changes in air pressure. The distance from the point of maximum compression to the next is the **wavelength** (λ), which can be calculated as the **velocity** (v) of movement divided by the **frequency** (f) of occurrence. Frequency is determined by the rate per second at which the pressure changes are generated at source, and is measured as **cycles per second**, or **Hertz** (**Hz**). The human ear is sensitive to a frequency range of around 20 Hz to 20 000 Hz. The **amplitude** (**A**) of the wave is the difference between the maximum, or peak, pressure and the mean pressure. This relatively simple wave is termed a **pure tone**, and the frequency of wave generation is appreciated by the auditory system as **pitch**. If two identical sinusoidal waves are generated at different times, they will be out of **phase**. The differences between their peaks and troughs are measured as an angle. If the two ears receive a single wave at different times, it may be appreciated as two separate pure tones.

Sound amplitude, or **sound pressure level**, is measured in **decibels** (**dB**) named after Alexander Graham Bell. These are expressed on a logarithmic scale because of the wide range of frequencies appreciated by the ear. They measure the maximum pressure change from mean to peak (or trough) pressure. A **standard pressure** (P_s) is chosen; this is near to threshold for the ear ($20 \, \mu\text{N}$ per m^2, where N = Newtons and m = meters). This is compared with the **test pressure** (P_t): dB = $20.\log_{10} P_s/P_t$. In humans, the dynamic range is about 120 dB. The pressure levels are also referred to as **sound intensities**. The human ear can detect movement of air molecules over the distance equivalent to the diameter of a hydrogen atom.

Pure tones are rare, and most sounds are complex mixtures of waves. **Fourier analysis** assumes that sounds are the sum of individual sinusoidal waves, whose frequencies are integral multiples of the frequency of the original wave. For example, a complex **waveform** can be **synthesized** by summing different sine waves of frequency f (fundamental frequency) + $f_2 \ldots f_n$. A **Fourier spectrum** represents the different frequencies graphically.

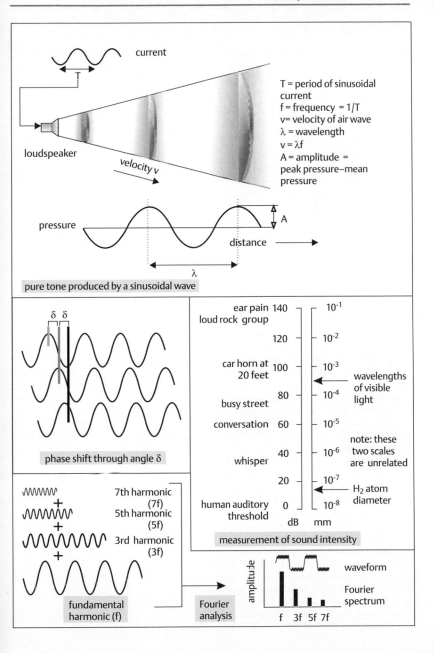

Sound and the Cochlea I

The receptor organ of hearing is the **organ of Corti**. These lie in the scala media within the cochlea in spiraling banks, supported on the basilar membrane. Each organ has pillar cells, which arch to form a **tunnel of Corti**. Adjoining the pillar cell is a single **inner hair cell**, which has **hair cells** (**stereocilia**) close to an overlying gelatinous **tectorial membrane**, but not attached to it. The scala tympani and media are filled with **perilymph**, which is high in Na^+. On the other side of the tunnel lies a triplet of **outer hair cells**, protruding from basal **Deiters' cells**. The outer hair cells, too, have stereocilia, the tallest of which are attached to the tectorial membrane.

The organ of Corti is **innervated** by **afferent** fibers from a **spiral ganglion**, which is housed in a bony **modiolus** around which the cochlear duct turns. The bipolar cells of the ganglion become unmyelinated as they pass through perforations in the bony sheath, and they synapse at the base of the inner and outer hair cells. **Type I** afferents terminate at inner hair cells, and **type II** synapse at outer hair cells. The cochlear portion of the **vestibulocochlear nerve** (cranial nerve VIII) provides **efferent** fibers to the cochlea. These are the central processes of the spiral ganglion. Medial **olivocochlear efferents** spiral on the inner side of the basilar membrane and terminate on inner hair cells; these may terminate presynaptically on the afferents. **Lateral** efferents cross the tunnel of Corti and terminate on outer hair cells.

The hair cells lie in the **cochlear duct**, in a fluid **endolymph**, which has high K^+ concentrations. When waves arrive at the vestibule and fluid is displaced in the scala tympani, the basilar membrane moves downwards and bends the taller stereocilia of outer hair cells against the tectorial membrane. Potassium ion channels at the tips of the stereocilia open, and K^+ from the endolymph flows through and depolarizes the inner hair cells. The depolarized hair cells open voltage-gated Ca^{2+} channels at their bases, and the Ca^{2+} influx causes fusion of synaptic vesicles with the cell membrane. The inner hair cells release transmitter into the cleft between the hair cell and the afferent nerve fiber. This generates an action potential on the cochlear afferent. The outer hair cells mechanically amplify movements of the basilar membrane and regulate the sensitivity of the acoustic apparatus when these cells and their stereocilia stiffen in response to efferent impulses. This is believed to lift the tectorial membrane away from the stereocilia of the inner hair cells. The inner hair cells transmit information to the acoustic nerve, and the Deiters' cells act as a viscoelastic coupling device between the basilar membrane and the outer hair cells.

The cochlea is a **tuning device**, since the basilar membrane has variable tension across its length, and stereocilia have varying length. It is not a simple Fourier analyzer because of the **non-linear** properties of basilar membrane wave transmission. Because of its variable tension, and thus its **frequency selectivity**, it is a more complex sound organ.

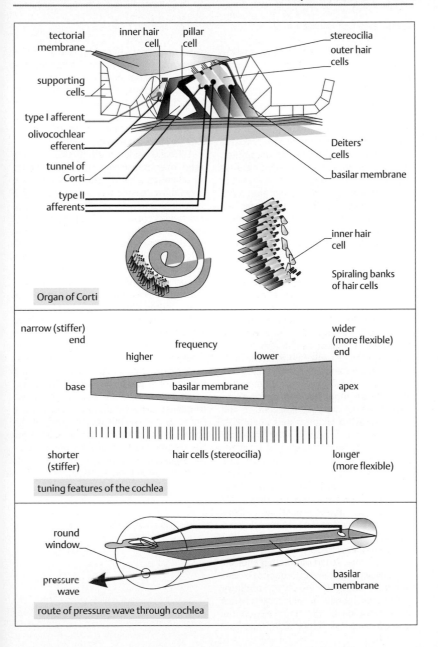

tectorial membrane

supporting cells

type I afferent

olivocochlear efferent

tunnel of Corti

type II afferents

inner hair cell

pillar cell

stereocilia

outer hair cells

Deiters' cells

basilar membrane

inner hair cell

Spiraling banks of hair cells

Organ of Corti

narrow (stiffer) end

wider (more flexible) end

frequency

higher

lower

base

basilar membrane

apex

shorter (stiffer)

hair cells (stereocilia)

longer (more flexible)

tuning features of the cochlea

round window

pressure wave

basilar membrane

route of pressure wave through cochlea

Sound and the Cochlea II

Different regions of the basilar membrane are responsive to different **sound frequencies**, and are able to perform a form of Fourier analysis. Damage to the basal end of the membrane causes selective loss of high frequency auditory processing. But the processing of sound is more complex than this, since there is also **longitudinal coupling** of the membrane components, with much so-called **nearest neighbor** interaction.

When a sine wave travels along the basilar membrane, the amplitude increases progressively to a maximum, which is reached at a point on the membrane dictated by the original frequency of stimulation. After the maximum, the amplitude falls off sharply. The lower the applied frequency, the nearer the maximum is to the helicotrema at the apex. There are also **lag phase** differences along the membrane; the lag phase between movement of the oval window and of the membrane is longest at the apex. These properties can be explained in terms of (i) **progressive widening** of the basal membrane towards the apex, (ii) interactions between **neighboring auditory components** of the auditory epithelium, and (iii) **innervation** of inner and outer hair cells. When sound waves enter the scala vestibuli, they take the route of **least resistance**. High frequency waves overcome membrane stiffness at the base and may short-circuit through the membrane into the scala tympani, where they exit through the round window. Lower frequency waves find it easier to overcome perilymph inertia and pass through the helicotrema. Presumably, the route taken is a compromise between the two choices.

Analysis of different frequencies into electrical impulses by the auditory epithelium depends on the characteristics and innervation of the hair cells. Outer hair cells have less **acuity** than inner hair cells, since each inner hair cell is innervated with several afferent fibers (**convergence**), while one outer hair cell may have only one afferent (**divergence**). About 90% of auditory fibers originate at inner hair cells. Outer hair cells respond mainly to membrane deflection, while inner hair cells respond to velocity of deflection.

Different auditory afferents also have different **response thresholds**, depending on where they lie on the membrane i.e. they show **frequency selectivity**. This frequency selectivity is reflected in central auditory receptive units in the inferior colliculus. Selectivity may also be due to a so-called **second filter** in the outer hair cell. This is an energy-dependent **resonance** between the hair cell and its cilia. If the second filter is removed with energy poisons such as cyanide, sharpness of tuning is lost through blunting of the threshold. Sharpness of tuning is also due to **lateral inhibition**. For each auditory unit, there is a central excitatory field, and an inhibitory outer field.

At lower frequencies, hair cell firing may become **phase locked** to the stimulating frequency; individual hair cells of a **frequency set** may not fire once during every wave cycle, but total activity of the units makes up for this. Phase locking increases the quality or timbre of the auditory signal at lower frequencies. This is important in sound **localization**.

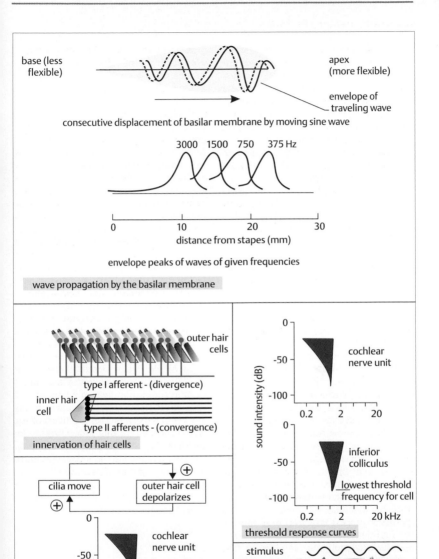

base (less flexible)

apex (more flexible)

envelope of traveling wave

consecutive displacement of basilar membrane by moving sine wave

3000 1500 750 375 Hz

0   10   20   30
distance from stapes (mm)

envelope peaks of waves of given frequencies

wave propagation by the basilar membrane

outer hair cells

type I afferent - (divergence)

inner hair cell

type II afferents - (convergence)

innervation of hair cells

cilia move → outer hair cell depolarizes ⊕

⊕

0

-50

-100

cochlear nerve unit

lost in absence of 2nd filter

second filter

0

-50

-100

sound intensity (dB)

0.2   2   20

cochlear nerve unit

0

-50

-100

0.2   2   20 kHz

inferior colliculus

lowest threshold frequency for cell

threshold response curves

stimulus

each fiber

total activity

phase locking

Ascending Auditory Pathways

Primary afferent fibers from the cochlea enter the brain stem at the level of the **cerebellopontine angle**. They synapse first in the ipsilateral **cochlear nuclear complex** in the medulla. The complex lies partly on the surface of the brain stem at the junction between the medulla and pons. The complex comprises three nuclei, the **dorsal, posterolateral**, and **anteroventral cochlear nuclei**. Each nucleus has a sonotopic representation of the basilar membrane frequency distribution. Lower frequency sounds are represented laterally in the cochlear nucleus, while higher frequency sounds are represented medially.

More ventrally situated cochlear nuclear fibers, such as the **spherical bushy cell**, have relatively simple responses to frequencies. This is because there is a one-to-one contact between incoming auditory fibers and the bushy cell. **Multipolar** cells, which are also ventrally situated, receive more than one incoming auditory fiber, and often show irregular 'choppy' responses. More dorsal cells have complex responses. **Octopus cells**, which integrate inputs from a wide array of cochlear afferents, fire only at the **onset** of a sustained tone, while **pyramidal cells** gradually build up firing amplitude to an incoming tone.

Central auditory pathways are still not fully understood. Dorsally situated cochlear nuclei cells project to the contralateral **inferior colliculus**, while simpler ventral cells project to the **superior olive**, which processes binaural (both ear) inputs, and appears to process **localization** of sounds. The superior olive lies in the caudal pons, near the facial motor nucleus. It is the first nucleus in the brain stem where auditory inputs from the two ears converge. Convergence is essential for localization of sound, and for the construction of the neural maps of contralateral auditory hemifields.

Cells in the **lateral superior olive** (LSO) are excited by the ipsilateral ear, and inhibited by the contralateral ear through fibers from the **trapezoid body**, which is a bundle of unmyelinated fibers that pass ventral to the superior olive. Ascending fibers from the trapezoid body decussate and terminate in the contralateral superior olive, or ascend in the lateral lemniscus. Cells in the **medial superior olive** (MSO) are fired more by low frequency inputs, and may be concerned more with **time** distinctions. All the ascending auditory inputs carried in the lateral synapse in the inferior colliculus. Here, MSO and LSO inputs are united in sonotopic organization. Every frequency point in the basilar membrane is represented here in an **isofrequency lamina**.

The next level up is the **medial geniculate nucleus** (sometimes called 'body'), which is visible as a small protuberance on the lower caudal surface of the thalamus. From here, cells project to the sonotopically organized **primary auditory cortex** (area AI). Ventrally situated cells in the medial geniculate nucleus project mainly to AI in the cortex; more medially placed cells in the medial geniculate nucleus, however, project to the secondary auditory cortex (AII); sound processing in this subsystem appears to be more complex. Cells may respond to more than one sound frequency, and may distinguish between different sound types, such as clicks or hisses, that are commonly encountered in speech sounds.

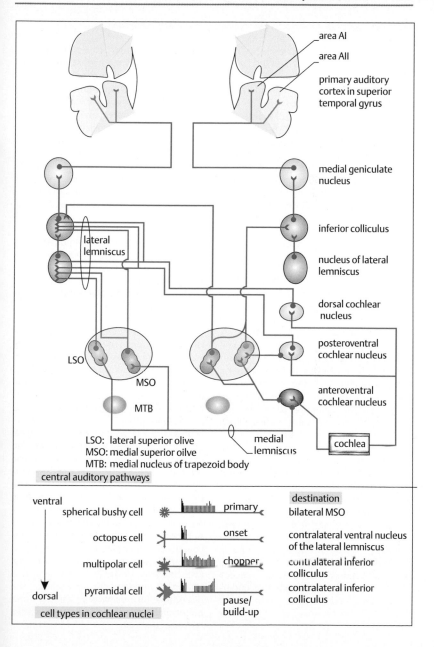

area AI

area AII

primary auditory cortex in superior temporal gyrus

medial geniculate nucleus

inferior colliculus

nucleus of lateral lemniscus

dorsal cochlear nucleus

posteroventral cochlear nucleus

anteroventral cochlear nucleus

lateral lemniscus

LSO

MSO

MTB

medial lemniscus

cochlea

LSO: lateral superior olive
MSO: medial superior oilve
MTB: medial nucleus of trapezoid body

central auditory pathways

ventral

destination

spherical bushy cell — primary — bilateral MSO

octopus cell — onset — contralateral ventral nucleus of the lateral lemniscus

multipolar cell — chopper — contralateral inferior colliculus

pyramidal cell — pause/build-up — contralateral inferior colliculus

dorsal

cell types in cochlear nuclei

Auditory Cortical Areas and Descending Auditory Pathways

The **primary auditory cortex** (area **AI**) includes the gyrus of Heschl, and lies in the inferior wall of the lateral sulcus. It is covered by parts of the parietal and frontal opercula, and is continuous with the **superior temporal gyrus**, which consists of anterior and posterior **gyri**. Area AI lies mainly in the anterior gyrus, but may also extend into the posterior gyrus. Area AI is distinguished by a dense granular cortex, with small granular cells in layer IV (see p. 38), and small pyramidal cells in layer VI. The **secondary auditory cortex** (**AII**) lies adjacent to the granular cortex in the posterior transverse gyrus. There are reciprocal connections between areas AI and AII. In addition, each auditory area has reciprocal connections with its corresponding area in the opposite hemisphere. Area AI is sonotopically organized into **isofrequency binaural response columns**, which run through it. Low frequencies are represented laterally, and high frequencies medially. Each auditory column has cell populations that are either excited by both ears (**E2**), or excited by the contralateral ear and inhibited by the ipsilateral ear (**E1**).

The primary auditory cortex is surrounded by an association cortex, which lies mainly in the posterior part of the superior temporal gyrus. It is connected with the primary auditory cortex by the **arcuate fasciculus**. This **speech reception area** is important in the integration of visual, somesthetic, and auditory inputs. It contains **Wernicke's area** (see also p. 342), which is often at least five times larger in the left hemisphere. If Wernicke's area is damaged, e.g. by stroke, this results in **Wernicke's** or **auditory aphasia**, when patients cannot understand speech sounds, although they usually can understand and discriminate non-speech sounds.

Association areas also extend into the **angular** and **supramarginal gyri**, which appear to be important in reading and writing. The **pars opercularis** and **pars triangularis**, in the inferior frontal gyrus, are called **Broca's area**, and are important for expressive language and speech. The arcuate fasciculus connects these two areas with the primary and association cortex. Damage to these areas by stroke or injury results in **Broca's aphasia**, which is non-fluent speech, although patients can still understand non-verbal and verbal sounds.

Descending auditory pathways constitute the descending component of a central feedback loop between the lower and higher auditory centers in the brain. The auditory cortex sends efferent fibers to the ipsilateral **medial geniculate nucleus**, and to the external nucleus of the **inferior colliculus**. Through their ascending fibers, these nuclei can in turn modulate the function of the primary, secondary and association cortices. The inferior colliculus sends efferents from its central nucleus to the ipsilateral and contralateral **olivary nucleus**, and to the **dorsal cochlear nucleus**. Fibers descend from the pericentral nucleus of the inferior colliculus to the ipsilateral and contralateral olivary nuclei. Fibers travel from the olivary nuclei in the **olivocochlear bundle**, in the vestibular part of the vestibulocochlear nerve. **Lateral olivocochlear fibers** terminate at ipsilateral **inner hair cells**, while **medial olivocochlear fibers** terminate on ipsilateral and **contralateral outer hair cells.** Descending pathways appear to be important in the filtering of auditory information at all levels of the CNS, and even down to the cochlea. This filtering is important in, for example, the discrimination between background noises and those that the listener wishes to concentrate on.

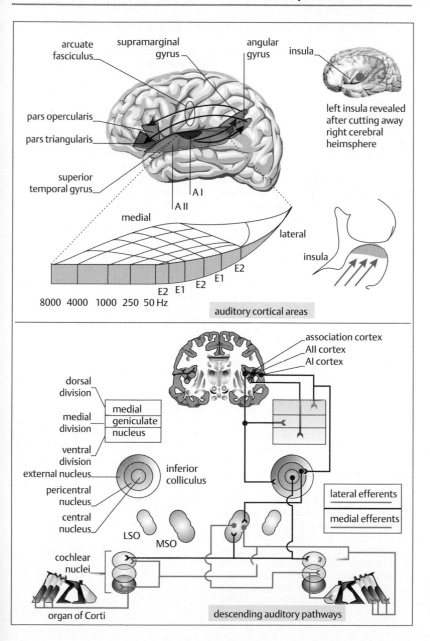

arcuate fasciculus
supramarginal gyrus
angular gyrus
insula

left insula revealed after cutting away right cerebral heimsphere

pars opercularis
pars triangularis

superior temporal gyrus

A I
A II

medial
lateral

insula

E2
E2 E1 E2 E1

8000 4000 1000 250 50 Hz

auditory cortical areas

association cortex
AII cortex
AI cortex

dorsal division
medial division
ventral division

medial geniculate nucleus

external nucleus
pericentral nucleus
central nucleus

inferior colliculus

lateral efferents
medial efferents

LSO MSO

cochlear nuclei

organ of Corti

descending auditory pathways

Localization of Sound

Basically, **sound localization** is made possible by the fact that sounds reach the two ears with different intensities and at different times. In other words, with only one ear, it is much harder to localize sounds. Sound localization has two main components, namely **distance** and **direction**. Accurate determination of distance is dependent on the presence of higher frequency components of sound waves. These tend to be more easily absorbed by intervening solids and liquids, and so the further away the source is, the more difficult it is to judge the distance.

Direction is determined by several mechanisms. In humans, the invaginated and indented vestigial pinna deflects different sounds in a characteristic way, and through repetitive hearing one learns to associates these angles of deflection with direction. The pinna allows direction to be determined to within a few degrees of accuracy. Both ears are not required, and the recruitment of the other ear (**binaural** listening) does not improve efficiency by more than 1° or 2°.

The ears often receive sounds at different **intensities** and different times or **phases**. **Intensity differences** are produced because when sound waves strike the head, they cast a 'sound shadow' that screens the ear from sounds coming from the opposite side. The head has to be turned to point it so that the two ears receive the same intensities. Clearly, animals that can rotate the pinna are more efficient at rapidly localizing sounds through intensity differences. The mechanism will not operate unless the head casts a sound shadow. For this, the wavelength of the incoming sound must be less than the order of magnitude of the head diameter.

Phase differences occur because sounds very often arrive at one ear earlier or later in time than at the other. This is a far more sensitive and accurate mechanism for determining localization of sound. Humans can detect movements of certain sounds by as little as 1° or 2°. It has been calculated that the brain is sensitive to interaural time differences of the order of 10 μsec. The mechanism is more accurate at lower frequencies, and once the frequency rises above 1-2 kHz, the wavelength is shorter than the distance between the ears. Perceived phase differences in these cases could be due to more than one sound direction. Note that the two mechanisms, namely intensity and phase differences complement each other, since intensity differences operate better at higher frequencies, while phase differences operate better at lower frequencies.

The initial central area for binaural sound localization most probably lies in the **superior olivary nucleus**, which is the lowest level where auditory inputs from both ears can be compared. Cells in the lateral part of the olive (LSO) are excited by higher frequency signals from the ipsilateral ear, and inhibited by those from the contralateral ear, due to a delay in the trapezoid body. Cells in the medial superior olive (MSO) respond to lower frequencies, and seem to be concerned with time differences. It is thought that time differences are resolved through a matching system, such that MSO cells will only respond to two **isofrequency** signals from the two ears if they arrive simultaneously and summate. This process is called **coincidence detection**.

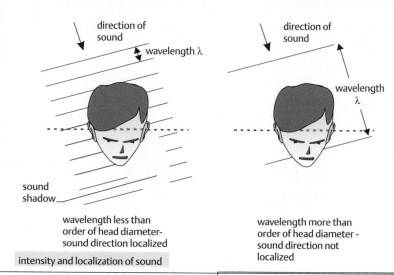

direction of sound

wavelength λ

sound shadow

wavelength less than order of head diameter- sound direction localized

intensity and localization of sound

direction of sound

wavelength λ

wavelength more than order of head diameter - sound direction not localized

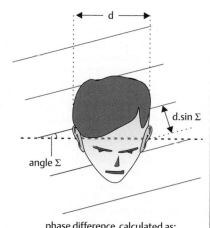

d

d.sin Σ

angle Σ

phase difference calculated as:
(d.sin Σ/λ) degrees
(d.sin Σ/v) msec.
where d = metres;
v = sound velocity (metres/sec)

phase differences in sound localization

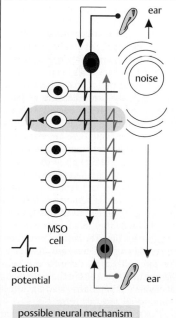

ear

noise

MSO cell

action potential

ear

possible neural mechanism

The Vestibular Apparatus

The **vestibular apparatus** is part of the **labyrinth** in the inner ear. It evolved partly from the lateral line organ, which in fish enables them to orientate in water and sense changes in water movement. The organ differentiated into the **cochlea**, which is **exteroceptive**, and senses air pressure changes, and the **vestibular apparatus**, which is **proprioceptive**, and senses head movements. Unlike the cochlea, the vestibular apparatus does not depend on the external ear. The vestibular apparatus is bilateral; each consists of three **semicircular canals** and two small vesicles, the **saccule** and **utricle**. These organs are oriented at different angles to each other, and together can sense changes in **angular** and **linear** velocity of the head.

Each **semicircular canal** is a looped tube, filled with endolymph, that communicates with the cochlear endolymph through the **ductus reuniens**. The **anterior**, **horizontal** (also called lateral) and **posterior** semicircular canals are oriented essentially orthogonally, representing the three dimensions of space. Each canal has a swelling, the **ampulla**, into which projects a **crest**, which is covered with a layer of **hair cells**. The cilia of the hair cells are embedded in a jelly-like **cupula**, a sort of flap that swings to and fro with movements of the endolymph in the canal. The bending of the cupula excites the cilia of the hair cells, which results in their discharge. The canals respond to **rotation** of the head; when the head turns, the fluid lags behind the head movement and pushes back onto the cupula, which bends. The cilia in a given crest are all oriented in the same direction. Turning the head to the right will fire cells in the right horizontal canal, and inhibit those in the left horizontal canal and *vice versa*.

The sensory epithelium of the vestibular apparatus consists of supporting cells and of sensory ciliated **hair cells** that are innervated by branches of the **vestibular nerve**. Hair cells are either **type I** or **type II**. The cell types are similar in both the semicircular canals and the otolith organs. Type I are goblet-shaped cells which are innervated by larger diameter afferent nerves whose endings are chalice-shaped, and which usually respond to stimulation with a phasic discharge. Type II cells are cylindrical, with smaller diameter afferent and efferent nerve endings at the base of each cell. The afferents respond, typically, with a tonic discharge. The cells are supplied by the vestibular ganglion (Scarpa's ganglion), which lies at the base of the external auditory meatus. Both cell types have **stereocilia** embedded in a **cuticle**; the stereocilia, of which there may be around 60-100, are relatively stiff, and increase in size toward a long, terminal **kinocilium**, which is a more complicated structure than are the stereocilia. Bending or deformation of stereocilia in the direction of the kinocilium increases ionic permeability of the cell, similar to that caused in cochlear hair cells, and causes excitation of the cilia. This results in release of a neurotransmitter, probably glutamate. Bending away from the kinocilium inhibits the stereocilia. The only major difference between vestibular and cochlear hair cells appears to be a permanent basal activity.

In the saccule and utricle there are patches of hair cells, the **saccular** and **utricular maculae**. These hair cells are covered by a jelly-like mass that contains **otolith** calcium crystals (see p. 270).

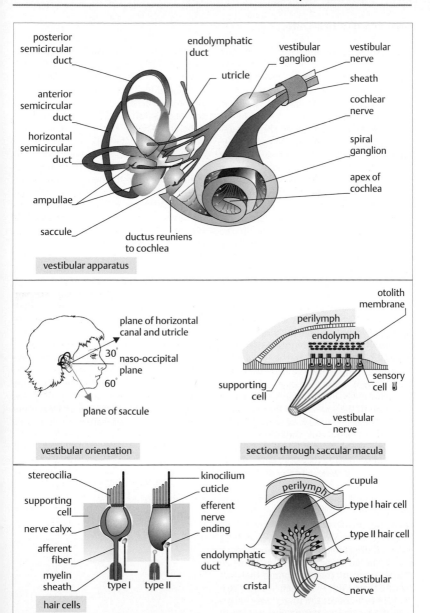

posterior semicircular duct

endolymphatic duct

vestibular ganglion

vestibular nerve

utricle

sheath

anterior semicircular duct

cochlear nerve

horizontal semicircular duct

spiral ganglion

apex of cochlea

ampullae

saccule

ductus reuniens to cochlea

vestibular apparatus

plane of horizontal canal and utricle

naso-occipital plane

30°

60°

plane of saccule

vestibular orientation

otolith membrane

perilymph

endolymph

supporting cell

sensory cell

vestibular nerve

section through saccular macula

stereocilia

kinocilium

supporting cell

cuticle

nerve calyx

efferent nerve ending

afferent fiber

endolymphatic duct

myelin sheath

type I   type II

cupula

perilymph

type I hair cell

type II hair cell

crista

vestibular nerve

hair cells

Orientation of Hair Cells

Hair cells fire off when their stereocilia are bent in the direction of the kinocilium. This phenomenon makes possible the sensing of head orientation and the initiation of appropriate postural and visual responses. The hair cells are oriented in the labyrinth of the ear through the orientation of the **canals** and of the **otolith organs**, the **saccule** and **utricle**. In the canals, the hair cells, which are the sensory receptors, are situated in the crista ampullaris, and in the otolith organs they are situated in the **maculae**.

The macula is a plate-like structure, which roughly follows the shape of the organ. It holds the **sensory epithelium**, which consists of the hair cells and supporting cells. On the macula, the hair cells are embedded in the otolith membrane, a gelatinous substance that contains **otoconia**, which are crystals of calcium carbonate. In both the saccule and utricle, the macula is roughly bisected by a **striola**, where the concentration of overlying otoconia is densest. In the utricle, the hair cells are polarized so that the kinocilium is always nearest the striola. This effectively divides the hair cells on each side of the striola into two morphologically opposed groups of sensory cells. Note that in the saccule, the stereocilia are polarized **away** from the striola. Since in both otolith organs the macula is curved, this enables a wide variety of hair cell alignments.

The otolith organs do not respond to the rotation of the head. Instead, they respond to **tilting** of the head and to its **linear acceleration**. These movements of the head displace the crystalline otoconia, due to the difference in density between the otoconia and the endolymph that surrounds them. The movement of the otoconia in turn moves the underlying gelatinous matrix on the macula. This results in the movement of the stereocilia, and depolarization of the hair cell, if the direction of movement is towards the kinocilium. If the movement is away from the kinocilium, this results in hyperpolarization of the hair cell. Hair cells situated on one side of the striola will be depolarized, while those on the other side will be hyperpolarized. The macula is curved, which greatly increases the versatility of the otolith organs in terms of their response to different degrees of tilt. Note that afferent fibers of the saccular and utricular nerves, which are branches of the vestibular nerve, each innervate hair cells of a relatively small area of the macular sensory epithelium. This greatly increases the acuity of the directional signal.

The otolith organs lie in different planes, essentially at right angles to each other, which makes possible the detection by the brain of many different directions of acceleration. Nevertheless, the brain is unable to distinguish between head tilting and linear acceleration purely through afferent inputs from the hair cells, because they respond only to displacement of the stereocilia in response to movement of the otoconia. Awareness of changes in the position of the head is provided by afferent inputs from the semicircular canals, and from the eyes.

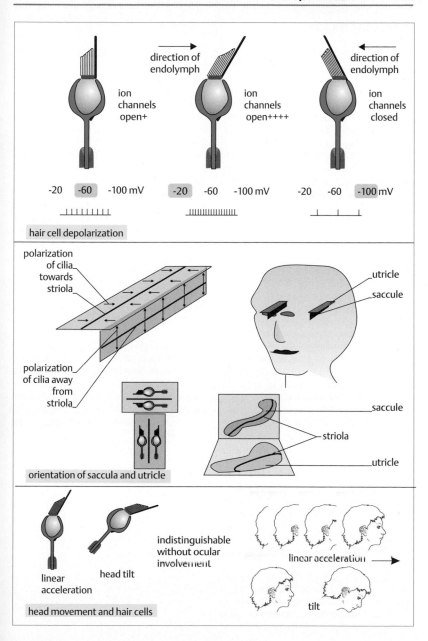

direction of endolymph

ion channels open+

ion channels open++++

direction of endolymph

ion channels closed

-20   -60   -100 mV

-20   -60   -100 mV

-20   -60   -100 mV

hair cell depolarization

polarization of cilia towards striola

utricle

saccule

polarization of cilia away from striola

orientation of saccula and utricle

saccule

striola

utricle

linear acceleration

head tilt

indistinguishable without ocular involvement

linear acceleration

tilt

head movement and hair cells

Structure of the Eye

The **eye** is structured to collect light and perform initial processing of visual inputs. The eyeball is a roughly spherical structure, with a strong outer layer of dense connective tissue, called the **sclera**, which protects the inner layers. The sclera is continuous with the dura mater of the brain. Beneath the sclera is the **choroid**, a vascular layer, and beneath the choroid is the **retina**, which contains the photoreceptors. The choroid is highly pigmented, which does not allow the light to penetrate it. At the front of the eye the sclera has an opening to let in light. The **cornea** covers the opening, which is a thin, transparent layer of connective tissue. The cornea is not vascularized, and is highly innervated with unmyelinated fibers, which make it very sensitive to touch. The lateral border of the cornea is continuous with the **conjunctiva**, a specialized epithelium that covers the sclera.

At the front of the eye the choroid thickens and forms rings, the **ciliary body**, that contain smooth muscles fibers, the ciliary muscles, which control the curvature of the eye. The choroid also forms the **iris**, a circular disk with a central opening called the **pupil**. The iris contains circular smooth muscle (sphincter pupillae), regulated by the parasympathetic division of the autonomic nervous system (ANS). When it contracts the pupil becomes smaller. The iris also contains radially arranged smooth muscles (dilator pupillae), which, when contracted in response to sympathetic stimulation, dilate the pupil. The choroid, ciliary body, and iris are collectively called the **uvea**, also called the vascular tunic. When this is inflamed the condition is called **uveitis**.

Light that enters the eye passes through and is refracted by the **lens**, a transparent crystalline structure held in place by **suspensory ligaments**, also called zonular fibers, situated just behind the pupil. Light is focused on to the retina by the lens, which can alter its shape by the action of the ciliary muscles through the mediation of the parasympathetic division of the ANS. This mechanism is called **accommodation**. In front of the lens, behind the pupil lies the **anterior chamber**, which is bathed with a fluid called aqueous humor, similar in composition to plasma, but with about 1% of its protein. Behind the lens is the larger posterior chamber, which is also bathed with aqueous humor, and which also contains a gel called the **vitreous body** or **humor**. Fluid drains away from the eye through the duct of Schlemm, and anything that blocks drainage causes **glaucoma**, which can lead to blindness.

The inner surface of the eye is covered with the retina, which consists of the **neural retina** and **retinal pigment epithelium**. In section, the retina is seen as a layered structure, whose outermost layer, the **pigment epithelium**, is in contact with the choroid. Internal to this layer is a layer of **photoreceptors**, followed by two further layers of neural cells. At the back of the eye is a yellow spot called the macula lutea, at the center of which is a shallow depression, called the **fovea centralis**.

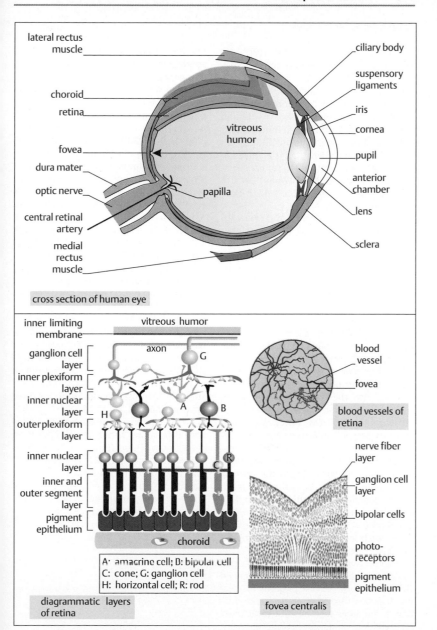

lateral rectus muscle

ciliary body

suspensory ligaments

choroid

retina

iris

cornea

vitreous humor

pupil

fovea

anterior chamber

dura mater

optic nerve

papilla

lens

central retinal artery

sclera

medial rectus muscle

cross section of human eye

inner limiting membrane

vitreous humor

ganglion cell layer

axon

G

inner plexiform layer

inner nuclear layer

A

B

outer plexiform layer

H

inner nuclear layer

R

inner and outer segment layer

C

pigment epithelium

choroid

blood vessel

fovea

blood vessels of retina

nerve fiber layer

ganglion cell layer

bipolar cells

photo-receptors

pigment epithelium

A: amacrine cell; B: bipolar cell
C: cone; G: ganglion cell
H: horizontal cell; R: rod

diagrammatic layers of retina

fovea centralis

Retina, Rods, and Cones

The retina has a layered structure consisting of the **neural retina** and the **pigment epithelium**. The pigment epithelium, which is adjacent to the choroid, consists of cuboidal cells bound by tight junctions that prevent passage of ions and plasma. It protects the retina from overexposure to light, passes glucose and certain ions to the neural retina, and is involved in the maintenance of neural retina structure. Bright light causes pigment cells to close up to photoreceptors and retract when light is dim.

The **neural retina** senses light through its **photoreceptors**, which convert photons into electrical impulses. Associated **retinal cells** perform the initial processing of light information and **ganglion cells** transmit the signals to the brain in their axons, which travel in the **optic nerve**. The retina can become **detached** from the pigment epithelium, and must be reattached as soon as possible since it is metabolically dependent on the pigment epithelium.

The neural retina has seven distinct **layers**. The outermost layer is the **photoreceptor inner** and **outer segment layer**, followed by the **inner nuclear layer**, which contains the nuclei of the photoreceptors. Next is the **outer plexiform layer**, which contains the synapses between photoreceptors and **bipolar** and **horizontal cells**. The **inner plexiform layer** is another layer of synaptic connections, followed by the **ganglion layer**, which contains cell bodies of **ganglion cells**. The innermost layer is made up of **ganglion cell axons**. The nerve layers are separated from the **vitreous humor** by the **inner limiting membrane**.

Photoreceptors are of two types: **rods** and **cones**. Both have similar general structures. Both convert photons to electrical signals through chemical transduction in the outer segments. In **rods**, these are cylinders containing stacks of membranous disks, which are filled with **rhodopsin**. When light strikes rhodopsin, it undergoes a conformational change that activates a **G-protein** called **transducin** which, together with another enzyme, **phosphodiesterase**, decreases intracellular levels of cyclic guanosine monophosphate (**cGMP**). In the dark, cGMP levels are high, and maintain a standing Na^+ current through open Na^+ channels into the outer segment of the rod, which results in a high resting potential. When cGMP falls, or Ca^{2+} increases, the Na^+ channels close, and the resting potential is driven towards the K^+ resting potential, and the rod cell is hyperpolarized. The outer segment is connected to a mitochondrion-filled inner segment by a **cilium**, made up of nine pairs of microtubules that project from a **basal body** in the inner segment.

Cones also have outer segments, although their disk stacks taper from the cilium to the tip, and the disks are exposed to extracellular fluid. The protein **opsin** in the disks undergoes conformational change in response to photons, which results in hyperpolarization. There are three types of cones: **L**, **M**, and **S**.

The synaptic terminals of rods and cones are called **spherules** and **pedicles**, respectively. These terminals have sheets of proteins called **synaptic ribbons**, which may have a 'conveyor belt' function for trafficking glutamate vesicles. Rods and cones release **glutamate** tonically in the dark. Glutamate release is decreased in response to light.

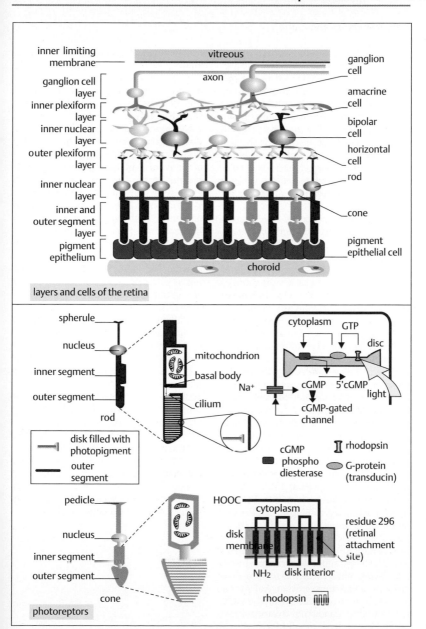

layers and cells of the retina

photoreptors

Photoreceptors and Light

Light is transduced into electrical signals through a primary **photoelectric** effect on the photopigment embedded in the disk membrane in the retinal photoreceptors. The pigment consists of a 40 000 molecular weight glycoprotein called **opsin,** which is associated with a chromophore called **retinal**. A chromophore is the part of a molecule that absorbs light and which gives the molecule its characteristic color. Opsin is a disaccharide-protein complex and retinal is a derivative of retinol (vitamin A).

Retinal is generated by the pigment epithelium in a specific isomeric form, **11-cis retinal**, which is bent into a conformation that allows it to bind covalently through a Schiff base linkage, to the protein opsin. When light strikes the complex, it isomerizes the retinal to a straight **all-trans** form, which cannot fit into the binding site in the protein. The protein opsin quickly passes through a series of unstable configurations to an unstable form called **metarhodopsin II**, and the Schiff base linkage is broken through hydrolysis. The all-*trans* form diffuses away. The 11-*cis* form is slowly regenerated through a recycling process in the pigment epithelium and recombines with free opsin. Retinal, which is poorly water-soluble, is transported between the photoreceptors and pigment epithelium by a retinal-binding protein. The slow rate of regeneration of the 11-*cis* form is given as the reason for the slow rate of dark adaptation. In bright light, most of the rhodopsin is bleached, and with time an equilibrium is established in which the rate of bleaching equals the rate of 11-*cis* retinal regeneration. The body cannot synthesize a 11-*trans* retinol (vitamin A), which is the precursor of 11-*cis* retinal; thus deficiency of vitamin A is associated with the syndrome called night blindness, and if not treated with vitamin A can lead to blindness due to degeneration of photoreceptor outer segments.

There are three types of cone, with differing wavelength optima for absorption of light. S-cones absorb at shorter wavelengths, M-cones absorb at medium wavelengths, and L-cones absorb at longer wavelengths. These three kinds are blue, green, and red absorbing, respectively. In other words, the three types are excited maximally by different wavelengths of light. In all three types, the chromophore is 11-*cis* retinal. The proteins, however, are different, although closely related. Humans have three genes for cone pigment proteins. The green and red absorbing proteins are closely linked on the X chromosome, and the blue absorbing protein is encoded on an autosome. The red and green absorbing cone pigment proteins differ in only 15 of their 348 residues, and about half of the amino acid sequence of rhodopsin is identical with those of the three cone pigment proteins. Interestingly, New World monkeys have only two cone pigments, one long wave and the other blue, whereas Old World primates, whose evolutionary path split from New World primates about 30 million years ago, have blue, green, and red.

Color blindness is caused by sex-linked mutations or deletions of genes encoding cone pigments. About 1% of men are red blind, and about 2% are green blind. Genetic analysis shows that a lack or defect in the gene encoding the green pigment protein causes color blindness.

11-*cis* retinal

all-*trans* retinal

Photoreceptors and Retinal Interneurons

Light is transduced by photoreceptors into a **hyperpolarization**, which is transmitted to the bipolar cells as a reduction in the tonic release of the neurotransmitter glutamate. The bipolar cells in turn transmit the information to the ganglion cells, from where the impulses are sent to the brain in the optic tract. Information about the illumination is extensively processed by **retinal interneurons** before it reaches the ganglion cells. These retinal interneurons are the **bipolar cells**, **amacrine cells**, and **horizontal cells**.

Rods synapse with specific **rod bipolar cells**, which receive converging inputs from several rods. The rod bipolars depolarize in response to light. A single **cone** may synapse with **invaginating** or **flat** bipolar cells. Photoreceptors are depolarized in the dark, presumably because their Na$^+$ channels are open. Also, photoreceptors produce graded changes in the membrane potential but not action potentials. When the cone hyperpolarizes in response to light, its Na$^+$ channels close. Unusually, glutamate, the transmitter of the photoreceptors, hyperpolarizes the bipolar cell. Some bipolar cells, however, are depolarized by glutamate. Bipolar cells have **receptive fields**. A cell with an **on-center field** will depolarize if a cone is stimulated which innervates the center of its field. Invaginating bipolars cells have **on-center fields**, which means they depolarize when light stimulates cones that innervate their centers. The **off-center field** of the invaginating bipolar cell is hyperpolarized by inputs from horizontal cells, which receive inputs from many cones, and can thus coordinate the status of bipolar cell fields. Flat (off-center) polar cells have off-center receptive fields; the cell hyperpolarizes in response to light. These cells are excited in the dark, when glutamate is released as an excitatory neurotransmitter, which is its more usual action on nerve cells.

The different actions of glutamate can be explained by its gating actions on different ion channels. The neurotransmitter depolarizes flat, off-center bipolar cells by opening Na$^+$ channels, which carry an inward depolarizing current. Glutamate may hyperpolarize invaginating, on-center bipolar cells by opening K$^+$ channels, and in others by closing Na$^+$ channels, which are normally open in the dark, and which normally keep the flat bipolar cell depolarized in the absence of light. The intracellular consequences of glutamate action are thought to be the same as those produced by light on photoreceptor disks. Glutamate may generate an intracellular cascade that lowers intracellular cGMP concentrations, which results in the closure of cGMP-gated ion channels.

Horizontal cells modulate transmission of light by actions on photoreceptors. Horizontal cells receive inputs from a wide range of photoreceptors, and synapse directly on to cones. They do not appear to synapse on to bipolar cells at all, but instead synapse with cones which affect the center of the bipolar cell's receptive field. When the surrounding area is illuminated, the horizontal cells depolarize the center of the field, which has the opposite effect to that produced when these cones are activated by light.

Horizontal cells also sharpen the borders of a receptive field by inhibiting photoreceptors adjacent to those that define the receptive field being sharpened (**lateral inhibition**). A photoreceptor serving the on-center of a receptive field synapses with a horizontal cell and depolarizes it. The horizontal cell in turn inhibits photoreceptors serving the surrounding area.

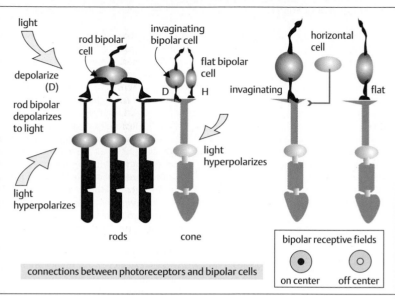

connections between photoreceptors and bipolar cells

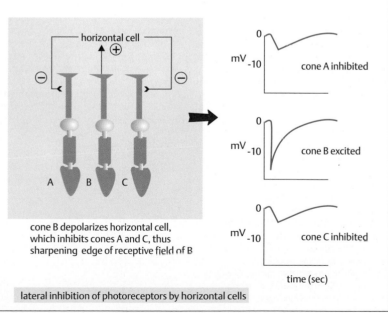

cone B depolarizes horizontal cell, which inhibits cones A and C, thus sharpening edge of receptive field of B

lateral inhibition of photoreceptors by horizontal cells

Retinal Ganglion Cells

Ganglion cells transmit electrical impulses generated by photon action to the brain through their axons, which make up the optic tract. Ganglion cells, like bipolar cells, have approximately circular **receptive fields** which can be defined as retinal areas where light stimulation causes an increase or decrease in the rate of impulse propagation of the ganglion cell. The receptive fields of ganglion cells increase in diameter with increasing distance from the fovea centralis.

There are two main types of ganglion cell, **M-cells** and **P-cells** (also termed A and B cells in some texts). M-cells are much larger than P-cells. There is evidence that M-cells are mainly concerned with **illumination** contrasts and movement, while P-cells transmit information about color and acuity. Different P-cells respond to different colors while M-cells do not. M-cells respond preferentially to moving objects, with bursts of activity at the start and end of movement, while P-cells fire continuously while an object is moving. About 80% of ganglion cells are P-cells. (Note that in studies of the cat retina, X, Y, and W retinal cells are described, but this terminology is not usually used in descriptions of primate retina.) Both types of cell send their axons mainly to the thalamus. A third type of ganglion cell has been described which is smaller than P-cells, and which sends its axons to the mesencephalon.

Ganglion cells, like bipolar cells, may have **on-center** or **off-center** receptor field with an antagonistic surrounding area. Ganglion cells fire off impulses tonically, even in the absence of light stimulation of the photoreceptors, and different ganglion cells respond to light depending on where it strikes the retina. On-center ganglion cells are less active in darkness, and their firing rate increases when light strikes the center of the receptive field. In contrast, light that strikes the surround inhibits electrical activity of the ganglion cell. Off-center ganglion cells decrease firing in response to illumination of the center of the field, and have bursts of activity when the light is turned off. When light strikes the surround of the off-center cell, its firing rate increases. Ganglion cells can **adapt** to light changes. In dim or bright light, after a time of continuous exposure to a fixed light intensity, the surrounding cells are unable to inhibit the effects of light on the center of the field. There are approximately equal numbers of on-center and off-center ganglion cells, and they provide parallel pathways for processing visual inputs, in that one photoreceptor transmits its information both to off-center and on-center ganglion cells.

The **transient** nature of some responses of ganglion cells, i.e. their bursts at start and ending of movement or light, may be due to modulating actions of **amacrine cells**. Much of this information comes from studies using cats. Amacrine cells have very similar responses to those of ganglion cells. There are many different morphological types of amacrine cell, with different neurotransmitters. **Sustained** responses appear to be controlled primarily by bipolar cells.

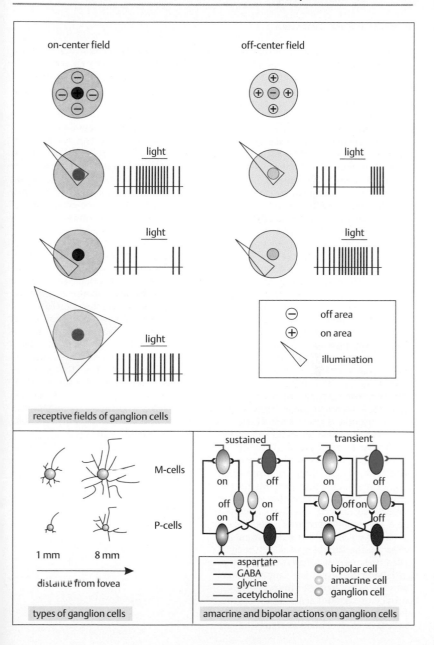

on-center field

off-center field

⊖ off area
⊕ on area
◁ illumination

light
light
light
light
light

receptive fields of ganglion cells

M-cells

P-cells

1 mm   8 mm

distance from fovea

types of ganglion cells

sustained   transient

on   off

off   on

on   off

on   off

off on

on   off

— aspartate
— GABA
— glycine
— acetylcholine

◉ bipolar cell
◉ amacrine cell
◉ ganglion cell

amacrine and bipolar actions on ganglion cells

Visual Fields and Pathways I

The accurate projection of visual inputs from the retina to the brain requires the preservation of the order of the original visual layout on the retina, the so-called **retinotopic map**. The map is plotted on the retina in terms of an orderly arrangement of photoreceptors and their associated ganglion cells. Thus, adjacent visual inputs are plotted by adjacent ganglion cells, somewhat analogous to the plotting of pixels by a computer.

The picture received by the retina when the subject looks at it with both eyes open is called the **visual field**. It consists of three zones: the **binocular zone**, the central zone constructed by inputs from right and left retinas, and crescent-shaped **monocular zones** (monocular crescents), constructed by each retina alone. Each retina has **nasal** and **temporal** fields. Light that passes through the pupil is focused on to the retina by the cornea and lens. Light that enters from the right strikes the nasal retina of the right eye and the temporal retina of the left eye, and *vice versa* if light enters from the left. Each field can be divided into nasal and temporal hemifields, and into upper and lower quadrants. This pattern of light entry is preserved faithfully throughout the CNS. The fovea is represented at the center of the field, where the greatest acuity is achieved, and adjacent to the fovea is the **optic disc**, where ganglion axons converge. It is also the **blind spot**, where ganglion axons pass through the sclera and become myelinated, so called because there are no photoreceptors in this area.

The main visual projection from the retina to the lateral geniculate body is called the **retinogeniculate projection**. On leaving the eyes, the ganglion axons form the **optic nerves**, which cross over partially (decussate) at the **optic chiasm**, after which the optic tracts travel, mainly, to the **lateral geniculate nucleus**. The vast majority of ganglion cell axons travel via the **optic nerve**, the **optic chiasm**, and the **optic tract** to the **lateral geniculate nucleus**. Some axons project to the **suprachiasmatic nucleus**, which governs diurnal rhythms, while others project to the **olivary pretectal** and **accessory optic nuclei**, which are involved in the pupillary light reflex (see also p. 244). Some axons terminate in the **superior colliculus** (see p. 9), which modulates visual reflexes and is involved in voluntary eye movements. The superior colliculus projects in turn to the **pulvinar** of the **thalamus** (see p. 285), which receives inputs also from the pretectum and the visual cortex.

Visual information is used to detect boundaries and edges of objects for recognition, which is a function of the cortex, and to locate objects in the external environment, primarily a function of the superior colliculus. It is used to assess our own position in relation to external objects in the world, a function of the pretectum (see below) and related nuclei and pathways in the brain stem. The visual system detects movement. It assesses the intensity of ambient light (i.e. tells the time of day), which involves accommodation and other eye reflexes concerned with the reception of light by the eye.

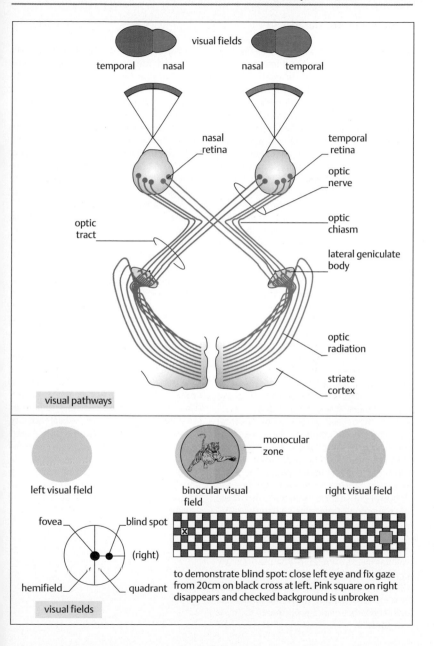

visual fields

temporal   nasal   nasal   temporal

nasal retina

temporal retina

optic nerve

optic chiasm

lateral geniculate body

optic tract

optic radiation

striate cortex

visual pathways

left visual field

binocular visual field

monocular zone

right visual field

fovea

blind spot

(right)

hemifield

quadrant

to demonstrate blind spot: close left eye and fix gaze from 20cm on black cross at left. Pink square on right disappears and checked background is unbroken

visual fields

Visual Fields and Pathways II

Visual information from each retina is first sorted for purposes of brain lateralization in the **optic chiasm**. In the optic chiasm, fibers are sorted according to their retinal origin. Visual field information from the left retina will be appreciated in the right hemisphere, and *vice versa*. In the chiasm, fibers originating in the **nasal** half of each retina (corresponding to the temporal hemifields) cross and enter the contralateral optic tract. In contrast, fibers from the **temporal** half (corresponding to the nasal hemifields) remain ipsilateral in the optic tract that emerges from the chiasm. Thus, each hemisphere receives visual information from both eyes. This anatomical arrangement is especially apparent after lesions in the vicinity of the optic chiasm.

A lesion to the optic nerve before it reaches the chiasm, caused usually by a cardiovascular aneurysm, will result in partial or complete blindness in the corresponding eye. Lesions in different parts of the chiasm have more complex effects on vision. The optic chiasm lies immediately above the pituitary gland, which renders the chiasm susceptible to pituitary tumors. A tumor pressing on the chiasm where fibers from the temporal visual halves meet will cause a **bitemporal hemianopia**. A lesion of the optic tract will cause a contralateral **homonymous hemianopia**. Note, however, that not all fibers decussate completely, and the point of greatest acuity, the fovea, is represented in both hemispheres, which results in the phenomenon of **macular sparing**.

Subcortical visual information is processed mainly in the **lateral geniculate nucleus** (**LGN**), which has six distinct cellular layers numbered 1 through 6. Layers 1, 4, and 6 process information from the contralateral eye, and 2, 3, and 5 process information from the ipsilateral eye. The functional significance of this is unknown.

Layers 1 and 2 of each LGN have cells with relatively large cell bodies, and are called **magnocellular** layers. Their axons project to the superior colliculus and other subcortical regions, although some axons do project to the cortex. The other layers are called **parvocellular** because of their smaller cell bodies, and project to the cerebral cortex. Magnocellular axons conduct at much higher velocities, which may be functionally significant in view of the need for rapid subcortical processing of visual inputs related to proprioception.

The ordering and arrangement of visual inputs to the LGN is kept strictly in register with that in the retina, and this ordering is sustained through to the occipital lobe of the cortex. Cells of the LGN have wavelength-dependent receptive fields similar to those of ganglion cells, with concentric on-center and off-center fields. LGN cells are modulated by nervous inputs from other brain areas, for example, during sleep.

Retinal inputs subserve different functional purposes, depending on where they are routed to in the brain. Those to limbic regions such as the hypothalamus subserve motivational behavior related to, for example, feeding or sexual activity. Those to the midbrain (pretectum, superior colliculus) subserve proprioception and localization. Those to the cortex subserve cognitive correlates such as recognition. These neural areas are, of course, interconnected, so that responses are coordinated.

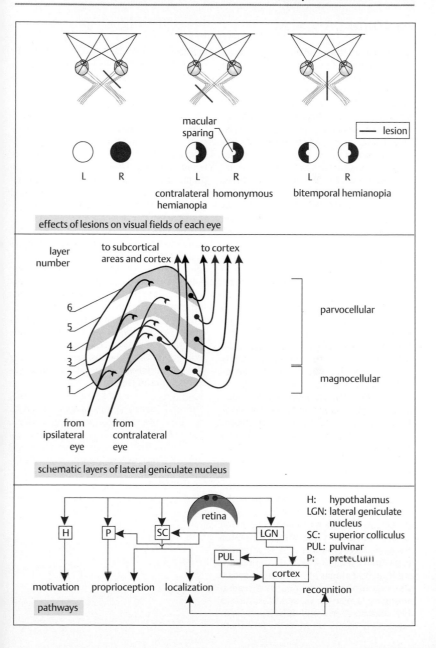

macular sparing

— lesion

L   R

L   R

contralateral homonymous hemianopia

L   R

bitemporal hemianopia

effects of lesions on visual fields of each eye

layer number

to subcortical areas and cortex

to cortex

6
5
4
3
2
1

parvocellular

magnocellular

from ipsilateral eye

from contralateral eye

schematic layers of lateral geniculate nucleus

H: hypothalamus
LGN: lateral geniculate nucleus
SC: superior colliculus
PUL: pulvinar
P: pretectum

retina

H   P   SC   LGN

PUL

cortex

motivation   proprioception   localization   recognition

pathways

Visual Cortex I

The **primary visual cortex** receives most of the efferent fibers from the lateral geniculate nucleus (LGN). It is a bilateral area lying almost entirely medially on either side of the **calcarine sulcus** in the occipital lobe. It is **Brodmann's area 17** (see p. 337), and is also referred to as area **V1**. It is also called the **striate cortex** because a thick stripe of afferent inputs, the **stripe of Gennari**, runs through it. It is surrounded by two other purely visual areas, area 18 (the **prestriate cortex**), and area 19 (**medial temporal cortex**). Area 18 has been subdivided into areas V2 through V4, and area 19 is area V5. Localization of visual inputs is achieved through projection to parietal areas, which address the question 'where?', and identification to temporal areas, which address the question 'what?'.

The **primary visual cortex** contains an ordered map of the **visual field**. Each hemifield is represented on the contralateral hemisphere. On each side, the upper quadrants are represented below the **calcarine fissure**, while the lower quadrants are represented above the calcarine fissure. In each hemisphere, a disproportionately large anatomical area of the visual cortex is devoted to the representation of the fovea, which is the retinal area of greatest acuity.

The visual cortex, in common with the rest of the cerebral cortex, consists of six layers. It is around 2 mm thick from the underlying white matter through to the overlying pia mater. **Layer 4** is especially prominent because it contains the stripe (or stria) of Gennari. The stripe consists of the very large numbers of myelinated fibers from the lateral geniculate nucleus, and from other areas of the cortex. **Layer 4** has been further subdivided into several subsidiary layers, **4A**, **4B**, and **4C**, which in turn consists of **4Ca** and **4Cb**. It has been found that axons of **M** cells terminate mainly in sublamina 4Ca, while axons of **P** cells terminate mainly in sublamina 4Cb. It will be recalled that P cells are concerned mainly with the detection of initial movement, while M cells are concerned with color and fine structure discernment. Layer 6, too, is especially prominent, and contains several efferent fibers, which form a feedback loop back to the LGN. The pyramidal cells of the visual cortex are the projection neurons, while the non-pyramidal stellate cells (see p. 39) are interneurons, whose processes are confined to the layers of the cortex.

The flow of visual information to the visual cortex starts with inputs to spiny stellate cells in layer 4, which project to layers 2, 3, and 4B. Cells in 2 and 3 project in turn to pyramidal cells in layer 5. These project to pyramidal cells in layer 6, and these project to inhibitory stellate cells in layer 4. The inhibitory stellate cells modulate the activity of excitatory stellate cells. Cells of the visual cortex, like those of the retina and LGN, have response fields, but of very different kinds. They may be **simple** or **complex**.

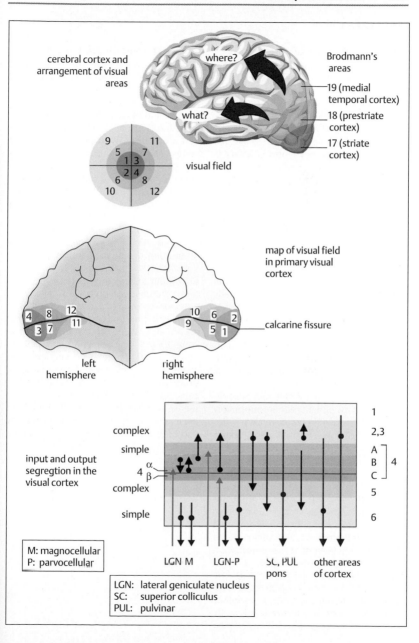

cerebral cortex and arrangement of visual areas

Brodmann's areas
- 19 (medial temporal cortex)
- 18 (prestriate cortex)
- 17 (striate cortex)

visual field

map of visual field in primary visual cortex

calcarine fissure

left hemisphere

right hemisphere

input and output segregation in the visual cortex

complex
simple
complex
simple

LGN M LGN-P SC, PUL pons other areas of cortex

M: magnocellular
P: parvocellular

LGN: lateral geniculate nucleus
SC: superior colliculus
PUL: pulvinar

Visual Cortex II

Some cells of the **visual cortex**, particularly those lying in layer 4 near the termination of afferent inputs from the lateral geniculate nucleus, show receptive field properties similar to those of retinal ganglion cells and cells in the lateral geniculate body (LGN). Most cells in area 17 (and all those in other cortical areas) have receptive field properties that are different from those in the retina and LGN.

Cells have been classified as **simple** or **complex**, depending on the nature of their receptive fields. **Simple** cells may not have a circular field, but a central strip, which is excited or inhibited by a strip of illumination of a particular orientation. For optimal firing, the incoming impulses generated by strip of light must activate not only a particular orientation but also a particular position on the cell. These simple cells have therefore also been called **line detectors**. The cells are part of the **recognition** system. They are generally more responsive to moving flashes of light, rather than to static, steady illumination, and respond poorly, if at all, to diffuse illumination of equivocal orientation.

Complex cells, like simple cells, also respond to strips of light, but are more versatile, in that they do not have clearly defined excitatory and inhibitory zones. Complex cells are specific for orientation of the light strip. Like simple cells, they will not respond to light strips not oriented for their configuration. As with simple cells, moving flashes of light are most effective in eliciting a response; complex cells often switch from being excited to being inhibited, or *vice versa*, if the direction of movement of the illumination is reversed. Apparently, therefore, complex cells are concerned more with the recognition of external objects than with their precise localization. There is another type of complex cell, which was originally called a hypercomplex cell but is now

termed the **end-stopped complex cell**. This cell responds selectively not only to strips of light of specific orientation, but also to an optimal **strip length**. (The properties of these various types of cortical cell have been defined in terms of strictly controlled experimental illumination types. At any one time, the response of the visual cortex to the irregular and constantly changing patterns of illumination is undoubtedly more complex than is suggested by experiments.)

Both simple and complex cells are aligned in the visual cortex in an orderly system of **columns**, which are arranged perpendicular to the cortical surface. The orientation is not haphazardly arranged, but changes systematically from column to column in repeating patterns. In addition, columns receive inputs from one eye only, which produces **ocular dominance** in the columns. Column segregation is not universal, however. In layer 4C there are complex cells that respond to both eyes.

Abnormal columnar development can cause visual problems. If there is inappropriate innervation of cortical cells by LGN cells during critical periods of development, **amblyopia** may result. Here, one eye is poorly represented in the columns, and binocular vision is lost. Development is generally complete by age 6 years.

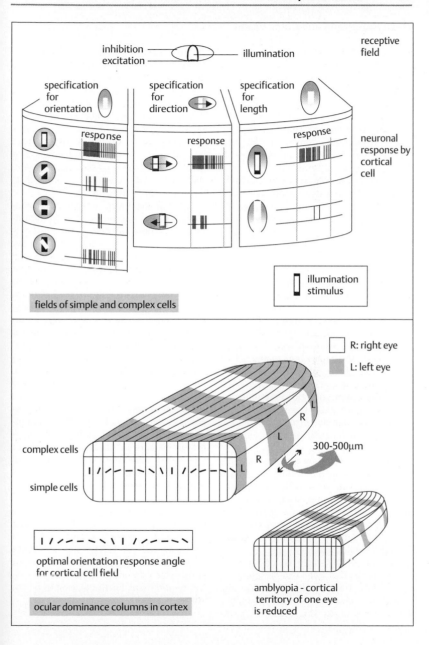

inhibition —
excitation —
illumination

receptive field

specification for orientation

specification for direction

specification for length

response

response

response

neuronal response by cortical cell

illumination stimulus

fields of simple and complex cells

R: right eye
L: left eye

complex cells

simple cells

300-500μm

L
R
L
R
L

optimal orientation response angle for cortical cell field

ocular dominance columns in cortex

amblyopia - cortical territory of one eye is reduced

Visual Processing and Color Vision

It is not known how the brain converts primary visual inputs to the striate cortex into meaningful images. There is little doubt, however, that the process involves integrative activity which recruits several cortical and subcortical structures.

There is evidence that information derived from inputs from retinal M and P cells diverges completely when it leaves the subregion **V2** of **Brodmann area 18** in the cortex. The **M pathway** (stream), which carries information almost exclusively from the rods and from relatively large retinal fields, passes to subregion **V3** of area 18, from there to the **medial temporal cortex**, and finally to the posterior parietal cortex (Brodmann's area 7a). This information enables the brain to analyze movement and the location ('where?'). The **P pathway** (stream) passes from subregion V2 to Brodmann's area 19, and thence to the inferior temporal cortex (area 37), where it is used to identify visual inputs (what?). This pathway was originally split in the lateral geniculate nucleus (LGN) into pathways specific for color and form. The color information originated from **color opponent** fields in retinal ganglion and LGN cells (see below). The P pathway mediating form originates in small field, high acuity receptor and ganglion cells.

Color perception by the brain is made possible through the ability of retinal cones to respond to specific wavelengths of electromagnetic radiation. Human vision is trichromatic, i.e. it responds to three wavelength peaks of the electromagnetic spectrum. These, commonly termed short (**S**), medium (**M**), and long (**L**), correspond to blue (B), green (G), and red (R), respectively. The eye can respond to wavelengths from about 400 to 700 nm. Cones may have one of three pigments, which respond to the different wavelengths. Deficiency of one or two (mono-

chromatopsia or dichromatopsia, respectively) will impair color perception. Since full color competence depends on the activation of three cone types, it follows that the colors of very small objects, whose reflected light falls on a relatively small retinal surface, may not be detected properly. Also, short wave stimulation (B) produces blurred images, a phenomenon called chromatic aberration. Color perception in the fovea is not trichromatic because of its dedication to acuity.

Color is perceived through **color constancy**, **color opponency**, and **simultaneous color contrast**. Color constancy enables the brain to identify the wavelength composition of light from an object regardless of the nature of the light source i.e. the color is the same regardless of the wavelength. Color opponency cancels mutually antagonistic primary color pairs such as red-green, and yellow-blue. Retinal and lateral geniculate nuclear (LGN) cells achieve this through the mutually antagonistic nature of concentric receptive fields, which respond differently to different wavelengths. Single opponent LGN color cells will respond either to red or green with depolarization or hyperpolarization. The LGN also has **coextensive single-opponent cells**, which block red-green while depolarizing to blue, or *vice versa*, and **concentric broad band LGN cells**, in which green and red cones cooperate to depolarize or hyperpolarize the cell.

The visual cortex has concentric double opponent cells in so-called **blob zones**, which respond preferentially to red-green contrasts, or to yellow-blue contrasts. There are also **complex double opponent cells**, which do not have such a rigid spatial requirement for the placing of a light stimulus within their receptive fields.

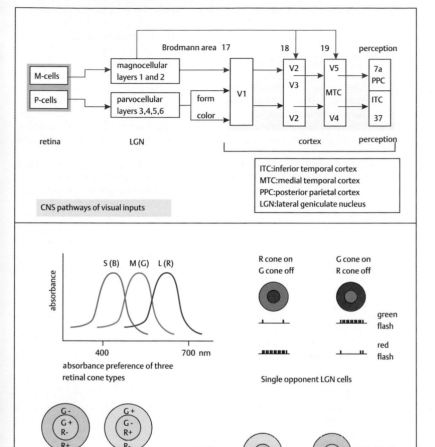

CNS pathways of visual inputs

ITC: inferior temporal cortex
MTC: medial temporal cortex
PPC: posterior parietal cortex
LGN: lateral geniculate nucleus

absorbance preference of three
retinal cone types

Single opponent LGN cells

concentric double opponent
cerebral cortical cells

concentric broad band LGN cells

coextensive single-opponent LGN cells

color vision

The Hypothalamus-Pituitary Axis

The hypothalamus is the brain center that controls much of the body's endocrine secretions, through its **portal blood** link with the **anterior pituitary gland** (adenohypophysis) and its neuroendocrine links with the **posterior pituitary** (neurohypophysis). Among its functions, the hypothalamus controls sexual function and behavior, thyroid secretion, the secretion of cortisol, and stress responses, appetite, temperature, and growth. It plays a crucial role in water and salt balance, and lactation.

The hypothalamus lies at the base of the diencephalon beneath the thalamus, from which it is separated by the hypothalamic sulcus. The rostral boundary of the hypothalamus is taken to be at the level of the lamina terminalis, while the caudal end is at the level of the **mamillary bodies**. These are arbitrary boundaries, since the hypothalamus runs rostrally into the **preoptic area**, and is continuous with the central gray matter.

The hypothalamus can be conveniently divided into the three main areas: the rostral supraoptic, middle tuberal and posterior mamillary areas. These three areas are associated with different groups of nuclei, or groups of cell bodies. The hypothalamus is also divided into the medial region, which contains well-defined nuclei, and lateral regions, in which nuclear organization is more diffuse. In the rostral region are the **supraoptic** and **paraventricular** nuclei, which project neurosecretory axons down into the neurohypophysis. As will be seen in more detail later, these nuclei control the secretion of oxytocin and vasopressin. The **suprachiasmatic nucleus**, which is also present in the rostral region, is important in the control of daily rhythms of hormone secretion, and in the generation of circadian rhythms of hormone secretion and behavior. In the middle region are the dorsomedial, ventromedial and **arcuate nuclei**. These regions are rich in steroid hormone receptors, and are involved in the feedback actions of several hormones such as thyroid, sex, and glucocorticoid hormones Functions mediated by these nuclei include responses to stress, the control of gonadotropin secretion, and the control of the thyroid gland. All these functions are dealt with in more detail later.

The arcuate nucleus projects neurosecretory axons to the **median eminence blood vessels of the portal system**, which carry the secretions down to the cells of the **adenohypophysis**. The cells of the hypothalamic nuclei also send projections to higher and lower brain areas. There are many connections between the hypothalamus and other brain areas, and a prominent pathway for ascending and descending fibers is the median forebrain bundle (see p. 295).

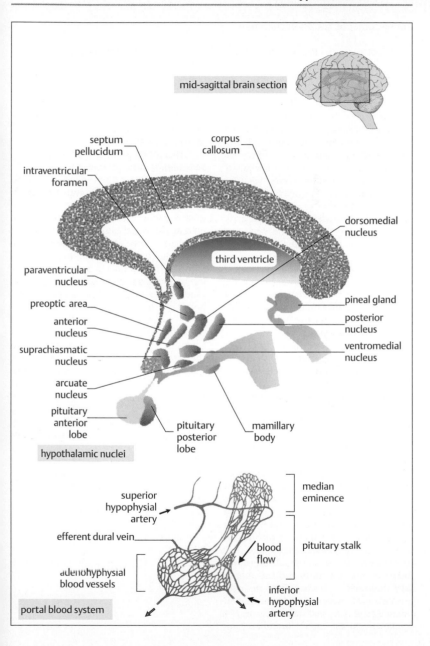

mid-sagittal brain section

septum pellucidum

corpus callosum

intraventricular foramen

dorsomedial nucleus

third ventricle

paraventricular nucleus

preoptic area

anterior nucleus

suprachiasmatic nucleus

arcuate nucleus

pituitary anterior lobe

pineal gland

posterior nucleus

ventromedial nucleus

pituitary posterior lobe

mamillary body

hypothalamic nuclei

superior hypophysial artery

median eminence

efferent dural vein

pituitary stalk

adenohypophysial blood vessels

blood flow

inferior hypophysial artery

portal blood system

Connections of the Hypothalamus

The hypothalamus, although anatomically relatively small, has extensive afferent and efferent connections with the rest of the brain. Some of these are well defined, while others are more diffuse and harder to define.

The afferent fibers that have been identified are (i) medial forebrain bundle, (ii) the hippocampo-hypothalamic fibers, (iii) precommissural fibers of the fornix, (iv) amygdalo-hypothalamic fibers, (v) brain stem reticular afferents, and (vi) retinohypothalamic afferents.

The **medial forebrain bundle** arises from the basal olfactory and periamygdaloid regions, and from the septal nuclei. It passes to and through the lateral hypothalamic and preoptic regions. It is smaller in man than in lower vertebrates. The hippocampo-hypothalamic afferents arise in the hippocampal formation, and form two tracts, the **fornix**, and the **medial corticohypothalamic tract** (not shown in figure). The fornix forms two distinct bundles in the septum, the compact fornix column, and the precommissural fibers (which project to the septal nuclei, the lateral preoptic region, the dorsal hypothalamus, and the nucleus of the diagonal band). The amygdalo-hypothalamic fibers are made up of the stria terminalis and another pathway, which lies ventral to the lentiform nucleus. The stria terminalis arises in the corticomedian region of the amygdaloid complex of nuclei, and projects fibers to the arcuate and ventromedial nuclei, the anterior hypothalamic nucleus, and to the medial preoptic nucleus.

Ascending fiber bundles include the brain stem reticular afferents, which climb to the hypothalamus through the **dorsal longitudinal fasciculus** and the **mamillary peduncle**. The mamillary peduncle arises from the ventral and dorsal tegmental nuclei of the midbrain and projects principally to the lateral **mamillary nucleus**. Some of these fibers pass through the hypothalamus and project to the forebrain. The ascending fibers of the dorsal longitudinal fasciculus arise in the midbrain central gray matter and they fan out over the dorsal and caudal regions of the hypothalamus, and become part of the periventricular system.

Other brain stem afferents to the hypothalamus arise in the midbrain raphe nuclei, the pons, and from the locus ceruleus. The raphe afferents are mainly serotonergic, originate in the dorsal and medial raphe nuclei, and ascend in the medial forebrain bundle to and through the lateral hypothalamus. Serotonergic terminals of this innervation have been found in the mamillary bodies, the preoptic region (which is concerned, among other things, with the regulation of sexual behavior) and the suprachiasmatic nucleus, which has been implicated in the regulation of body rhythms. The nucleus solitarius projects ascending afferents to the thalamus and to the hypothalamic **paraventricular nucleus**. This latter pathway is involved in the regulation of vasopressin secretion. The locus ceruleus also projects noradrenergic pathways in the dorsal tegmental bundle to the dorsomedial, paraventricular, and **supraoptic nuclei**.

The **retinohypothalamic fibers** arise in the retinal ganglion cells and project bilaterally through the optic nerve and optic chiasm to the suprachiasmatic nuclei.

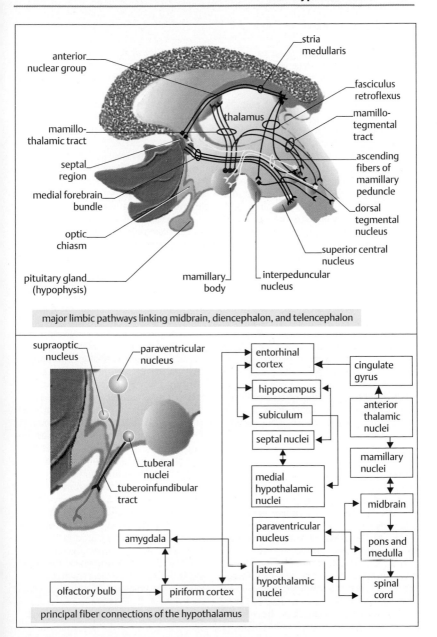

major limbic pathways linking midbrain, diencephalon, and telencephalon

principal fiber connections of the hypothalamus

Neuroendocrine Axis

The neuroendocrine axis for a particular endocrine gland consists of the brain, pituitary, and end target organ, together with the chemical mediators involved in the operation of the gland. The anterior lobe of the pituitary gland (also called the adenohypophysis) receives releasing factors from the brain via the portal system, and these in turn release **tropic hormones**, which target the endocrine glands. These release their **hormones**, which exert their physiological actions, and also feed back to the brain and pituitary gland, which possess receptors for the hormones. The posterior pituitary receives **oxytocin** and **vasopressin** from the supraoptic and paraventricular nuclei, and releases these in response to afferent stimuli from lower and higher brain centers. There is, in addition, an **intermediate pituitary lobe** in man, which releases the **endorphins** and **melanocyte-stimulating hormone** (**MSH**).

The major **anterior lobe tropic hormones** are (i) **ACTH** (**adrenocorticotropic hormone**) whose major target is the adrenal cortex, where it stimulates hypertrophy of the organ, and the release of the steroid hormones, notably cortisol and the androgens (see p. 300), (ii) **GH** (**growth hormone**, somatotropin), which targets a number of tissues to stimulate muscle protein synthesis, bone elongation, and lipolysis (see p. 304), (iii) **LH** (**luteinizing hormone**) and **FSH** (**follicle-stimulating hormone**), which act primarily on the gonads to stimulate steroid hormone secretion and germ cell production (see pp. 302, 303), (iv) **TSH** (**thyroid-stimulating hormone**), which acts on the thyroid cell to stimulate the production of thyroxine (T_4) and thyrotropin (T; see p. 306); (v) **prolactin**, which stimulates milk production, and is also released during stress (see p. 328).

The major **posterior lobe hormones** are **oxytocin** and **vasopressin**. Oxytocin has a number of actions, including the release of milk from the breast and contraction of the smooth muscle of the endometrium (see p. 310), and vasopressin is an antidiuretic hormone, acting on the kidney, and also has important CNS functions, affecting, for example, memory (see p. 312).

The **anterior lobe** (also called the pars intermedia), is present in many vertebrates, and secretes the **endorphins** and **MSH** (**melanocyte-stimulating hormone**), which stimulates melanin production.

Autoradiographic and receptor-binding studies have revealed the presence in the brain of **receptors** for many of the endocrine hormones. These receptors reveal the sites in the brain where these hormones act to regulate the production and release of neurotransmitters and releasing hormones. They may also be the sites where several of these hormones act to modulate many types of behavior. **Estrogen receptors**, for example, are highly localized in the diencephalon, and particularly in the hypothalamus, where they have negative and positive feedback effects on the release of gonadotropin-releasing hormone (Gn RH). There are high concentrations of estradiol in the preoptic area (where, in lower mammals, they mediate the regulation of sexual behavior), in the amygdaloid nuclei, and in the basal hypothalamus. There are also very high concentrations of estradiol receptors in the gonadotroph cells of the anterior pituitary, where they mediate the negative feedback effects of estradiol on gonadotropin release. Sensitive binding studies have also showed the presence of estrogen receptors in cells of the neocortex, where their function is unknown, but may involve mediation of estrogen action on sexual behavior.

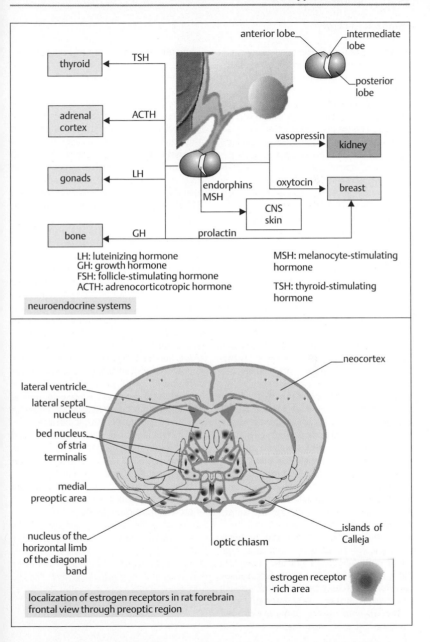

LH: luteinizing hormone
GH: growth hormone
FSH: follicle-stimulating hormone
ACTH: adrenocorticotropic hormone

MSH: melanocyte-stimulating hormone

TSH: thyroid-stimulating hormone

neuroendocrine systems

localization of estrogen receptors in rat forebrain
frontal view through preoptic region

estrogen receptor-rich area

Feedback Control

Feedback control is part of the body's homeostatic mechanisms. Living organisms have developed tight control over their internal environment, which in mammals includes temperature regulation, appetite, water and salt balance, blood pressure, sexual function and behavior, and regulation of the thousands of biochemical and electrochemical changes that occur. Internal control of all the different systems is achieved through the integration of physical, biochemical, and neural events. In all cases, feedback control is composed of several fundamental components: (i) **signals**, which may be physical (such as pressure), chemical (such as antigens or neurotransmitters), or electrical; (ii) **sensors**, which may be structures which respond electrically to a physical or chemical stimulus; sensors may also contain a complex of receptor proteins linked to ion channels or to second messenger systems; (iii) **transducers**, which convert the signal into one which can be understood by the body; transducers are coupling systems which convert one form of energy into another (for example a physical pressure into a train of electrical impulses, or an electrical impulse into a quantum of neurotransmitter release); (iv) **responders**, the cellular or multicellular apparatus that responds to the stimulus to produce a response, which may be a train of electrical impulses, a biochemical reaction, hormone release, a muscle twitch, or a mood change; a complex response might involve several different responders.

In the neuroendocrine system, feedback control is achieved through hormonal and neural integration. The hormone is the signal that binds to a sensor receptor, which may be on the cell surface (e.g. epinephrine), or internal (e.g. estradiol); transducers may involve ion channels, second messengers, or both (epinephrine), and a physical reaction between the hormone receptor and the genome which initiates transcription (estradiol).

Feedback is commonly termed negative or positive. An example of negative feedback is the action of **cortisol**, released into the general circulation from the **adrenal cortex**, on the hypothalamus and **anterior pituitary** corticotrophs, where it acts to limit further release of corticotropin-releasing hormone (**CRH**) and **ACTH**, respectively (see also p. 300). An example of positive feedback is the action of estradiol, released from the ovary, on the hypothalamus, where it acts through a poorly understood mechanism to cause the dramatic preovulatory surge of **LH** release from the anterior pituitary (see also p. 303). Virtually all of the endocrine hormones released through the neuroendocrine system modulate their own release through feedback actions at the hypothalamus and, possibly, other brain areas, and directly on the pituitary cells. The neuroendocrine hormones of the hypothalamus are peptides, which are termed releasing or release-inhibiting hormones, and those released by the pituitary gland are termed tropic hormones.

The elucidation of the components and mechanisms of neuroendocrine feedback systems has led to major medical developments, including the oral contraceptive, fertility treatments, and diagnosis and treatment of thyroid disorders, and those of growth hormone and ACTH.

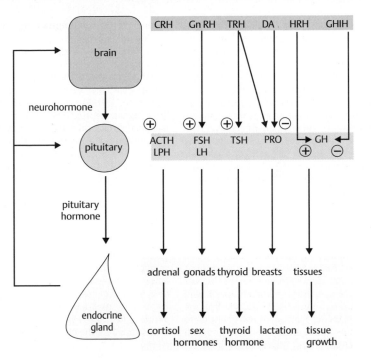

GHRH: growth hormone-releasing hormone
GHIH: growth hormone-inhibitory hormone
TSH: thyroxin-releasing hormone

CRH: corticotropin-releasing hormone
Gn RH: gonadotropin-releasing hormone
TRH: thyrotropin-releasing hormone
DA: dopamine
PRO: prolactin
LPH: lipotropic hormone
ACTH: adrenocorticotropic hormone

neuroendocrine systems

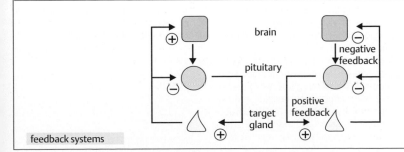

feedback systems

Control of Adrenocorticotropic Hormone Release

The anterior pituitary corticotroph cells synthesize **adrenocorticotropic hormone** (**ACTH**), which is released after stimulation of the cell by corticotropin-releasing hormone (**CRH**), or by **vasopressin** (arginine vasopressin, **AVP**). Human CRH is a 41-amino acid peptide found throughout the brain, but is most concentrated in the hypothalamus in paraventricular nucleus parvocellular neurons which project axons to the median eminence portal blood system. Human CRH is often referred to as CRH-41. The role of vasopressin in the release of ACTH is poorly understood.

CRH-41 release from parvocellular neurons is controlled by several neurotransmitter systems. Both acetylcholine (ACh) and 5-HT stimulate CRH release, while GABA and norepinephrine inhibit release. Influences from other brain centers, for example stress-related stimuli, will affect CRH release. CRH acts on specific membrane receptors of the corticotroph to activate G-proteins and the cAMP second messenger system. This in turn stimulates transcription and also opens voltage-gated Ca^{2+} channels. AVP acts on receptors to activate the IP_3 (inositol 1,4,5-triphosphate) system, which opens receptor-gated Ca^{2+} channels. The net result in both cases is ACTH release.

Release of both CRH and ACTH is modulated through a negative feedback effect of cortisol, a glucocorticoid, which acts on specific receptors in the hypothalamus and anterior pituitary corticotroph. There is evidence that the negative feedback of cortisol on CRH release is biphasic, consisting of fast and delayed feedback mechanisms. The negative feedback mechanism provides a useful tool to test the integrity of the axis, and to diagnose diseases such as tumors of the adrenal cortex, the anterior pituitary or of the hypothalamus.

ACTH is derived from an important precursor peptide called propiomelanocortin (**POMC**). POMC is the precursor of a number of peptides, which are differentially expressed. POMC possesses a 26-amino acid signal peptide followed by three principal structural domains: (i) an **N-terminal sequence**, whose function is not fully understood, (ii) **ACTH**, and (iii) β-lipotropin (β-**LPH**) at the C-terminal end. POMC is first cleaved to yield β-LPH and ACTH, which is attached to the N-terminal fragment. Inside the corticotroph, ACTH is released at the second cleavage stage. Several molecules of β-LPH are also cleaved to yield β-**endorphin** and γ-**LPH**. Further cleavage results in the release of smaller peptides, e.g. melanocyte-stimulating hormone (**MSH**), an anterior pituitary hormone involved in melatonin release and **met-enkephalin**, an opioid neurotransmitter. There is evidence that CRH stimulates the cleavage of POMC and release of all the peptides held in the same secretory granule.

Cortisol release from the adrenal cortex exhibits a daily (diurnal) rhythm (in some books the term circadian rhythm may be used.) The rhythm is determined largely by central mechanisms that in turn are influenced by sleep patterns, and patterns of light-dark cycles. The rhythm of cortisol release is reflected by a similar rhythm of ACTH release. The suprachiasmatic nucleus is an endogenous 'time clock' whose rhythms may also be synchronized by the external influences of light and dark.

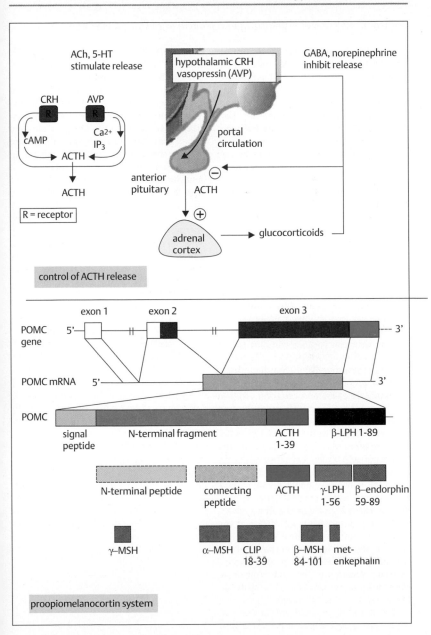

ACh, 5-HT
stimulate release

hypothalamic CRH
vasopressin (AVP)

GABA, norepinephrine
inhibit release

CRH   AVP

R   R

cAMP   Ca²⁺
IP₃

ACTH

ACTH

R = receptor

portal
circulation

anterior
pituitary   ACTH

⊖

adrenal
cortex   ⊕   → glucocorticoids

control of ACTH release

POMC
gene   5'   exon 1   exon 2   exon 3   ---- 3'

POMC mRNA   5'   3'

POMC

signal
peptide   N-terminal fragment   ACTH
1-39   β-LPH 1-89

N-terminal peptide   connecting
peptide   ACTH   γ-LPH
1-56   β-endorphin
59-89

γ-MSH   α-MSH   CLIP
18-39   β-MSH
84-101   met-
enkephalin

proopiomelanocortin system

Control of Release of Luteinizing and Follicle-stimulating Hormones

Luteinizing hormone (**LH**) and **follicle-stimulating hormone** (**FSH**) are glycoproteins produced by the gonadotroph cells of the anterior pituitary gland. They are released in response to the hypothalamic gonadotropin-releasing hormone, **Gn RH**. Together, LH and FSH control sex hormone release from the gonads, the maturation of the ovarian follicles, and the production of the ovum and spermatozoa.

In the human and other primates, there is an endogenous **90 minute pulse** rhythm of Gn RH secretion into the portal system, where it is carried to the gonadotroph cells of the anterior pituitary gland to release the gonadotropins LH and FSH. These in turn cause the release of the sex hormones, which feed back to the hypothalamus and anterior pituitary to limit further release of LH and FSH. In the male, only the negative feedback effects of the sex hormones appear to be operational, but the situation is more complex in the female, largely through the effects of estradiol and progesterone on the brain.

In the female, there is a regular cycle of hormone release and ovarian follicle development, which is on average 28 days in length, although this may vary with the individual, age, or health. During the follicular phase of the menstrual cycle, the negative feedback effects of estradiol on gonadotropin release appear to dominate. At about mid-cycle, however, there is a surge of estradiol concentration in the plasma; these high levels apparently overcome the negative feedback effects of the hormone in brain, and cause a massive release of LH. This is due, perhaps, to increased Gn RH release, and probably to increased sensitivity of the pituitary gonadotrophs to Gn RH, also probably caused by the estradiol surge.

The situation is different in the rat, which has a 4-5 day estrous cycle also characterized by surges of estradiol and LH release prior to ovulation. A clear surge of Gn RH has been detected in the portal blood of the proestrous rat, but it is not certain whether a surge of Gn RH is necessary to induce the LH surge in humans. Unlike the situation in the human and many other primates, however, the rat will not receive the male except during the period of proestrus, during the hours of about 2-4 a.m. on the morning of the day of estrus. The receptivity of the female is absolutely dependent on the presence of estradiol, which apparently governs sexual behavior in the female rat through its interaction with its receptors in the preoptic region of the brain (see p. 293). The male rat is not constrained by its hormonal status and is always free of constraints in terms of sexual behavior.

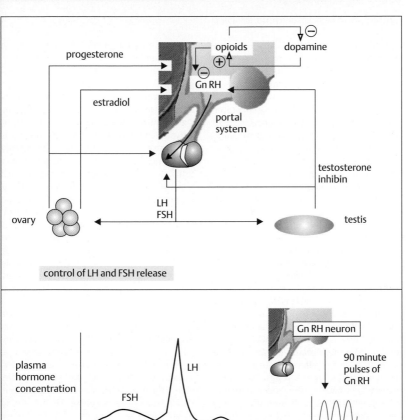

control of LH and FSH release

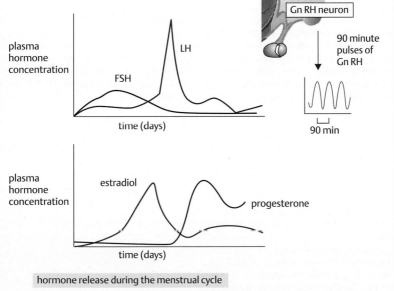

hormone release during the menstrual cycle

Control of Growth Hormone Release

Growth hormone (GH), also called **somatotropin (STH)**, is a glycoprotein secreted by the anterior pituitary, and needed for normal growth. Without somatotropin the individual would develop to be a dwarf. The hormone has both direct and indirect actions. It has a direct diabetogenic, anti-insulin action, causing lipolysis in adipocytes, and is catabolic in muscle and liver, generating glucose from glycogen and amino acids. Directly, GH acts on the liver to stimulate production of the **somatomedins**, which promote lipolysis, protein synthesis in muscle, and bone growth and cartilage synthesis. Like many other anterior pituitary hormones, GH secretion is controlled by the hypothalamus.

Many hypothalamic neurons in the arcuate nucleus synthesize and secrete a peptide, a releasing hormone called **growth hormone-releasing hormone (GH RH)** or **somatocrinin** into the portal blood. In humans, GH RH is a 44-amino acid peptide which binds to specific receptors on the membrane of the anterior pituitary somatotroph cells, causing somatotropin (STH) release through the mediation of the cAMP second messenger system, and possibly also through the IP_3 system. In addition, there are arcuate nucleus neurons which synthesize another peptide, **somatostatin**, a 14-amino acid peptide, which **inhibits** STH release. There is evidence that the feedback control of STH release is effected by an insulin-like growth factor, IGF-1, released by the liver. IGF-1 stimulates the release of somatostatin.

The release of STH is episodic. That is it fluctuates, in this case daily with the light-dark cycle. Plasma concentrations peak twice daily, and peak during the first hour of sleep in children and adults. Chemically, STH is a single chain 191-amino acid member of a family of polypeptide hormones. Other members include prolactin (PRL) and placental lactogen (PL), all of which are derived from a single ancestral precursor; nevertheless, each hormone is expressed by a separate gene.

Deficiency of STH secretion in children, as mentioned above, causes dwarfism. Dwarfism may be genetic, transmitted as an autosomal recessive, which produces an insensitivity of the liver to STH, possibly through defective STH-receptor interactions. In hypothalamic dwarfism, which may be caused by hypothalamic injury, tumors, or from asphyxia during birth, no somatocrinin is released into the portal circulation,. STH is an example of a natural therapeutic agent, also referred to as hGH (human growth hormone), which has been used to promote growth. Originally derived from human pituitaries, it is now genetically engineered to circumvent problems of infection.

Excess STH secretion in children results in giantism, and in adults causes **acromegaly**, and is commonly caused by pituitary adenoma. Acromegaly is manifested in the patient as exaggerated growth of the lower jaw or mandible, giving the face a characteristic appearance. Facial skin becomes coarse. Diabetes may result, from a lowering of the glucose tolerance, in about 10% of patients with acromegaly. Treatment may be chemical, with drugs such as bromocriptine, which lowers STH secretion, irradiation of any tumor, or by hypophysectomy (removal of the pituitary).

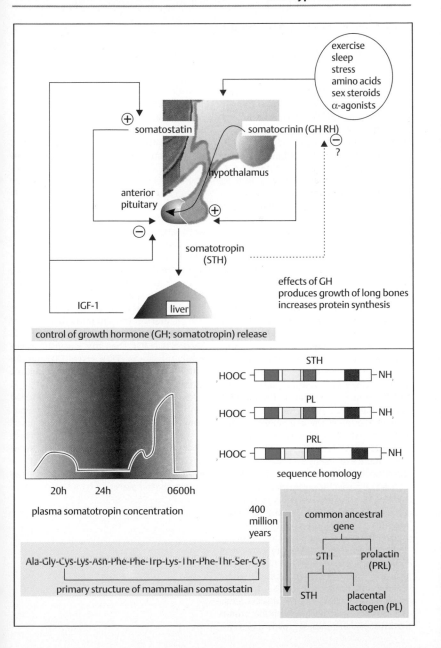

control of growth hormone (GH; somatotropin) release

plasma somatotropin concentration

sequence homology

Ala-Gly-Cys-Lys-Asn-Phe-Phe-Trp-Lys-Thr-Phe-Thr-Ser-Cys

primary structure of mammalian somatostatin

400 million years

common ancestral gene

STH   prolactin (PRL)

STH   placental lactogen (PL)

Control of Thyroid Hormone Release

The follicle cells of the thyroid gland secrete the thyroid hormones tri-iodothyronine (T_3) and thyroxine (T_4). The hormones increase the activity of the $Na^+/K^+ATPase$ pump. They enable homeotherms to generate their own heat through stimulation of mitochondrial oxygen consumption and the production of ATP, which is needed for the sodium pump. The **hypothalamus** and **pituitary** tightly control the control of hormone release through negative feedback mechanisms.

The hypothalamus synthesizes and secretes into the portal circulation a peptide called **thyrotropin-releasing hormone** (**TRH**). TRH is synthesized from a hypothalamic precursor protein preprohormone. In the rat, the preprohormone contains 255 amino acids, and each molecule generates five TRH molecules. TRH acts on specific receptors on **thyrotroph cells** in the anterior pituitary, causing them to release **thyroid-stimulating hormone** (**TSH**), and on lactotroph cells, which release prolactin. Prolactin and the thyroid hormones act together in several mammalian systems. For example, both are required for normal development of the mouse mammary gland.

In the pituitary thyrotroph, the mechanism of action of TRH appears to involve both the **cAMP** and **IP$_3$** systems. Overall, the influence of the hypothalamus on TSH secretion is powerfully stimulant. TSH in turn acts on specific **receptors** on the follicle cell membrane, and triggers a host of changes, including the uptake of iodine into the cell, the synthesis of T_3 and T_4, and their release from colloid.

The thyroid hormones are carried in the general circulation to the anterior pituitary and the hypothalamus, where they **inhibit** the release of TSH and TRH, respectively. In addition, there is evidence that another hypothalamic peptide, **somatostatin**, which inhibits growth hormone release from the anterior pituitary (see p. 304), also inhibits TSH release, and may together with TSH and the thyroid hormones form part of a physiological system that regulates thyroid hormone release.

As with other neuroendocrine feedback systems, the availability of TRH, TSH, and the thyroid hormones provides a powerful means of testing the functional integrity of the hypothalamic-pituitary-thyroid axis. Hyperthyroidism can occur through excessive prescribing of T_4 or TSH-secreting tumors or in Graves' Disease, where the patient has long-acting TSH antibodies in the circulation. These stimulate thyroid hormone release from the thyroid. An abnormally raised serum TSH level together with raised serum T_3 and T_4 suggests that there is an ectopic production of TSH, since raised thyroid hormone should inhibit further TSH release from the pituitary. If the patient with suspected hyperthyroidism is given TRH and the TSH response is flat, then this suggests an ectopic release of TSH, since TRH should stimulate TSH release from the pituitary gland.

In hypothyroid patients, TSH will also be high, due to the reduced negative feedback on TRH and TSH release. If the pituitary is functional, then TRH administration should elevate TSH in plasma. If thyroid hormone levels fail to rise after TSH administration, then the problem may reside in the thyroid gland.

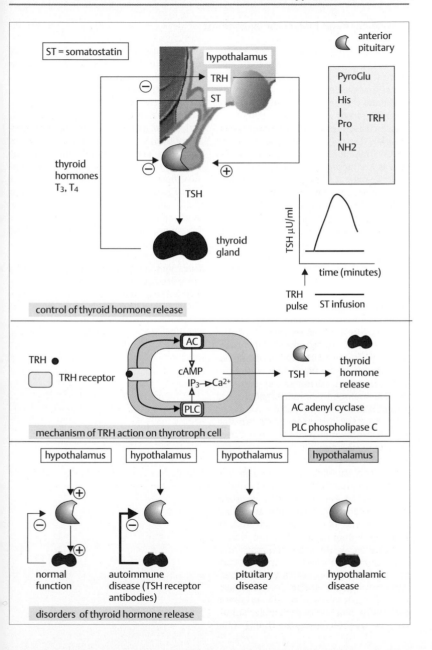

ST = somatostatin

anterior pituitary

hypothalamus
TRH
ST

PyroGlu
|
His
|
Pro
|
NH2

TRH

thyroid hormones T$_3$, T$_4$

TSH

thyroid gland

TSH μU/ml

time (minutes)

TRH pulse   ST infusion

control of thyroid hormone release

TRH ●

TRH receptor

AC

cAMP
IP$_3$ ►Ca^{2+}

PLC

TSH → thyroid hormone release

AC adenyl cyclase

PLC phospholipase C

mechanism of TRH action on thyrotroph cell

hypothalamus   hypothalamus   hypothalamus   hypothalamus

normal function

autoimmune disease (TSH receptor antibodies)

pituitary disease

hypothalamic disease

disorders of thyroid hormone release

Parvicellular and Magnicellular Systems

The nuclei of the hypothalamus can be distinguished not only in terms of their anatomical location and size, but in terms of the size of the cell bodies, and the neurohormones they secrete. Two main types of systems have been described, and classified as the **magnocellular** and **parvicellular** secretory systems, based on the observation that the magnocellular system is composed of relatively large cell bodies, while those of the parvicellular system are relatively smaller. Both magnocellular and parvicellular systems can coexist with the same anatomical nucleus.

The **supraoptic** and **paraventricular nuclei** of the anterior hypothalamus contain large cells, which project axons down to the posterior pituitary or **neurohypophysis**. The bundle of axons which makes up this neural tract is called the **hypothalamo-hypophysial tract**, and the large cell bodies are collectively termed the **magnocellular secretory system**. The cell bodies of the magnocellular system are very richly vascularized. The magnocellular cells of the supraoptic and paraventricular nuclei elaborate the neuroendocrine hormone peptides **oxytocin** and **vasopressin**, which are transported as larger inactive precursors along the **hypothalamo-hypophysial tract** to the **neurohypophysis**, where they are released as endocrine hormones into blood vessels of the general circulation as oxytocin and vasopressin. Oxytocin contracts uterine small muscle and causes milk ejection, while vasopressin controls salt and water balance, and has been implicated in memory, among various other functions.

Scattered within the paraventricular nucleus there are several groups of smaller neuronal cell bodies, which together constitute the **parvicellular secretory system**. The cells of the parvicellular system control the function of the anterior pituitary, or **adenohypophysis**, through the neurohormones they secrete. The axons of the parvicellular neurons project their nerve endings to the blood vessels of the **median eminence**, and from their terminals secrete into it the 'releasing hormones' which are peptides that control the function of the anterior pituitary (adenohypophysis). These releasing hormones include the gonadotropin hormone-releasing hormone (Gn RH; see also p. 303), corticotropin-releasing hormone (CRF; see p. 301), thyrotropin-releasing hormone (TRH; see p. 307), and somatostatin and somatocrinin, which modulate the secretion of growth hormone from the anterior pituitary (see p. 305).

The secretion of the hypothalamic peptides into the portal circulation is under complex feedback control, and the peptide-secreting cells are therefore responsive to circulating levels of the hormones whose release they control, through receptors for the hormones.

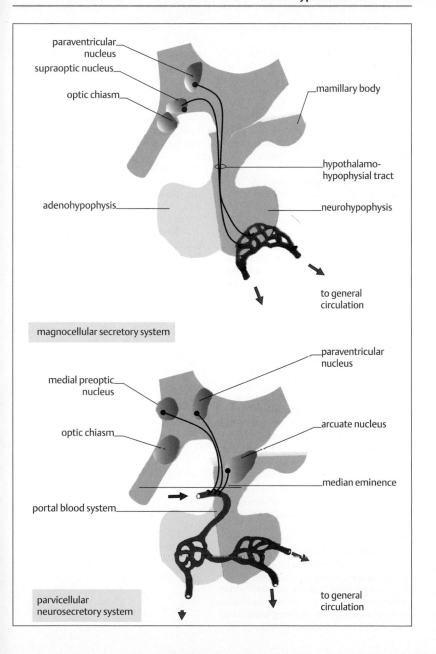

paraventricular nucleus

supraoptic nucleus

optic chiasm

mamillary body

hypothalamo-hypophysial tract

adenohypophysis

neurohypophysis

to general circulation

magnocellular secretory system

paraventricular nucleus

medial preoptic nucleus

arcuate nucleus

optic chiasm

median eminence

portal blood system

to general circulation

parvicellular neurosecretory system

Control of Oxytocin Release

Oxytocin and **vasopressin** were the first peptide hormones structurally identified and chemically synthesized *in vitro*. They are structurally similar and have a common mechanism of transport to the posterior pituitary gland. Both are synthesized in nerve cells in the hypothalamic **paraventricular** and **supraoptic nuclei** and transported down axons whose terminals lie in the posterior pituitary (neurohypophysis). The two hormones are, however, produced in different nerve cells. This spread deals with oxytocin, and the next with vasopressin.

Oxytocin has many functions, some of which are still poorly understood, and many, especially in the brain, doubtless await discovery. Its better-understood physiological actions include the **contraction of uterine smooth muscle** and the **ejection of milk** from the **mammary glands**. Oxytocin is a nonapeptide synthesized from a precursor called prepro-oxyphysin. It is produced together with associated **neurophysin 1** protein. The neurophysin acts as a carrier for oxytocin, and transports it in vesicles along the axon at a rate of 2-3.5 mm/hour. The time from synthesis of oxytocin (and vasopressin) to arrival in the posterior pituitary is around 11-13 hours in humans. Oxytocin is released from the axon terminal in response to the arrival of an axon potential. This causes an increase in intracellular Ca^{2+}, and consequent exocytosis of the granule which releases oxytocin together with neurophysin 1 into the extracellular space from which it diffuses into the bloodstream through the blood vessel wall.

A stimulus for oxytocin release from the posterior pituitary is physical suction on the nipple. In the rat, nipple suction produces a stream of action potentials that are conducted to the spinal cord and up to the **tractus solitarius** (**solitary tract**), and from there to the hypothalamus, where they initiate a synchronized activation of magnocellular oxytocin neurons and a pulsatile release of oxytocin. Acetylcholine is an excitatory neurotransmitter mediating oxytocin release. Oxytocin release may also be initiated during intercourse in women. Oxytocin is released from the neurohypophysis prior to **suckling** in the absence of suction. It has been found that the sound of the baby's cry is sufficient to elicit a pulse of oxytocin release, which suggests that there are inputs from perhaps higher centers to the magnocellular neurons.

Oxytocin is a powerful uterine smooth muscle contracting agent. Its potency in this regard is lower during the follicular phase of the menstrual cycle, but increases markedly in the luteal phase. Oxytocin's contractile potency also increases greatly during the last 10-14 days of pregnancy. There is evidence that this is due to estrogen, which stimulates the synthesis of oxytocin receptors on uterine smooth muscle plasma membranes shortly before parturition.

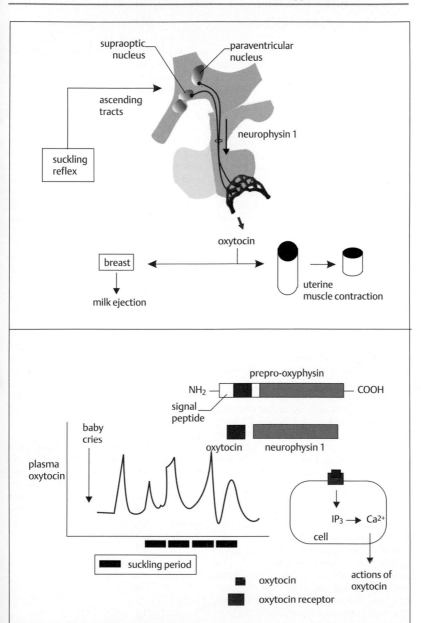

Control of Vasopressin Secretion

The major physiological role of **vasopressin** (**antidiuretic hormone, ADH**) is in the control of water excretion by the **kidneys**. It is therefore crucially important in the determination of **osmotic pressure**. Its synthesis in the hypothalamus is an indicator of the importance of the hypothalamus in the control of salt and water balance. Vasopressin is also intimately concerned with the regulation of blood pressure. Vasopressin is a potent vasoconstrictor (hence its name), but it is more potent as an antidiuretic hormone (hence the term ADH). There is evidence that vasopressin is involved in higher brain function, including memory, and is a potent releaser of **ACTH**.

Like oxytocin, ADH is synthesized mainly in the supraoptic and paraventricular neurons, although other hypothalamic centers such as the suprachiasmatic nucleus, and extrahypothalamic areas, notably the limbic system, possess vasopressin-synthesizing neurons. The hormone is derived from a precursor, **prepropressophysin**, a 166-amino acid polypeptide, which contains not only the sequence of vasopressin, and of the transport protein neurophysin II, but of a glycopeptide of unknown function (if any). The axons of vasopressinergic neurons project mainly to the posterior pituitary, although some axons terminate in the median eminence on the fenestrated capillaries of the pituitary portal system that carries the releasing factors to the anterior pituitary gland.

Vasopressin acts through two main **receptor types**, **V1** and **V2**, although there appear to be several subtypes of receptor 2. The kidney alone appears to possess only subtype V2, while subtype 1 and its various subclasses occur in many other tissues, including brain. Type I acts through the IP_3 system, while type 2 acts through cAMP.

Vasopressin acts in the kidney mainly on the ascending loop of Henle and on the collecting ducts. During hemorrhage or dehydration, for example, when the plasma volume drops, vasopressin makes the walls of the ducts permeable to water and the urine becomes hyperosmotic. Vasopressin increases the insertion of water channels called **aquaporins** into **apical cell membranes** of the collecting ducts. Normally, in the healthy individual, vasopressin regulates the changes in the osmotic gradient as urine travels through the tubule, and plays a vital role in the conservation of body water. Changes in osmotic pressure are detected by sensitive osmoreceptors near the supraoptic and paraventricular nuclei in the hypothalamus. These osmoreceptors are very sensitive to changes in sodium or glucose, whose concentration increase when blood volume is reduced.

Vasopressin also modulates blood pressure through a reflex arc. When blood volume rises, this is detected by pressure-sensitive receptors in the left atrium, the aortic arch, and the carotid sinus. These send afferent impulses through the vagus and glossopharyngeal nerves to the brain stem and vasopressin release is suppressed.

As mentioned above, vasopressin causes **ACTH** release, and also potentiates the actions of corticotropin-releasing hormone (see p. 301). The functional significance of this is not well understood, however. In brain, vasopressin has been shown to inhibit the loss of learned avoidance behavior in rats.

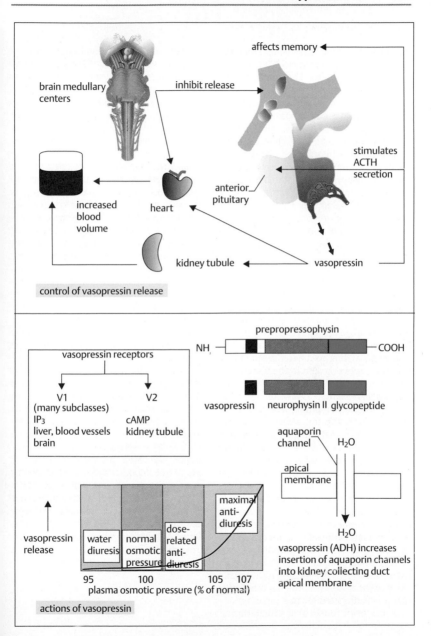

affects memory

brain medullary centers

inhibit release

stimulates ACTH secretion

anterior pituitary

increased blood volume

heart

kidney tubule

vasopressin

control of vasopressin release

prepr_propressophysin

NH₂ ——— COOH

vasopressin receptors

V1 (many subclasses)
IP₃
liver, blood vessels
brain

V2
cAMP
kidney tubule

vasopressin   neurophysin II glycopeptide

aquaporin channel   H₂O

apical membrane

H₂O

vasopressin (ADH) increases insertion of aquaporin channels into kidney collecting duct apical membrane

vasopressin release

maximal anti-diuresis

water diuresis

normal osmotic pressure

dose-related anti-diuresis

95   100   105 107
plasma osmotic pressure (% of normal)

actions of vasopressin

Thermoregulation

The **hypothalamus**, despite its relatively small size, is an important component of **homeostatic systems**. Through its receptors, it detects changes in body **temperature**, osmotic pressure, and circulating hormones. In addition, it has massive connections with the limbic system (see p. 295), which feed the hypothalamus with processed information about external stimuli. Through its efferent connections the hypothalamus can cause autonomic, endocrine, and behavioral changes, to enable the maintenance of homeostasis. It is, in effect, an important **interface** between the **blood and the brain**, and is both a **need detector** and a **response generator**. Examples of the hypothalamic control of circulating hormones have already been given, and this spread deals with the control of **temperature**.

Temperature is a **controlled variable**, and needs to be kept within strict limits. Information about body temperature is collected together by a **feedback detector**, consisting of the peripheral temperature sensors on the skin, and in the viscera and spinal cord, and centrally in the hypothalamus. The hypothalamus possesses a temperature **set point**, and is able to compare incoming temperature information with the signal using an **error detector**, or **integrator**. If the two values do not match, the hypothalamus can generate an **error signal**, which is sent to and drives centers controlling behavior, endocrine hormones, and the autonomic nervous system. The stimuli which generate an error signal may be internal, or **external** (also termed **incentive**). Temperature regulation requires the integration of autonomic, behavioral and skeletomotor responses, and it is readily apparent from a study of the anatomy of the hypothalamus that it is well suited for this task.

It has been found that stimulation of the anterior hypothalamus in conscious animals generates heat dissipation responses. These include the suppression of shivering, cutaneous vasodilatation, panting in dogs, and reduced locomotion. The animal tries to reduce energy expenditure. Conversely, stimulation of the posterior hypothalamus causes cutaneous vasoconstriction, shivering, and increased locomotor activity.

Recordings made from neurons in temperature-regulating areas of the hypothalamus suggest that the neurons themselves are sensitive to changes in temperature. Neurons in the preoptic region of the anterior hypothalamus increase firing if they are warmed, and are termed **warm-sensitive neurons**. These neurons will also fire off if the skin or spinal column is warmed, and firing is inhibited if the skin or spinal cord are cooled. Conversely, cold-sensitive neurons in the posterior hypothalamus respond to direct cooling and to inputs from other cooled areas by firing off, and are inhibited by warming.

The hypothalamic areas that determine the temperature set point are regulated chemically as well as electrically. The set point can be altered by **pyrogens**, which cause disease-associated fever. Macrophages release the peptide interleukin-1 (IL-1), which enters the brain at, for example, the area postrema (see p. 53), where the blood-brain barrier is not as complete as elsewhere, and IL-1 acts at the preoptic area to raise the set point. In other words, the preoptic area is a **pyretic area**. In addition, there is pharmacological evidence that this region possesses an **antipyretic area**, where vasopressin may be the endogenous neuromodulator.

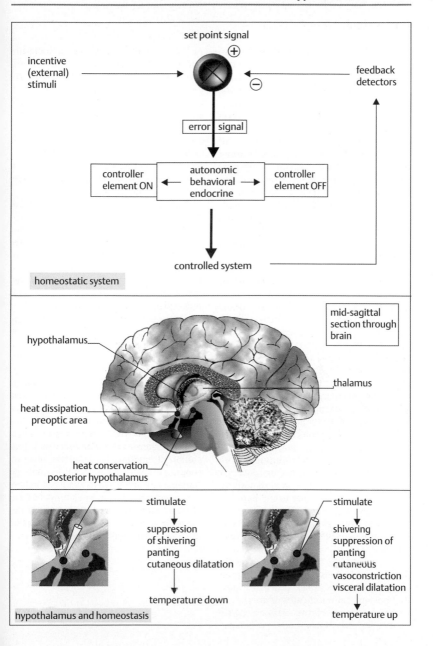

Limbic System 1: Introduction

The term **limbic system** is derived from the Latin word *limbus*, meaning a border, and was introduced by the neuroanatomist Pierre Paul Broca to describe the ring of gyri that surround the brain stem. In 1937, **James Papez** described a circuit that he suggested formed the anatomical site for **emotion**. His circuit consisted of the **hypothalamus, mamillary bodies, anterior thalamic nuclei, cingulate gyrus**, and **hippocampal formation**. His basic proposal still stands, although the circuitry has been extended to include other structures. His circuit has been enlarged to include the **septal area, the nucleus accumbens**, and **neocortical areas** including the **amygdala**, and **orbitofrontal cortex**. The limbic structures are phylogenetically very ancient, and the hippocampal formation includes a primitive form of cortex underlying the evolutionarily newer neocortex.

The limbic system includes the following areas of gray matter: the limbic lobe, the hippocampal formation, the amygdaloid nucleus, and the anterior nucleus of the thalamus. The **connecting pathways** of the system are the **alveus, fimbria, fornix, mamillothalamic tract**, and the **stria terminalis**. Papez originally suggested that emotion is appreciated by higher cognitive centers, and that there must therefore be reciprocal communication between the hypothalamus, an area that generates emotions such as rage, and the higher centers. According to his hypothesis, the hypothalamus feeds emotional information to the cingulate gyrus through the mamillary bodies and the mamillothalamic tract, via the anterior thalamic nuclei. The cortex in turn modulates hypothalamic function through the hippocampal formation, which processes information and communicates it to the hypothalamus via the fornix. This essentially correct hypothesis has been extended to include pathways from the **association cortex** to the **cingulate gyrus** and the **entorhinal cortex**. The hippocampus receives major inputs from the entorhinal cortex through the **perforant path**, which passes through the **subiculum**. The subiculum is a cortical area that has major reciprocal innervation with other areas of neocortex and receives important inputs from the hippocampus. Fibers of the fornix that innervate the hypothalamus originate in the subiculum.

Functional correlates of anatomical designation of limbic system come principally from studies of electrical stimulation, recording, and ablation. For example, the hypothalamus has been found to be profoundly associated with **emotional responses** (as distinct from **emotional sensations**). If a cat or dog has the entire cerebral cortex, basal ganglia and most of thalamus removed, **sham rage** consisting of biting, scratching, and snarling can be elicited by stimulation of the hypothalamus. In contrast to rage in intact animals, the rage cannot be directed against any particular target. Therefore, it appears that the hypothalamus integrates and coordinates behavior expressing rage i.e. a final common pathway from higher centers. Interference with higher centers appears to suppress the experience or appreciation of emotion. For example, bilateral removal of the cingulate gyrus in monkeys tames them, and patients whose cingulate gyrus had been partially lesioned to treat chronic pain reported alleviation of depression, although the results of this form of surgery are highly variable.

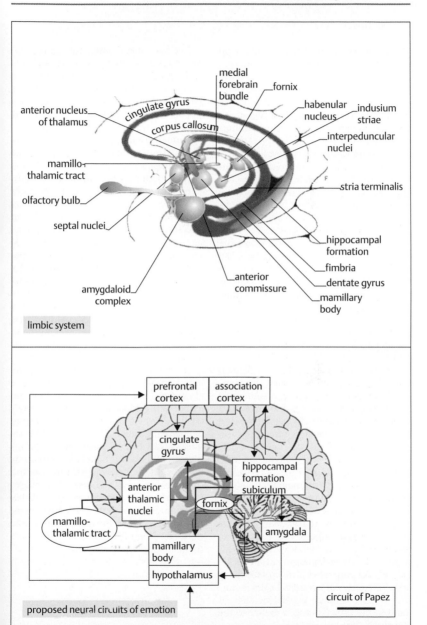

limbic system

proposed neural circuits of emotion

The Hippocampus

The **hippocampal formation** is made up of the **hippocampus**, and the neighboring temporal regions, namely the **dentate gyrus** and the **subiculum**. The subiculum is located in the parahippocampal gyrus. In addition, the **hippocampal region** includes the entorhinal area in the parahippocampal gyrus.

The **hippocampus** is recognized anatomically as a medial bulge in the temporal horn of the lateral ventricle. The bulge is caused by the invagination (turning in) of the ventricular wall. This invagination is the result of the infolding called the hippocampal fissure. The **dentate gyrus** is a narrow band along the medial aspect of the hippocampus. The dentate gyrus and hippocampus are part of the **allocortex**, which has a laminar (layered) structure similar to the neocortex, although with less layers and somewhat more simplified. The allocortex is phylogenetically older than the neocortex, but is still nevertheless highly complex.

The hippocampus has a clearly defined layer of large **pyramidal cells**, which communicate extensively through GABAergic basket cell interneurons. The pyramidal cells communicate with layers above and below the pyramidal layer through extensive axonal and dendritic processes. The hippocampus has been subdivided into three areas termed **CA1**, **CA2**, and **CA3**. The dentate gyrus consists mainly of smaller neurons termed **granule cells**, which synapse with the dendrites of the pyramidal cells. The axons of the granule cells are termed **mossy fibers** and terminate mainly on the apical dendrites of the pyramidal cells of the hippocampal area CA3. Cells of CA3 project **Schaffer collaterals** to apical dendrites of pyramidal cells in area CA1. From CA1, there is a major efferent input to the subiculum, and thence to the entorhinal area.

The main inputs (**afferents**) to the hippocampus come from the entorhinal area of the hippocampal gyrus, and there is a smaller input from the septal nuclei. The pathway from the entorhinal area to the hippocampus is termed the **perforant path**, and has three synaptic interruptions *en route* to the hippocampus, where many axons terminate in the dentate gyrus. The hippocampus projects **efferent** fibers mainly to the entorhinal area, the subiculum, and the septal nuclei. Therefore the hippocampus acts directly mainly on neighboring brain areas. However, it can indirectly influence more distant regions such as the hypothalamus, mamillary bodies, and the neocortex, particularly the cingulate gyrus, through its connections with the subiculum and the entorhinal area. The hippocampus is a bilobate structure; the two sides communicate through the commissural fibers. The pathways that constitute the hippocampus-entorhinal area-hippocampus circuit are all excitatory.

Some of the neurotransmitters of the hippocampal formation pathways have been identified. The fibers from the septal nuclei to the hippocampus release acetylcholine, which causes a long-lasting depolarizing action. Stimulation of septal nucleus cell bodies causes prolonged increased excitability of hippocampus pyramidal cells without necessarily causing them to fire off action potentials. Therefore these cholinergic fibers are probably neuromodulators of hippocampus pyramidal cell function. The raphe nuclei of the midbrain (see p. 210) project 5-HT fibers to the hippocampus, and noradrenergic afferents project to the hippocampus from the locus ceruleus.

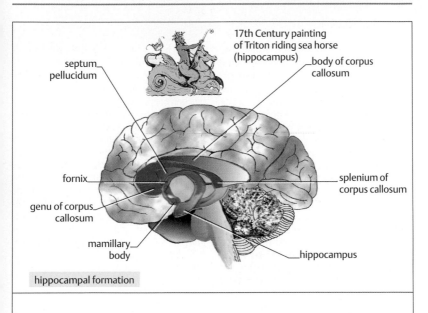

septum pellucidum

17th Century painting of Triton riding sea horse (hippocampus)

body of corpus callosum

fornix

genu of corpus callosum

mamillary body

splenium of corpus callosum

hippocampus

hippocampal formation

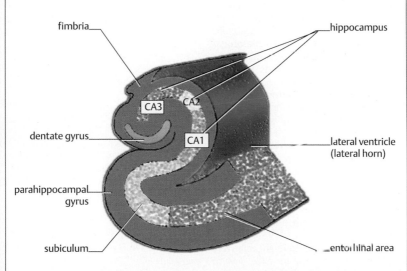

fimbria

hippocampus

CA3   CA2

CA1

dentate gyrus

lateral ventricle (lateral horn)

parahippocampal gyrus

subiculum

entorhinal area

frontal section through medial temporal lobe, showing hippocampus

The Septal Nuclei

The septal nuclei (septal region) consists of a small area of brain in the telencephalon, in the medial wall of the cerebral hemisphere rostral to the anterior commissure and medial to the lateral ventricles. (The septal nuclei should not be confused with the **septum pellucidum**, which is a thin sheet of tissue dorsal and caudal to the anterior commissure, and which separates the lateral ventricles.)

The septal nuclei have been subdivided into two main parts, the **medial** and **lateral** septal nuclei. The medial septal nucleus consists of relatively large neuronal cell bodies, while the lateral nuclear cell bodies are smaller. The septal region also includes the **bed nucleus of the stria terminalis**, the **triangular septal nuclei**, the **septohippocampal** and the **septofimbrial nuclei**, and the **diagonal band of Broca**.

The medial septal nuclei receive major **reciprocal inputs** from the hippocampus via the fornix. The septal nuclei also receive afferent inputs from the **amygdaloid nuclei** via the **ventral amygdalofugal pathways** and the **stria terminalis** (see p. 317) and also receive inputs from the ventral tegmental nuclei in the midbrain. They also receive afferents from the **cingulate gyrus**, and reciprocal inputs from the **hypothalamus** and preoptic region via the **medial forebrain bundle** (see p. 317). The principal septal nuclei **efferents** are those to the hippocampus via the **fornix**, to the ventral tegmental nuclei via the medial forebrain bundle, to the habenular nucleus, to the medial thalamic nuclei via the stria medullaris thalami, and there are also efferents to the lateral hypothalamus and preoptic region.

The septal area, although relatively small in size, appears to have several diverse and important functions. The human septal nuclei have been stimulated and this is reported to produce intensely **pleasurable sensations**, and a sensation of well being. In other species, this area is possibly an important site of reward reactions. In animals such as cats and rats the septal area is disproportionately large. It has been reported that rats will repeatedly press a bar to stimulate this area to the exclusion of all other activities, to the point of death from starvation. If the septal area is destroyed, this seems to remove an inhibitory influence on rage, and the animal responds with signs of displeasure, so-called '**septal rage**'. The neurotransmitter that may mediate the pleasurable response in this area is **dopamine**. There is evidence from studies in humans that antipsychotic drugs may produce their effects by modifying the dopaminergic inputs to the septal nuclei.

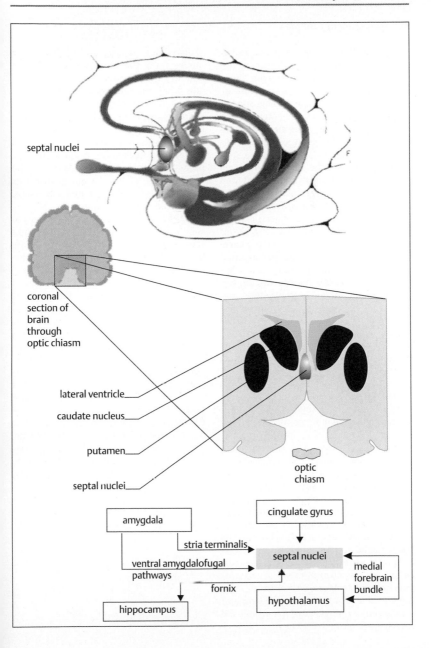

septal nuclei

coronal
section of
brain
through
optic chiasm

lateral ventricle

caudate nucleus

putamen

septal nuclei

optic
chiasm

amygdala

cingulate gyrus

stria terminalis

septal nuclei

ventral amygdalofugal
pathways

medial
forebrain
bundle

fornix

hippocampus

hypothalamus

The Amygdaloid Complex

The **amygdaloid complex**, or the **amygdala**, an almond-shaped collection of nuclei, is found in the temporal lobe, beneath the uncus. It comprises the **basal**, **central**, **lateral**, and **superficial** groups of nuclei. In addition to the afferent and efferent connections, there are several intrinsic connections between the amygdaloid nuclei.

In some texts the nuclei have been grouped as the larger **basolateral** and smaller **corticomedial** nuclei, which include the **central nucleus**. This grouping is based on function and connections; the basolateral nuclear group has connections with the striatum, thalamus, and the **cerebral cortex**, while the corticomedial group is connected mainly with the **hypothalamus**, **central visceral nuclei**, and the **olfactory bulb**. The basolateral nuclear group increases in size up the evolutionary ladder, and is relatively large in the human brain. The corticomedial group may be more concerned with autonomic function, while the basolateral group may mediate some conscious processes related to frontal and temporal lobe activity.

The **intrinsic** connections within the amygdaloid complex suggest that the nuclei are connected in series, although there are recent reports of reciprocal intrinsic connections as well. The **afferent** and **efferent** connections of the amygdaloid nuclei include major inputs from the **olfactory bulbs** to the **superficial nucleus**, which sends back reciprocal efferents; it appears that other nuclei, with the exception of the central nucleus, receive indirect olfactory inputs as well. The **lateral** and **basal nuclei** receive inputs from several unimodal **sensory areas** of the cerebral cortex, and several multimodal sensory inputs from the temporal cortex. In addition, the lateral and basal nuclei receive major somatosensory inputs from the orbital and insular parts of the cortex.

The lateral and central nuclei receive inputs from **thalamic nuclei**, including auditory afferents from the medial geniculate body, and gustatory inputs from the ventral posterior medial nucleus. There are also reciprocal connections between the lateral and ventromedial **hypothalamic** nuclei and the central and basal amygdaloid nuclei. The **brain stem**, too, projects important afferents into the amygdaloid nuclei, including afferents from the diagonal band of Broca, the pons, and the ventral tegmental area.

Major **amygdalofugal efferents** to subcortical destinations include the **stria terminalis**, which travels medial to the body and the tail of the caudate nucleus, and terminates in the bed nucleus of the stria terminalis, which lies just dorsal to the anterior commissure. This nucleus projects in turn to the anterior hypothalamus and to the brain stem via the median forebrain bundle. Another important pathway is the ventral amygdalofugal tract, which terminates in the lateral preoptic nucleus and the lateral hypothalamus. The amygdala also sends fibers from the central nucleus to the **midline thalamic nuclei**. Another major amygdalofugal pathway travels from the basal nuclei to the **striatum**, particularly the nucleus accumbens (so-called 'limbic striatum'), and to the putamen and the ventromedial caudate nucleus. There are also connections between the amygdala and the reticular formation, the periaqueductal gray matter and the parasympathetic cranial nerve nuclei.

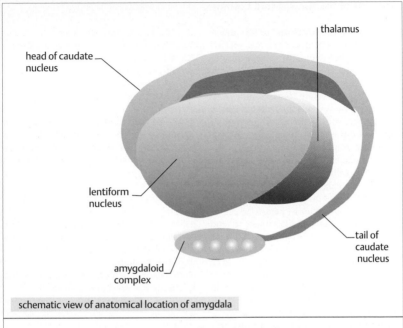

schematic view of anatomical location of amygdala

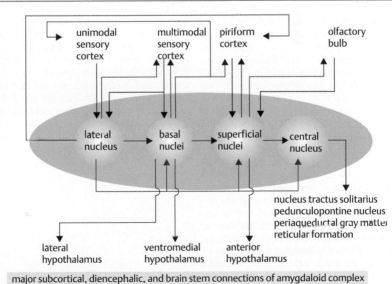

major subcortical, diencephalic, and brain stem connections of amygdaloid complex

Functions of the Amygdaloid Complex

Knowledge of the **functions** of the amygdaloid nuclei has been derived from observations of behavior after **ablation** or **stimulation** of the amygdala in animals or after **damage** to the amygdala in humans. It is difficult precisely to assess the contribution of the various amygdaloid nuclei to any behavioral or autonomic response, due to the diffuse anatomical relationships within the amygdala.

In animals, stimulation of the amygdala produces stereotyped behavioral responses. For example, stimulation of the basolateral group of nuclei produces signs of increased attention in cats. The pupils dilate and the animal lifts its head and looks around with what appears to be increased curiosity about its immediate surroundings. In particular, it turns its head to the side opposite from that in which the electrode is implanted. Concomitant with these behavioral signs, there are activational changes in the EEG. If the intensity of the stimulus is increased, this produces aversive behavior. The animal snarls, backs away, or may even attack.

Ablation (bilateral surgical removal) of the temporal lobes, which include the hippocampal formations as well as the amygdala, results in docile behavior in monkeys. There is an apparent deletion of any rage or fear response to stimuli which evoked these responses prior to the operation. The operation produces aberrant behavior as well. Monkeys exhibited increased, and, in some cases, apparently bizarre sexual behavior. They attempted to mount others of the same sex, of other species, and inanimate objects. If the lesions were confined to areas within the amygdala, without discernible damage to the hippocampal formation, the animals exhibited docility without the expression of aberrant sexual behavior. The aberrant sexual behavior may have been due to destruction of brain areas adjacent to the amygdala. It should be noted, nevertheless, that the amygdaloid nuclei of both sexes are rich in estrogen receptors, which strongly suggests that the amygdaloid nuclei are targets for the sex hormones.

Experiments with monkeys suggest a memory role for the amygdala. If the amygdala are lesioned, then monkeys lose the ability to associate objects and their implications. For example, if monkeys are taught that an object is associated with a punishment, they lose this memory after lesions of the amygdala.

In humans, stimulation of the amygdala during brain surgery under local anesthesia produces sensations of anxiety and fear. Similar feelings are elicited if the temporal lobe is stimulated; it is known that the temporal lobe projects to the amygdala. There is in humans a condition called the **Klüver-Bucy syndrome**, caused by the bilateral lesioning of the amygdaloid nuclei. Lesions may be caused through temporal lobe surgery for epilepsy, or through trauma. It is unclear whether the syndrome is due purely to injury to the amygdala or to adjacent areas as well. The patient may no longer recognize objects by sight (visual **agnosia**), touch (tactile agnosia), or by hearing (auditory agnosia). Patients are generally docile. They may eat to excess (**hyperphagia**), and eat objects that are not food. There is also sometimes overt, and inappropriate and antisocial, **hypersexuality**.

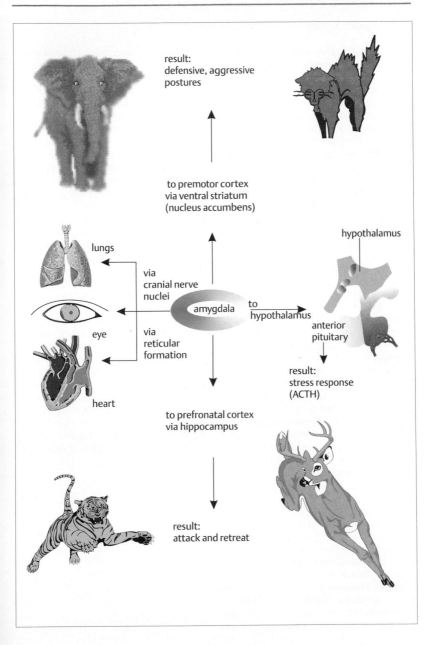

result:
defensive, aggressive
postures

to premotor cortex
via ventral striatum
(nucleus accumbens)

lungs

via
cranial nerve
nuclei

eye

via
reticular
formation

heart

amygdala

hypothalamus

to
hypothalamus

anterior
pituitary

result:
stress response
(ACTH)

to prefronatal cortex
via hippocampus

result:
attack and retreat

The Cingulate Gyrus

The **cingulate gyrus** is continuous with the **parahippocampal gyrus**, and runs around the splenium of the **corpus callosum**. The cingulate gyrus lies below the cingulate sulcus. The cingulate gyrus and the parahippocampal gyrus are linked by the fibers of the **cingulum**. The cingulate gyrus is a form of primitive cortex, with three layers instead of the six layers of the neocortex. It is a major part of the circuit of Papez (see p. 317).

The cingulate gyrus has connections with the other members of the limbic system, and is intimately involved in the functions of the system. The main efferent outputs of the **anterior thalamic nuclei** are to the cingulate gyrus. Information about the functions of the cingulate gyrus comes mainly from experiments in which the gyrus was stimulated at various points. The responses were **autonomic**, **somatic**, or **behavioral**, depending on the site of stimulation.

One of the most marked autonomic responses that has been noticed in anesthetized animals after stimulation of the cingulate gyrus is the **inhibition of respiration**. This effect was reversed, and respiration was **stimulated** if the electrode was moved posterior to the point where respiration was inhibited. Stimulation of the anterior cingulate cortex resulted in both depression and elevation of **blood pressure**; the electrodes needed to be shifted only a few mm to change from depression to elevation of blood pressure. Other autonomic responses reported include salivation, pupillary dilatation, bladder contraction, and inhibition of peristalsis. Nevertheless, removal of the cingulate gyrus does not noticeably affect autonomic or visceral function.

Several behavioral reactions to stimulation have been observed in unanesthetized animals. These are sometimes referred to as **arrest reactions**. The animal immediately ceases all activity and appears to be surprised. This is often accompanied by movements of the head and eyes to the side opposite from that in which the stimulus was applied. Stimulation of the anterior cingulate gyrus often produces **aggressive** behavior, and bilateral removal of the cingulate gyrus makes monkeys docile. They sometimes become **socially indifferent** in that they apparently lose interest in members of the social group of which they are a part. Stimulation of the posterior cingulate gyrus appears to produce pleasurable emotions, in contrast to the aversive behavior observed after stimulation of the **amygdala**. Animals display sexual activity and grooming.

In humans, the cingulate gyrus has been removed in operations to treat chronic, chemically untreatable pain. Results were inconclusive, although some patients reported partial relief from the pain. In some cases, patients reported alleviation of clinical depression. These operations have not generally found favor for the treatment of chronic pain, or for clinical depression. **Somatic** effects reported after stimulation of the anterior cingulate gyrus include inhibition of spontaneous activity, swallowing, licking and chewing movements, and inhibition or facilitation of reflex responses.

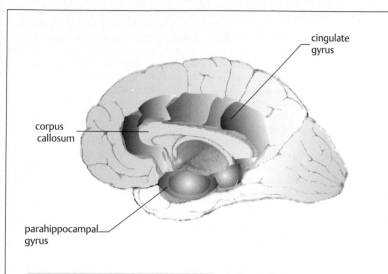

anatomical location of the cingulate gyrus

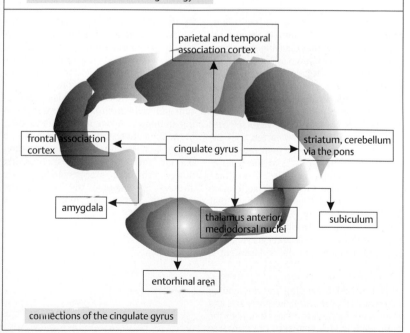

connections of the cingulate gyrus

Limbic System and Stress

Stress is a physiologic phenomenon that occurs in response to a perception of apparently threatening physical or environmental change. The response is presumably adaptive to the organism, and is designed as a relatively short-lived change. In experimental animals and in humans, conditions that produce prolonged stressful responses also produce pathological changes. One of the most immediate and noticeable adaptive responses to stress is the activation of the system that releases glucocorticoids from the adrenal gland, and the inadequate or inappropriate activation of this system is possibly the first step in the cascade of pathological changes which result from prolonged stress.

The release of cortisol in humans is controlled by the activity of a part of the neuroendocrine system, the hypothalamo-anterior pituitary-adrenal cortex (HPA) **axis** (see p. 300). The **hypothalamus** releases **corticotropin-releasing hormone** (**CRH**), previously known as corticotropin-releasing factor (CRF), into the blood portal system. The portal system carries CRH to the **anterior pituitary** corticotroph cell, which responds by releasing adrenocorticotropic hormone **ACTH**. ACTH releases cortisol from the adrenal cortex, and the cortisol in turn limits its own release by means of feedback effects at the level of the hypothalamus, the anterior pituitary, and possibly also through its actions on the hippocampus. There is evidence that after adrenalectomy in animals and humans, there is atrophy of neurons in hippocampal areas CA1 and CA3, which is reversed if glucocorticoid replacement is given.

Release of ACTH during stress is controlled by both ascending and descending pathways. Hypertension, hemorrhage, and respiratory distress activate centers in the brain stem, which results in the discharge of **catecholaminergic** fibers projecting to the hypothalamic paraventricular nucleus, which expresses CRH. The **amygdala**, too, activates the axis, by projecting a **GABAergic** inhibitory pathway to neurons in the preoptic area, which themselves inhibit CRH release from the paraventricular nucleus. Injury to the central or medial amygdaloid nuclei results in a reduced stress-induced release of ACTH and cortisol. ACh-containing hypothalamic neurons stimulate CRH release, but the wiring of this input is unknown.

The limbic system acts also to limit the stress response, perhaps through the **hippocampus** and **prefrontal cortex**. The hippocampus is an important brain target for glucocorticoids, since it has high concentrations of glucocorticoid receptors. Electrical stimulation of hippocampal nuclei has been shown to cause a reduction in HPA activity in humans and other species, while lesions of the hippocampus result in the potentiation of stress-induced ACTH and glucocorticoid secretion in primates and rats. In experimental animals, the induction of stress generates a large increase in early mRNA synthesis in the septum and in the prefrontal cortex, suggesting an important role for these structures in the mediation of the stress response. It should be noted, however, that hippocampal and prefrontal cortex responses, like others in the brain, are specific for certain stresses. For example, the hippocampus does not respond to hypoxia-induced stress.

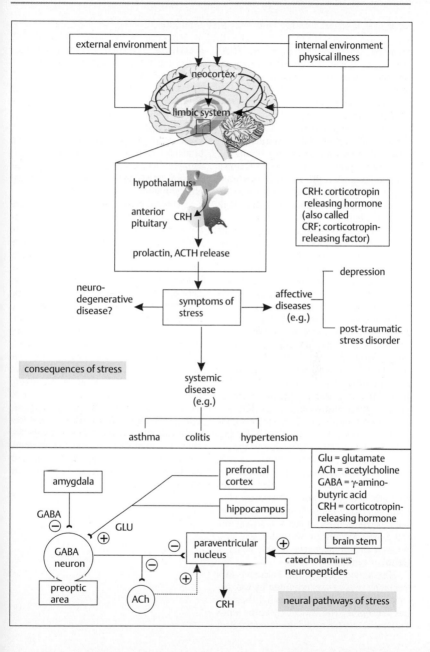

Neuronal Mechanisms for Learning and Memory

Memory can conveniently be classified into three main subdivisions, namely **sensory**, **motor**, and **central** (and also as short- or long-term memory). **Sensory memory** is the ability of, for example, the visual and associated cortical areas to assemble and retain spatial and color patterns for later recall. **Motor memory** is the ability of the brain to learn and retain the memory for execution of ballistic actions. **Central memory** is the ability of the brain to assemble, integrate and attach meaning to sensory inputs, and store them for recall at will.

A unifying theme in all three types of memory is the ability of the brain to **associate**. A graphic demonstration of association was provided by **Pavlov**, who trained a dog to associate a ringing bell ringing with food; the dog **salivated** on hearing a **bell**. Here, the brain associated different sensory inputs with food. Clearly, a dual pathway was created to a common neuronal unit (CNU) that triggered salivation. It may be assumed that before the conditioning experiment, the pathway from the original stimulus to the CNU (S_1) was already functional, and the pathway carrying the auditory input was dormant or perhaps nonexistent. During the conditioning process, the second pathway (S_2) became functional, perhaps due to the activity of association areas of the cortex. Thus, the often repeated concomitant firing of the two presynaptic systems strengthened the auditory pathway, a phenomenon that was predicted by the neuroscientist **Hebb** over 50 years ago; we now call a synaptic system in which one presynaptic input strengthens the other a **Hebbian synapse**.

Direct evidence for the existence of a Hebbian synapse was provided by the discovery of the **NMDA** (n-methyl-d-aspartate) **receptor**. The NMDA receptor binds the excitatory central neurotransmitter **glutamate**, and is both voltage and ligand-gated. For the receptor channel to open, the postsynaptic cell must be depolarized, and the receptor must have glutamate bound to it; calcium ions will then flow through into the cell. Depolarization at these synapses is provided by the release from presynaptic sites of glutamate, which binds also to other receptors on the postsynaptic surface, the so-called **quisqualate/kainate (Q/K) receptor**, a more common glutamate receptor in the CNS.

Hebbian synapses of this sort have been found on the dendritic spines of hippocampal neurons, of neocortical stellate and pyramidal cells, and of Purkinje cells of the cerebellum. If the terminal opposite the NMDA receptor fires off, glutamate binds to the NMDA receptor, but it does not open the channel, which is blocked by Mg^{2+} ions. But if the terminal opposite the Q/K receptor fires as well, the postsynaptic membrane becomes depolarized. This removes the Mg^{2+} block, the NMDA channel opens and Ca^{2+} ions flow into the cell. The intracellular calcium triggers protein kinases in the postsynaptic cell, leading to the generation of (perhaps) nitrous oxide (NO), which diffuses into the presynaptic cell (retrograde diffusion) and induces more glutamate release. Alternatively, the NO may generate the synthesis of more postsynaptic Q/K receptors. The process has been called **long term potentiation**, or **LTP**.

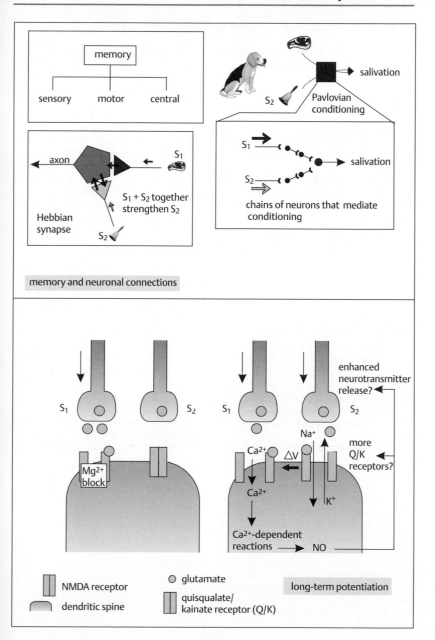

memory and neuronal connections

long-term potentiation

Long-term Potentiation in the Hippocampus

There is evidence that **long-term potentiation** (**LTP**) occurs in the **hippocampus**, and that the hippocampus is a site for the transition of memory from short to long term. The connections of the hippocampus, the electrical behavior of its neurons, and the results of accidental or deliberate interruption of pathways and destruction of nuclei, especially in area **CA1**, all support this.

The hippocampal cortex exhibits a regular sequential arrangement of **pyramidal cells**. Each pyramidal cell in the **entorhinal cortex** projects to a series of pyramidal cells in the dentate gyrus, and each of these in turn projects to pyramidal cells in area **CA3**. These cells in turn project to the pyramidal cells of CA1. Branches of CA3 cells also unite to form the **fornix**, which projects to the septum and the mamillary bodies. Pyramidal cells of CA1 form an efferent pathway, which projects to the **subiculum**, and from there to the anterior and central thalamus. The subiculum projects the excitatory **perforant pathway** to the granule cells of the dentate gyrus. These cells in turn form the **mossy fiber** bundles to the pyramidal cells of CA3, and these send excitatory collaterals, the **Schaffer cells**, to the pyramidal cells of CA1.

LTP can be demonstrated in CA1 cells by stimulating any of the three sequential afferent pathways to the cells and recording excitatory postsynaptic potentials. After stimulation, there was increased excitatory postsynaptic potential (EPSP) activity in CA1 cells, which lasted several weeks. This may be regarded as a form of neuronal memory within a single nerve cell. The properties of hippocampal CA1 LTP fit with the properties of a Hebbian synapse (see p. 331). LTP of a CA1 cell will not occur unless the cell is depolarized at the same time that electrical activity occurs in the presynaptic cell.

The neuronal synaptic unit that produces LTP exhibits certain properties. Firstly, LTP will not occur unless the presynaptic fiber and the postsynaptic cell are coincidentally active; this property is called associative activity. Secondly, more than one presynaptic fiber needs to be active; this is cooperativity. Thirdly, LTP that is produced at a given synapse is specific for a given site. In other words, fibers that produce LTP at a certain synaptic location will not produce LTP at another.

More than 95% of pyramidal CA3 cells exhibit another property, that of being multimodal. This means that they will respond to virtually any combination of sensory modalities. This suggests that the hippocampus may be a unifying or final pathway for the output of neocortical sensory integrators. Another interesting property of pyramidal cells is that they appear to respond more readily to novel stimuli. In memory terms, this means they are more sensitive to new information. They may thus be a gateway for new memories into the brain. This possibility is supported by the consequences of a famous surgical operation that went wrong. An epileptic patient had the tips of both temporal lobes removed, and as a result was no longer able to remember anything **new** i.e. anterograde amnesia.

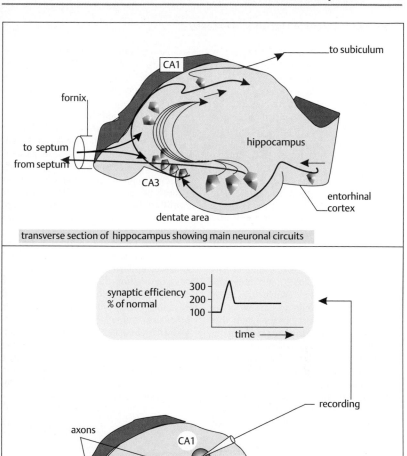

transverse section of hippocampus showing main neuronal circuits

long term potentiation in the hippocampus

The Limbic System in Health and Disease

The limbic system is important in the mediation of **affective behavior** in health and disease. Affective behavior is behavior usually dominated by a single emotion, or a set of emotions, that defines the behavior of an individual. Ever since the proposal of the circuit of Papez (see p. 317), evidence has grown implicating components of the limbic system in the mediation of fear, aggression, sexual behavior, and pleasurable responses. The limbic system is also involved in the etiology of several **disease states** of central origin.

The limbic cortex has been implicated in **autism**. Autism presents in children, usually before age 3, and presents as difficulties in relating to others and communicating with them. Autistic children have enlarged temporal lobes and abnormal EEG patterns. Autistic behavior can be induced experimentally in monkeys by lesioning the temporal lobes when they are very young. **Schizophrenia** is characterized by severe behavioral abnormalities, and is often associated with abnormal CA hippocampal neurons in patients, together with noticeably smaller parietal and temporal cortices. Dopamine neurotransmission may be abnormal in schizophrenic patients, particularly in the projections to anterior limbic structures.

Emotional disturbances of behavior generally appear to be due to dysfunction of **anterior** limbic structures such as the amygdala and anterior portions of the cingulate gyrus. But dysfunction associated with **memory and learning** loss appears to be associated more with **caudal structures** such as the hippocampus and posterior part of the cingulate gyrus. Memory has been classified as **declarative** i.e. memory of facts that can be recalled into conscious awareness, and **procedural** memory, which is memory of learned motor skills. It is likely that the limbic system is important in the conversion of declarative memory from short-term to long-term. Mention has already been made of the importance of the **temporal lobe** in the reception and retention of declarative memory.

The diencephalon is important in acquisition and retention of declarative memory. Patients with the **Korsakoff syndrome** demonstrate this. These patients are chronic alcoholics whose thiamine deficiency leads to anterograde amnesia. In these patients, there is damage to the **mamillary bodies**, frontal cerebral cortex, and medial dorsal nucleus of the thalamus.

Certain forms of **epilepsy** are associated with the limbic system. In temporal lobe epilepsy (see p. 362), post-mortem examination often shows damage to area CA1 of the hippocampus, which is presumably the epileptogenic focus. In some cases, surgical ablation of the damaged area abolishes seizures, but can adversely affect memory. Repetitive seizure activity actually causes more damage to pyramidal neurons in the hippocampus. Alzheimer's disease is associated with limbic dysfunction (see also p. 376).

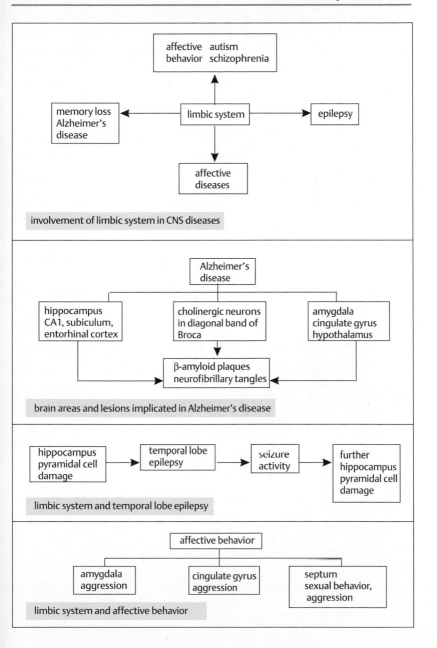

involvement of limbic system in CNS diseases

brain areas and lesions implicated in Alzheimer's disease

limbic system and temporal lobe epilepsy

limbic system and affective behavior

Brodmann's Maps of the Cerebral Cortex

A German neuroscientist, Korbinian Brodmann, produced a cytoarchitectural map of the human cortex early in the 20th Century. The cortex was divided by numbers into different regions, based on the cytoarchitecture of the cells, i.e. their structure as seen on microscopic examination, and their arrangement in groups or layers in the cortex. The numbering system simply represents the order in which the different areas were studied. The coordinates of this map are still used today in reference to cortical areas that are studied both structurally and functionally.

Brodmann layers 1, 2, and 3 are the somatosensory cortex, which lies in the postcentral gyrus of the parietal lobe (see p. 338). Layer 4 is the motor cortex, which lies in the precentral gyrus of the frontal lobe. Earlier, in the 19th Century, neurophysiologists had discovered that stimulation of the motor cortex elicited movements of the limbs, and had begun to construct a forerunner of the motor homunculus (see p. 78).

The cerebrocortical visual system is located in the lateral wall of the occipital lobe and the walls of the calcarine sulcus, and Brodmann was able to distinguish areas 17, 18, and 19, which we now know subserve different visual functions (see p. 286). The auditory cortex, which lies in the transverse gyri of the superior temporal gyrus, is often referred to as Brodmann's areas 41 and 42.

Based on the cytoarchitectural properties of the areas studied, the prefrontal association cortex was designated as areas 8, 9, 10, and 11, and parietal-temporal-occipital cortex as areas 19, 21, 22, 37, 39, and 40. The cortical area that controls speech, the motor speech area, was first described by Broca in the nineteenth century, and is called Broca's area. This is Brodmann's area 45, which lies in the posterior part of the frontal lobe. Patients in whom area 45 is lesioned can understand speech but cannot speak. The lesion may extend to area 44 as well. At about the same time, Wernicke described a brain area in the posterior part of the temporal lobe, which when lesioned eliminated the patient's ability to understand speech, although they could still speak (Wernicke's aphasia; see also p. 342). This is Brodmann's area 22. The lesion may also extend to areas 39 and 40 in the superior region of the temporal lobe, and to area 37, which is located inferior to the other areas. Areas 22 and 45 are connected by the arcuate fasciculus (see also p. 265).

Brodmann's areas are still used to describe areas involved in the integration of visual inputs and motor decisions. The posterior parietal cortex is important in the integration of sensory and somatosensory inputs with the decision-making apparatus, which includes the focusing of attention on to external objects, emotional and cognitive components, motivational factors, and the initiation of purposeful movement. In humans, the posterior parietal cortex includes areas 5 and 7, the angular gyrus (area 40) and the submarginal gyrus (area 39).

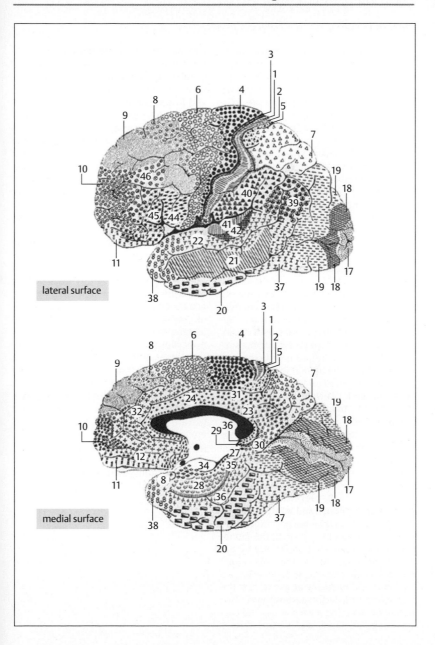

lateral surface

medial surface

Surface Features of the Cerebral Cortex

The surface of the human cerebral cortex is extensively folded, which greatly increases the surface area of cortex that can be accommodated by the skull. The extensive folding is due to the unequal rate of evolution of the cortex and of the cranium, which has resulted in the deep infolding of the cortex. The raised ridges of cortex are termed **gyri**, (*singular*: gyrus), and the infoldings are termed **sulci** (*singular*: sulcus). The pattern of folding is relatively constant and certain sulci and gyri are used to divide the brain into four **lobes**. The **central** and **parieto-occipital sulci** are used to divide the cortex into the four lobes. The lobes are named after the cranial bones that lie over them, and are the **frontal, occipital, parietal**, and **temporal** lobes.

The **central sulcus** lies immediately behind the motor cortex, and immediately in front of the somatosensory cortex (see pp. 189 and 177). The **lateral sulcus** occurs principally on the lateral and inferior surfaces of the cortex. It splits into three **rami**, which divide the temporal lobe into three gyri, the **superior, middle**, and **inferior temporal gyri**. The term *ramus* is used to describe any branch-like structure. The **occipital lobe**, which contains the primary visual cortex, lies behind the parieto-occipital sulcus.

The **frontal lobe** is the cortical area anterior to the central sulcus, and superior to the lateral sulcus. Three sulci divide the frontal lobe into the **precentral gyrus** and the **superior, middle**, and **inferior frontal gyri**. The **parietal lobe** lies posterior to the central sulcus and superior to the lateral sulcus, and is bounded posteriorly by the parieto-occipital sulcus. The lateral surface of the parietal lobe is divided by two sulci into the **postcentral gyrus**, and the **superior** and **inferior parietal gyri** (also called lobules). The posterior parietal cortex integrates visual and somatosensory

information. The **temporal lobe** lies inferior to the lateral sulcus. The **superior** and **middle temporal sulci** divide the temporal cortex into the **superior, middle**, and **inferior temporal gyri**. The temporal cortex holds the primary cortical auditory areas. The various cortical lobes and areas form associative relationships in order to perform the three principal cortical functions, namely **perception, motivation**, and **movement**. The frontal lobe is important in the planning of voluntary movement.

In medial section, the large **corpus callosum**, which joins the two hemispheres, is very prominent. Most of the fibers of the corpus callosum connect symmetrical areas of the two hemispheres. Its main function is to transfer information from one hemisphere to the other, and its integrity is important for the normal function of sensory experience, memory, and learned behaviors. Sectioning of the corpus callosum does not, however, impair intelligence, although it does affect certain discriminatory functions. Several gyri can be distinguished in medial section. These, for example the **parahippocampal gyrus**, are concerned mainly with more primitive cortical and subcortical function, such as emotional behavior (see p. 319). They are part of the limbic system, and the nature of the infolding of the cortex brings them in close proximity with the hippocampus, a major part of the limbic system.

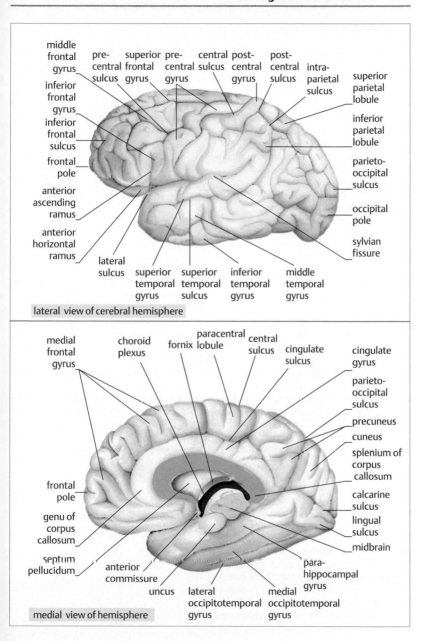

middle frontal gyrus
pre-central sulcus
superior frontal gyrus
pre-central gyrus
central sulcus
post-central gyrus
post-central sulcus
intra-parietal sulcus
superior parietal lobule
inferior frontal gyrus
inferior frontal sulcus
frontal pole
anterior ascending ramus
anterior horizontal ramus
lateral sulcus
superior temporal gyrus
superior temporal sulcus
inferior temporal gyrus
middle temporal gyrus
inferior parietal lobule
parieto-occipital sulcus
occipital pole
sylvian fissure

lateral view of cerebral hemisphere

medial frontal gyrus
choroid plexus
fornix
paracentral lobule
central sulcus
cingulate sulcus
cingulate gyrus
parieto-occipital sulcus
precuneus
cuneus
splenium of corpus callosum
calcarine sulcus
lingual sulcus
midbrain
frontal pole
genu of corpus callosum
septum pellucidum
anterior commissure
uncus
lateral occipitotemporal gyrus
medial occipitotemporal gyrus
para-hippocampal gyrus

medial view of hemisphere

Cortical Association Areas

The **association areas** of the cerebral cortex are those that are not believed to receive direct sensory inputs nor to send motor outputs to motoneurons. This is in contrast to the primary visual, auditory, somatosensory, and motor cortices, which do have direct afferent and efferent connections with sensor and effector systems. The association areas increase in size relative to the total cortex up the evolutionary scale, and the relative size is largest in humans. The functions of the association areas are not known with certainty, but they are believed to integrate inputs from other cortical areas, including the **limbic cortex**, and modulate activity in other cortical areas. The vagueness of this description is indicative of our poor understanding of these areas. From metabolic and other studies of brain activity, it is evident that very many, if not most of these association areas are activated and 'busy' during cognitive activities such as problem solving, purposeful ambulation, and verbal activity.

In the parietal cortex, areas associated with the primary somatosensory and motor areas have been particularly well studied, especially in primates. Brodmann areas 5 and 7 are together termed the parietal association cortex. Both of these areas integrate information from the somatosensory and visual cortices. Information is transmitted from these areas to the motor and premotor areas. The parietal association cortex also communicates with the prefrontal cortex and the cingulate gyrus, and this link may provide the functional two-way traffic connections between brain areas subserving emotional and reasoning components of motivation and motivational behaviors. There is evidence that area 7 integrates somatosensory and visual inputs to coordinate the hand and the eye. Area 5 appears to use somatosensory inputs for proper manipulation of objects and for goal-oriented voluntary movements. Lesions of areas 5 and 7 in humans result in **agnosia**, when the patient apparently does not convert a sensory input into an appropriate motor response. The patient may also exhibit **apraxia**, which is the inability to use familiar tools.

The association areas have also been divided arbitrarily into **unimodal** and **multimodal** association areas. Unimodal association areas are usually adjacent to primary areas of sensory input. Thus, Brodmann areas 18 and 19 and part of the inferior gyrus of the temporal lobe, which are adjacent to area 17, the primary visual cortex, are together called the **visual unimodal association cortex**. These areas are presumed to provide a 'picture' of the visual world as it is presented to the eyes. Similarly, the **auditory association cortex** in the superior temporal gyrus (area 22) is adjacent to the primary auditory cortex, and ascribes meaning to signals picked up by the cochlea.

Multimodal association areas are those which are assumed to use a number of diverse inputs for reasoning and intelligent communication. Multimodal associative activity is expressed, as far as is presently known, in the forms of spatial awareness, attention, language, and planning. Space and attention appear to be controlled in the parietal cortex, while planning is a function of the prefrontal cortex. Language is a function mainly of two well-defined cortical areas (see p. 343).

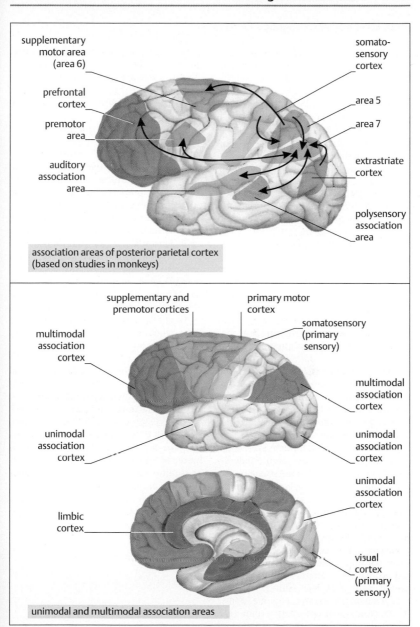

supplementary motor area (area 6)

prefrontal cortex

premotor area

auditory association area

somato-sensory cortex

area 5

area 7

extrastriate cortex

polysensory association area

association areas of posterior parietal cortex (based on studies in monkeys)

supplementary and premotor cortices

primary motor cortex

multimodal association cortex

somatosensory (primary sensory)

multimodal association cortex

unimodal association cortex

unimodal association cortex

unimodal association cortex

limbic cortex

visual cortex (primary sensory)

unimodal and multimodal association areas

Brain Laterality and Language Centers

The first evidence of **brain laterality** and its connection with speech was given in 1861 by **Broca**, who described a lesion in the frontal lobe of the left hemisphere of a patient who could understand speech but could not speak. The patient could sing a song, but could not put a sentence together verbally or in writing, despite having no obvious motor problems with vocal or manipulative effector organs. The area described is now called **Broca's area**. Another area involved in speech was described by **Wernicke** in 1876, who described a patient who could speak, but did not understand what was said. The patient had a cortical lesion in the posterior region of the temporal lobe, an area now called **Wernicke's area**. Disorders of language understanding or generation are called **aphasias**. Wernicke's aphasia may be caused by thalamic tumors, which invade the subcortical white matter, or by occlusion of the parietal and temporal branches of the middle cerebral artery. Broca's aphasia is caused, usually, by occlusion or tumors of the frontal branches of the middle cerebral artery.

More gross evidence of brain hemispheric laterality was the discovery that the **planum temporale** is much larger in the left hemisphere. This area is seen in a horizontal section through Wernicke's area. Further functional evidence of dominance of the left hemisphere was given by the Sodium Amytal test. Sodium Amytal (amylobarbitone) is a barbiturate sedative. If injected into the left carotid artery, the drug is carried preferentially to the left hemisphere. By this route it prevented a conscious patient from speaking or replying to questions. Injection on the right side did not have this effect. Patients also reported feelings of depression if the drug was given on the left side, and of euphoria if the drug was given on the right side, which suggests the existence of laterality of emotional function. This is supported by the observation that patients with lesions of Broca's area are very aware of their condition and upset by it, while those with a lesion in Wernicke's area seem relatively unconcerned.

Lateral hemispheric asymmetry and handedness also appear linked. Left hemisphere dominance is associated with right-handedness, as well as a preference for use of the right foot and even the right eye. A small proportion of the population have right hemispherical dominance, and most (but not all) of these are left-handed. In the latter group, right-handedness may have been socially imposed, which suggests that the right hemisphere can adopt functions of the left hemisphere. It is possible that naturally occurring left-handedness may reflect developmental abnormalities in the left hemisphere.

Laterality is also associated with other, less clearly defined functions. The left hemisphere is associated with more logical thought patterns, analytical approaches to problem solving, and verbal fluency in the articulation of ideas. Right hemispheric dominance is associated with intuitive reactions, creativity, and relatively less skill in articulation of thought. The extent to which dominance is exerted over the functioning of the individual is hinted at also by experimental, accidental, or surgical severance of the corpus callosum (see p. 361).

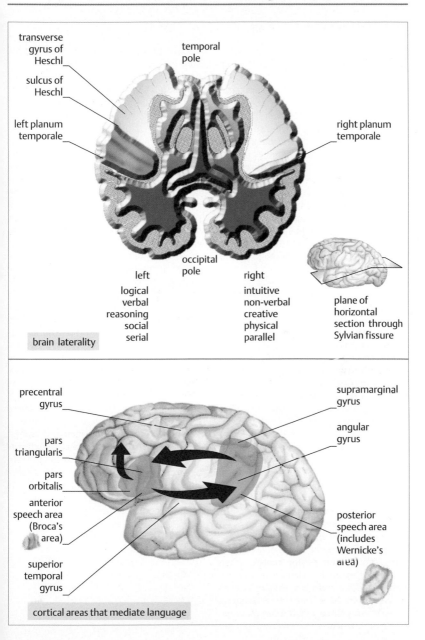

transverse gyrus of Heschl

sulcus of Heschl

left planum temporale

temporal pole

right planum temporale

occipital pole

left
logical
verbal
reasoning
social
serial

right
intuitive
non-verbal
creative
physical
parallel

plane of horizontal section through Sylvian fissure

brain laterality

precentral gyrus

pars triangularis

pars orbitalis

anterior speech area (Broca's area)

superior temporal gyrus

supramarginal gyrus

angular gyrus

posterior speech area (includes Wernicke's area)

cortical areas that mediate language

Neural Processing of Language

Language (in humans) is a learned form of **communication with the external environment**. It encompasses the sensory appreciation of symbols, their central interpretation, and the verbal or non-verbal expression of the symbols in a manner intelligible to others who have also learned the language. It is used for the expression of cognitive activity, which ranges in complexity from simple repetition of received language to the expression of thought processes. Language processing should not be confused with the expression of sounds that are semantically meaningless (such as a cough, or a baby's gurgle, which may be a form of communication that expresses pleasure, but is arguably not language processing).

At the moment we have a very poor understanding of the neural processing of language, and virtually all information comes from observing the results of damage to brain areas (see p. 346). Language involves the processing of visual, auditory, and (as in the case of the blind) tactile inputs. **Auditory inputs** travel from the ear to the **auditory cortex**, and from there to the auditory association cortex in the angular gyrus. From the association areas, the signals are projected to **Wernicke's area**, the left posterior part of the temporal lobe (Brodmann's area 22), where comprehension of the inputs is effected. The information is then projected to Broca's area (Brodmann's areas 44 and 45), where the semantic 'dictionary' is stored, and where the stored words are assembled meaningfully. This information is sent to the frontal cortex and the **premotor areas** for associative motor processing prior to being sent to the **motor cortex**, where vocal and manual articulation are controlled, and the word is spoken or written.

Visual language inputs travel from the retina to the **primary visual cortex**, where electrical impulses are converted into raw visual information. This is projected to the adjacent **extrastriate cortex** for further processing, before it is sent to Broca's area for assembly into grammatical form, and is projected from there to the prefrontal and premotor areas. There are thus independent pathways for the auditory and visual processing of language. Very little is known about how a tactile input is translated into language by the brain.

These postulated pathways are undoubtedly vast simplifications, but they do explain why damage to Broca's area still permits the understanding of language, even if it cannot be expressed. They also explain why the interruption of the arcuate fasciculus, which connects Wernicke's area with Broca's area, prevents the conversion of auditory language inputs into verbal expression of words. They do not take into account the fact that subcortical structures and cortical white matter are also involved in the processing of language. The left caudate nucleus, thalamus, and some interconnecting pathways in the left hemisphere participate in language processing. The pathways also do not explain the mechanisms whereby patients with severe damage to left hemisphere areas involved in speech are still able to sing and express sounds (including words) in melodic form. This process, called **prosody**, is more emotional than cognitive in performance, and is thought to be a function of the right hemisphere, which is more concerned with intuitive and nonreasoning cortical function.

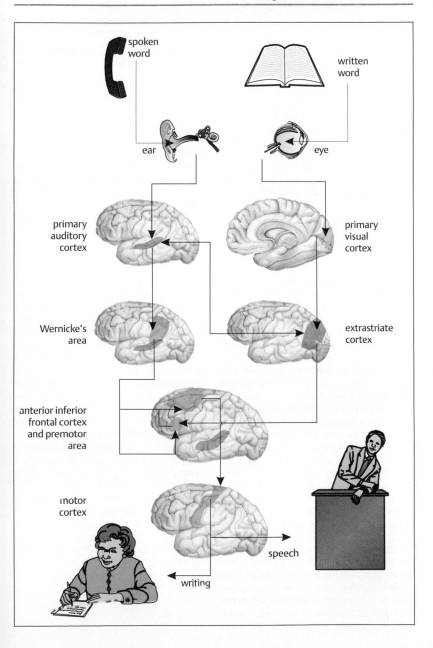

Language Disorders

Disorders of language, which are the failure or impairment of understanding, speaking, reading, or writing, may be associated with damage to brain areas that control language. The type and degree of the problem reflects the anatomical location and extent of the lesions. Individuals may be able to read, write and speak perfectly but be unable to understand language, or they may be able to understand and speak language perfectly, but present with complete or partial failure to read and write.

Aphasias are disturbances of comprehension or verbalization of language, due, mainly, to damage to cortical or subcortical brain areas involved in language processing. Aphasias have been classified principally according to the severity of the lesion. **Global aphasia** is a virtual loss of the ability to understand and verbalize language, and results from extensive damage to the perisylvian area, including **Broca's area**, **Wernicke's area**, the inferior parietal cortex, and underlying white matter. **Broca's aphasia** results from damage to areas 44 and 45 (see p. 344). The patient understands language, but is rendered *non-fluent*, saying, for example, 'manifent' instead of 'magnificent'. Patients with **Wernicke's aphasia** are fluent, but have impaired comprehension. Repetitive and semantic skill is poor; for example, the patient may say 'director' instead of 'conductor'. The aphasia, and its severity, are caused by variable degrees of damage to Wernicke's area in the left posterior superior temporal gyrus and adjacent areas.

Conduction aphasia is characterized by a failure to repeat. The patient comprehends, but cannot write dictated language. Written language can, however, be copied. The aphasia is associated with lesions in the supramarginal gyrus (area 40). **Transcortical aphasia** differs from the other aphasias described in that patients have unimpaired ability to repeat verbal language. The lesion may be anterior to Broca's area, when the patient presents with symptoms similar to Broca's aphasia, but can repeat. This is called **transcortical motor aphasia**. Lesions posterior to Wernicke's area produce a syndrome reminiscent of Wernicke's aphasia, except that repetition is spared. This is called **transcortical sensory aphasia**. **Subcortical aphasia** is caused by damage to the left basal ganglia, particularly to the head of the caudate nucleus, and is also called basal ganglia, or atypical aphasia. Patients may present with dysarthria (impaired articulation), variable degrees of fluency, impaired auditory comprehension, and right hemiparesis (body paralysis).

Failure to read and write are called **alexia** and **agraphia**, respectively, and there is a significant occurrence of **dyslexia** and **dysgraphia**, which are impaired reading and writing, respectively. Alexia can occur without agraphia. Patients with alexia and agraphia usually have lesions in the angular or supramarginal gyri; these form part of an association area that integrates visual, auditory, and tactile inputs, before passing the information to the speech areas of the temporal lobe and thence to those of the frontal lobe. Patients with these lesions cannot associate language symbols with their sounds. Pure alexia is associated with lesions in the splenium of the corpus callosum, which carries visual information from area 18 of one hemisphere to that of the other. Lesions to more anterior parts of the corpus callosum impair the ability to write with the left hand.

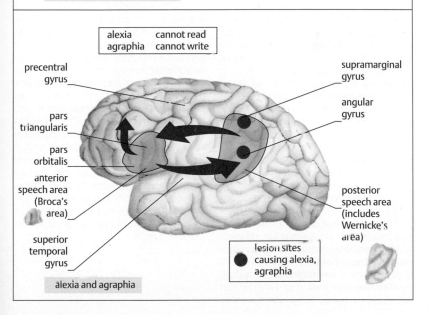

name	area	symptoms
Broca's aphasia	Broca's area	non-fluency
Wernicke's aphasia	Wernicke's area	non-comprehension
conduction aphasia	area 40	non-repetitive
global aphasia	all language areas	severe impairment
subcortical aphasia	left basal ganglia	variable impairment
transcortical aphasia	left prefrontal cortex or left posterior temporal inferior to Wernicke's area	verbatim repetition spared
anomic aphasia	areas 21, 22, 37	cannot name
aprosodia	right perisylvian area	loss of intonation

disorders of spoken language

alexia   cannot read
agraphia   cannot write

precentral gyrus

supramarginal gyrus

angular gyrus

pars triangularis

pars orbitalis

anterior speech area (Broca's area)

posterior speech area (includes Wernicke's area)

superior temporal gyrus

lesion sites causing alexia, agraphia

alexia and agraphia

Learning: Classical Conditioning

Learning is a process whereby the brain acquires information from the external environment. This definition excludes instinctive (intrinsic) knowledge, with which we are born, or the possible postnatal accumulation of information from internal sources, such as the process of denervation supersensitivity. It is not to be confused with **behavior**, which is the motor expression of motivation, derived from the integration of intrinsic and learned information, usually in response to environmental cues. Numerous tests of learning ability have been devised to assess normal and pathological brain function. These tests range in complexity from the **conditioning** of a relatively simple organism to a noxious stimulus, to the application of complex social scenarios in primates. Learning has been classified as **non-associative** and **associative**.

Non-associative learning has been further divided as **habituation** and **sensitization**. Habituation is the attenuation of a behavioral response to repeated application of a non-noxious stimulus. We may initially jump when a door is slammed, but soon cease to react when the door is slammed during a given test period. Sensitization (pseudoconditioning) is an increased response to a noxious or intense stimulus. For example, a gentle touch on a skin area previously given a painful pinch will elicit a pain response.

Associative learning derives from the experimental procedure of pairing two events and the assumed pairing formed by the animal. The term implies that the association cortices are important mediators, and this is highly likely. In experimentation, two forms are prominent: **classical** and **instrumental conditioning**. **Classical conditioning** is the creation of an association between a **conditioned** and an **unconditioned** stimulus. The concept was first given credence by **Pavlov**, who created an association in the mind of a dog between two stimuli, one conditioned and the other unconditioned. The conditioned stimulus is an applied stimulus, and might be auditory (e.g. a voice or a ringing bell) or visual (e.g. a light flash). The unconditioned stimulus (also called reinforcement) is one that was not devised by the experimenter. An unconditioned stimulus produces an **unconditioned response**. The sight of food (unconditioned stimulus) reflexly elicits salivation (unconditioned response). The response is unconditioned because it is innate and not acquired through learning. An association between conditioned and unconditioned stimuli is made by the animal's brain if the conditioned stimulus (light) is repeatedly followed by the unconditioned stimulus (sight of food); eventually the conditioned stimulus alone elicits the conditioned response (salivation).

The physiological mechanism which underlies the association between the conditioned stimulus and the unconditioned response is not permanent, and will become ineffective if the unconditioned stimulus is not periodically applied as well, a process called **extinction**. The light flash alone will eventually fail to elicit reflex salivation. This is probably not merely the dissipation of the neural associative pathways, but an active learning process, in which the animal gradually realizes that light alone will not bring food. It has been suggested that classical conditioning, and possibly all forms of associative learning, enable the animal to recognize causal relationships in the external environment, instead of randomly associating coincident external events.

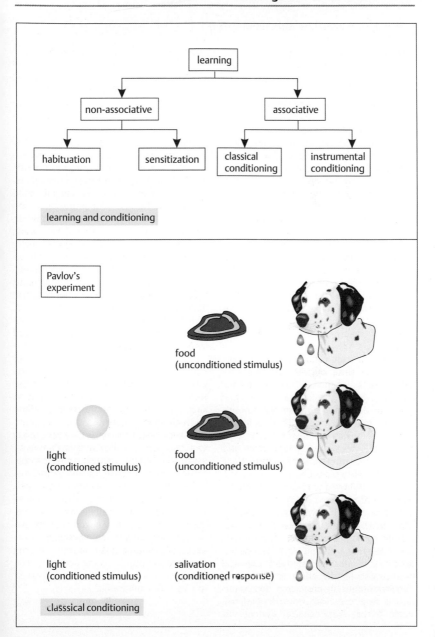

learning
non-associative
associative
habituation
sensitization
classical conditioning
instrumental conditioning

learning and conditioning

Pavlov's experiment

food (unconditioned stimulus)

light (conditioned stimulus)
food (unconditioned stimulus)

light (conditioned stimulus)
salivation (conditioned response)

classsical conditioning

Learning and Instrumental Conditioning

Instrumental conditioning is an important form of associative learning. It is also sometimes called trial-and-error or operant conditioning. The animal learns that a certain behavior (the **operant behavior**) elicits an **outcome** from the machine, either a **reward** or something **noxious**. If the reward is pleasant, for example food, then the animal will repeat the operant behavior. If the reward is unpleasant for the animal, it will not repeat the behavior. In addition, operant behaviors that are rewarded tend to be repeated at the expense of those that are not rewarded. This is called the **law of effect**. Notice that in instrumental conditioning, unlike classical conditioning, the operant behavior is often a **randomly selected** one. The animal learns by chance that the pressing of a lever results in the appearance of a banana, whereas the operation of some other lever does not. The animal will subsequently selectively press the lever that results in the reward.

The time scale of instrumental conditioning has **time optima** for reinforcement. This is also the case in classical conditioning. There are critical 'time windows' for the period between the operant behavior and the reward. There is an inverse relationship between the time that elapses between the operant behavior and the **efficiency of response learning**. Conditioning will be weaker, the longer the time that is allowed to elapse between the operant behavior and the reward or noxious outcome. Similarly, there are optimal time relationships between the conditioned and unconditioned stimuli. The longer the time difference between conditioned and unconditioned stimuli, the weaker will be the effect of the conditioned stimulus in producing the conditioned response. This time dependence suggests that both classical and instrumental conditioning might have neural mechanisms in common.

Both instrumental and classical conditioning as behavioral expressions of neural activity may have biological, and particularly evolutionary, significance. In other words, they are possibly not purely the consequences of laboratory-engineered behavior. It could be argued that taste, for example, evolved as a reward mechanism to protect animals from the consequences of eating plants or other animals that tasted bitter because of their poisonous ingredients. Many poisonous plant alkaloids are very bitter. In humans, child rearing has historically been associated with punishment-reward behavior, which is often associated with **taste**. Sweet-tasting foods are rewards for socially acceptable behavior, while in some societies bitter or noxious tastes have been forcibly applied. In many countries, a child's fingers have been coated with bitter aloes to discourage nail biting.

Instrumental and classical conditioning are used clinically in many situations. Chronic alcoholics are conditioned to associate alcohol consumption with nausea and vomiting by administering alcohol and an emetic together. This so-called aversive training teaches the patient to associate the taste of alcohol with nausea. In psychiatric clinics, patients who exhibit socially unacceptable behavior are rewarded with prizes or compliments if they refrain from such behavior. Patients who exhibit phobias are trained, while in a relaxed state, to envisage a scenario in which they are exposed to the phobia. This repetitive conditioning eventually attenuates the impact of the actual phobia, and may be a type of extinction observed in classical conditioning.

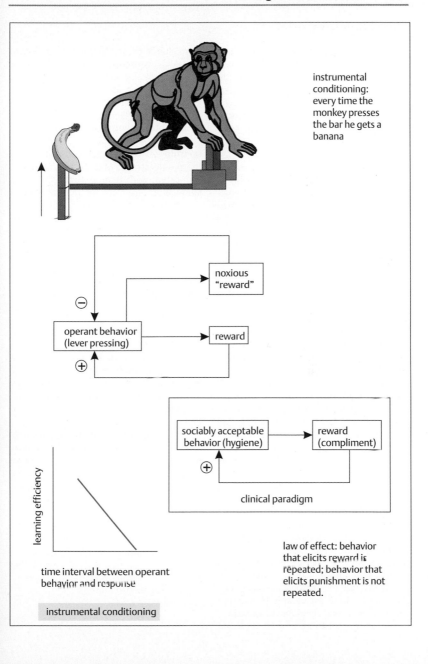

instrumental conditioning: every time the monkey presses the bar he gets a banana

noxious "reward"

$\ominus$

operant behavior (lever pressing) → reward

$\oplus$

sociably acceptable behavior (hygiene) → reward (compliment)

$\oplus$

clinical paradigm

learning efficiency

time interval between operant behavior and response

law of effect: behavior that elicits reward is repeated; behavior that elicits punishment is not repeated.

instrumental conditioning

Parietal Association Areas

The **posterior parietal cortex** contains Brodmann areas 5 and 7, the so-called **parietal association areas**. Area 5 lies in the upper, and 7 in the lower, parietal lobule. They are sandwiched between the **visual cortex** and **premotor** and **motor** areas, and process visual inputs, which are transmitted to the premotor and motor cortices. The parietal association areas are essential for appropriate use of somatosensory inputs, efficient manipulation of objects, and for proper execution of goal-directed **voluntary movements**. Area 5 may be more concerned with the control of manipulative movements, while area 7 integrates coordination between hand and eye. Hence, lesions in areas 5 and 7 will affect these functions to variable extents, depending on the size and location of the lesion. Lesions may affect the processing of emotional inputs from the cingulate gyrus, causing inappropriate motor responses to emotional states.

From experiments with monkeys, it seems that areas 5 and 7 coordinate **intention** and **purposeful movement**. Thus, certain cells in these areas will fire only if the animal decides to perform a specific act, for example to reach for an item of food. Cells are activated that ensure that the task can be executed effectively i.e. the hand grasps the food instead of grasping the space next to it. These cells will not fire if a hand swings aimlessly at the animal's side, only when it is moved to an object of interest.

Most, if not all, of what is known about the function of areas 5 and 7 in humans is derived from observations of patients with lesions in these areas. Lesions may impair understanding of the meaning of sensory inputs, a condition called **agnosia**. Agnosias may be, for example, visual or tactile. Patients may not be able to manipulate objects, a condition labeled **apraxia**. A patient may want to pick up an apple but be unable to do so, despite the absence of visual or muscular defects. The same patient may be able to tie a shoelace without looking at it. Patients may have trouble assessing distances between objects, or from themselves. Patients may have trouble drawing objects, possibly because they cannot arrange the spatial relationships between the components of these objects. The objects are drawn disconnected, with inappropriate spatial relationships, and often highly simplified.

There are various types of agnosias, most of which affect the hands, and particularly the fingers (finger agnosia). This is because a disproportionally large volume of the parietal cortex is devoted to finger manipulation. There is also a **laterality** to the manifestation of symptoms of posterior parietal damage. Lesions in the right parietal lobe may produce a condition in which the patient loses awareness of the left side of the body (**contralateral** neglect). The patient may, for example, disclaim ownership of his or her own left hand or foot. Similar symptoms have been observed after lesions in the prefrontal cortex, and in subcortical structures, including the basal ganglia and the thalamus.

There is evidence that many of the neuronal systems in areas 5 and 7 learn to associate visual and somatosensory inputs during development, and that deprivation of sight shortly after birth severely and perhaps permanently blocks the development of these associations.

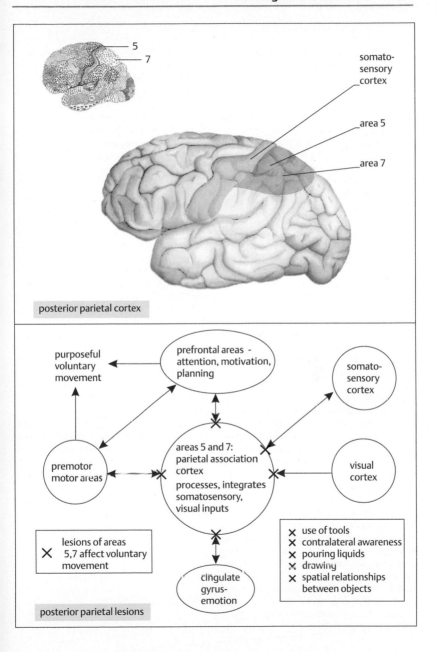

5
7

somato-sensory cortex

area 5

area 7

posterior parietal cortex

purposeful voluntary movement

prefrontal areas - attention, motivation, planning

somato-sensory cortex

premotor motor areas

areas 5 and 7: parietal association cortex

processes, integrates somatosensory, visual inputs

visual cortex

× lesions of areas 5,7 affect voluntary movement

× use of tools
× contralateral awareness
× pouring liquids
× drawing
× spatial relationships between objects

cingulate gyrus- emotion

posterior parietal lesions

Prefrontal Association Cortex

The **prefrontal association cortex** lies in front of **Brodmann areas 6** and **8**, the premotor area and frontal eye field, respectively. This area occupies a far higher proportion of cortical area than in any other species, and is the largest single cortical subdivision in humans. The prefrontal association cortex receives a vast input from the occipital, parietal and temporal lobes, and from the cingulate gyrus. It also receives subcortical inputs from the medial dorsal (dorsomedial) nucleus of the thalamus. The prefrontal cortex is thus continuously aware of all sensory inputs to the brain, and about the emotional and motivational condition of the brain. The prefrontal cortex in turn sends efferent fibers to virtually all of the cortical areas from which it receives inputs, and to many subcortical areas, including the subthalamus, the hypothalamus, and to the caudate nucleus in the striatum. Lesions of the prefrontal cortex may cause motor disturbances, but most commonly produces changes in **mood** and **personality**.

Classically, the prefrontal cortex was (erroneously) considered to be the seat of intelligence. But lesions to the prefrontal cortex do not support this assumption. The most famous case is that of an American railway worker called Phineas Gage, who had an iron bar blasted accidentally through his brain in 1848. Amazingly, he survived, but with virtually his entire prefrontal association cortex destroyed. The result was not a loss of reason or intelligence, but a change in personality. He lost restraint, used language and behavior generally considered improper, and was described as having no deference for authority. His doctor described his behavior as 'capricious' and 'obstinate'. His friends and acquaintances said that he was more carefree and less inhibited.

This case prompted the experimental ablation of the prefrontal cortex in monkeys, which attenuated anxiety in these animals. That observation led to the use in depressed or anxious patients of prefrontal ablation, **prefrontal leucotomy**, from about 1935 onwards. The operation was routinely used until the 1960s, when antidepressants, such as the monoamine oxidase inhibitors, and muscle relaxant drugs, for example the benzodiazepines, were introduced. Drugs were preferable to an irreversible operation, which in some cases produced extremes of mood and behavior, including inattention, euphoria, and antisocial habits. The operation nevertheless produced noticeable relief from anxiety, improved performance at work, and increased energy. The operation also provided relief from intractable pain. The relief was not an analgesic effect; the patient still felt the pain, but did not seem to care.

The only apparent loss of reasoning observed after frontal leucotomy was a **loss** of certain **performance skills**. Patients appeared unable to carry out more than one intellectual task simultaneously. For example, if a patient was asked to count to ten, interrupted and asked to recite the alphabet from A to G, they would forget how far they had counted in the first test. Similar results were obtained in animal tests. Monkeys with frontal lesions will not remember to complete tasks when interrupted, while normal animals complete these tasks easily. It is as though the frontal cortex stores the program of action as a form of memory.

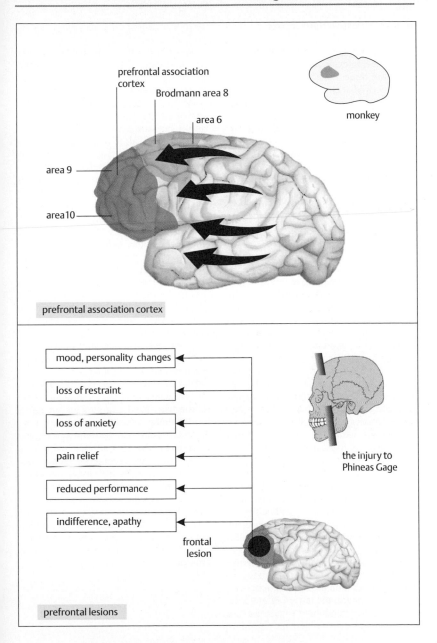

prefrontal association cortex

Brodmann area 8

area 6

area 9

area 10

prefrontal association cortex

monkey

prefrontal association cortex

mood, personality changes

loss of restraint

loss of anxiety

pain relief

reduced performance

indifference, apathy

frontal lesion

the injury to Phineas Gage

prefrontal lesions

Temporal Association Cortex

The **temporal association cortex** consists mainly of Brodmann **areas 20**, **21**, and **22**. There are three main functions known to be associated with the temporal association cortex: **memory**, **auditory learning**, and the learning of **visual tasks**.

Lesions of the **inferior temporal** area result in a dramatic reduction in the rate of learning of complex visual tasks. The patient (or experimental animal) is not blind, but has difficulty learning and improving a set of visually related tasks, for example fitting together differently colored and shaped wooden blocks. In addition, the retention of memory of the learned set is severely impaired. The lesioned cortex is unable to process inputs from the extrastriate cortex normally. Damage to the inferotemporal region typically produces **visual agnosia** ('psychic blindness'), when patients cannot recognize people or objects previously well known to them. The inferotemporal cortex appears to be important in the processing of complex visual inputs, for example the features of the face.

Lesions of the superior temporal gyrus, on the other hand, interfere with normal processing of **auditory** inputs. The superior temporal gyrus has strong reciprocal connections with the primary auditory cortex. Damage to the auditory association areas does not produce deafness, but an impaired ability to learn sets of sounds. The patient, for example, has difficulty learning and remembering the musical set *do, ray, me, fah, so, la, te, do*, and being able to distinguish different sound patterns. The patient, for example, may not be able to distinguish *do, ray, me* from *do, me, ray*.

The temporal lobes are also concerned with **memory**. Unilateral lesions may produce relatively mild memory deficits, particularly long-term memories. Bilateral lesions to the temporal lobes cause more serious memory deficits, and may produce amnesia. This is due, mainly, to damage to the hippocampal formation. In addition, patients are easily distracted, and have an **attention deficit**.

Much of the information about the known effects of temporal lobe **stimulation** in humans comes from the results of surgical removal of damaged temporal lobe tissues in patients suffering from epilepsy. A Canadian surgeon, Wilder Penfield, electrically stimulated temporal lobe areas in patients under local anesthesia prior to removal of tissue. Stimulation of the primary auditory cortex produced ill-defined noises, while stimulation of the superior temporal gyrus produced distortions of sound perception and **hallucinations**. Interestingly, these were often vivid recollections of past events. Bilateral removal of temporal lobe tissue resulted in variable loss of long-term memory that was invariably more severe than after unilateral ablation.

There was also laterality of effects of surgery. Ablation of left temporal cortex resulted in a loss of ability to remember **verbal** information, for example a list of objects. Removal of right temporal tissue, on the other hand, caused a loss of ability to remember sensory input patterns. Patients could not remember irregular patterns such as faces, although they could remember regular geometric shapes such as squares, triangles and circles. Cells have been found in monkey temporal cortex that will respond only to one particular face, while others will respond to any face presented to the animal. Damage to temporal parts of the limbic cortex may render patients more susceptible to emotional arousal.

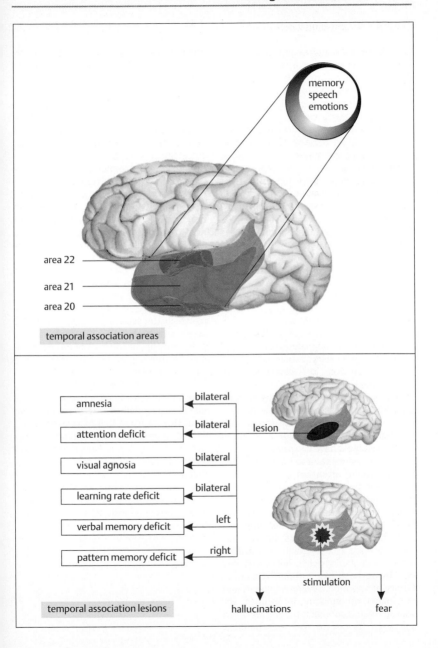

memory
speech
emotions

area 22
area 21
area 20

temporal association areas

amnesia — bilateral
attention deficit — bilateral — lesion
visual agnosia — bilateral
learning rate deficit — bilateral
verbal memory deficit — left
pattern memory deficit — right

stimulation

temporal association lesions

hallucinations   fear

Theories of Consciousness

Consciousness is a term used to describe the state of awareness of the brain, its degree of attention, and the ability of the organism to respond to external stimuli. Basically, no one knows really what consciousness is, and it is perhaps an unhelpful term, describing a condition that does not exist. To address the problem, it is necessary to separate states such as **sleep-wakefulness**, **attention**, and **responses to sensory and somatosensory stimuli** from each other, despite the possibility that all these are components of 'consciousness'. The brain areas involved in these different states have to some extent been localized and partially characterized. The term also raises complex philosophical issues, not least the difference between **brain** and **mind**.

In some texts, consciousness is contrasted with sleep, a condition of the brain that renders it relatively unresponsive to external stimuli. Sleep is characterized by an altered EEG, unresponsiveness, and dreams that are usually contextually enigmatic. Alternations between sleep and **wakefulness** (consciousness?) are controlled by the **reticular activating system**, which is a phylogenetically ancient brain stem system. It could thus be argued that all creatures that alternate between sleep and wakefulness have consciousness.

Consciousness has also been described as a degree of **attention**. This, too, is a complex issue. Attention is considered to be an ability to keep focused on one object, group of objects, activity or idea. The temporal lobe appears to be important in achieving this, and disorders such as schizophrenia are characterized by variable disorders of attention. In other words, it is possible to be awake without having the facility of attention. Several analogies and metaphors of attention have been advanced. The conscious brain has been compared to a stage with a searchlight playing over it, the so-called **theater of attention**. The cortex selects information and plays it under the 'searchlight'. It is suggested that the searchlight is controlled by the thalamus, which filters sensory information to the cortex. The anatomical location of the stage is unknown, and is probably not the frontal cortex, since almost complete destruction of this brain region, as happened to Phineas Gage (see p. 354), does not abolish consciousness. The theater analogy requires that the events on stage have an audience i.e. a brain mechanism for witnessing the events. It is suggested that limbic areas, the basal ganglia and cerebellum 'witness' the play and provide feedback (stay to watch or switch off?). The metaphor also proposes several plays simultaneously performed, for example in auditory, somatosensory, or other ill-defined areas, to which the searchlight can switch. The content of each 'play' is determined by prevalent inputs from all brain areas, including intercommunicating inputs from each hemisphere.

Consciousness has been described as a condition of sensory receptiveness and the ability to respond to external sensory inputs. This is very similar to a classically accepted definition of wakefulness, as opposed to sleep. Yet it is well known that when awake, subjects may be so immersed in thought (a particular stage play?) that they are unaware of all visual and auditory inputs. Clearly this is a brain issue whose scientific status lags well behind other aspects of neuroscience.

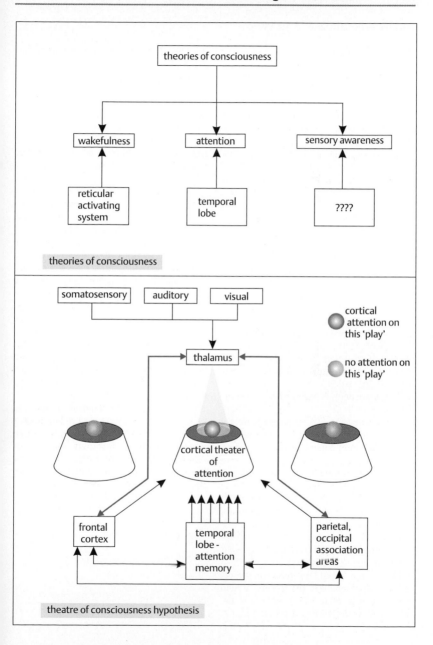

theories of consciousness

theatre of consciousness hypothesis

Corpus Callosum and 'Split Brain'

The **corpus callosum** is a thick mass of white matter that in the main connects corresponding areas in the two **cerebral hemispheres**. The fibers connect cortical areas that control bilateral body parts that work together, such as the back. Parts such as the hands, which can operate independently, are poorly represented through commissural connections. The striate cortices, also, are virtually unconnected. Much of what is known about the role of the corpus. callosum comes from observations of experimental animals and patients, in whom the corpus callosum has been surgically severed.

The American surgeon, Roger Sperry and his colleagues provided the first important information about the functional significance of the corpus callosum. They sectioned the corpus callosum (commissurotomy) and, in some patients, the anterior commissure as well, to prevent the spread of **epileptic seizures** from one hemisphere to the other. In these patients the two hemispheres could operate independently, and patients were referred to as '**split brain**' patients. The operations also provided further evidence of brain lateralization.

'Split brain' patients managed perfectly well in everyday life situations. One reason is that each hemisphere received an accurate representation of the patient's gaze through their intact optic fiber systems. But these patients could not verbally *name* an object if it was seen only from the left visual field, even though the patient still knew what the object was and could touch or pick it up. This is because the visual information could not travel from the right to left hemisphere where language is controlled. Patients could not read and understand text presented to the left visual field unless it was relatively simple, for example the word *CAT*. It was concluded that the right hemisphere is almost devoid of the ability to emit any verbal output.

The right hemisphere was, however, able to perform certain tasks more efficiently than the left. Patients found it easier, for example, to assemble colored wooden models of known objects with the left hand. This supports the idea that the **right hemisphere** is specialized for **spatial tasks**. These experiments also suggested the curious possibility that the two hemispheres acted as two independent minds in these patients. If the patient was asked to perform a manual task using one hemisphere, the other hand would often intervene, indicating that the other hemisphere was aware of the task and was trying to contribute. In principle, however, it was found that the hemisphere best suited to a particular task would control the execution of it. Some experiments suggested that after commissurotomy both hemispheres lost efficiency in the carrying out of both **verbal** and **spatial tasks**, which suggests that in normal, intact brains, both hemispheres contribute to the efficient execution of tasks which may be lateralized to one hemisphere or the other.

Hemispheric lateralization appears to be laid down prenatally before language is first verbalized. Nevertheless, children who suffer left hemisphere damage, or whose corpus callosum is poorly developed, do learn to use language with the right hemisphere later in life.

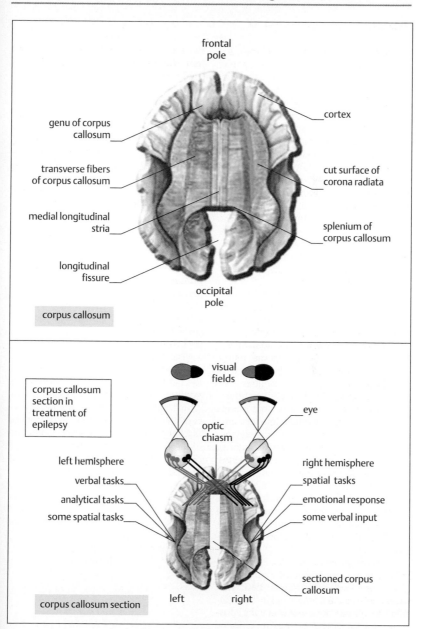

frontal pole

genu of corpus callosum

cortex

transverse fibers of corpus callosum

cut surface of corona radiata

medial longitudinal stria

splenium of corpus callosum

longitudinal fissure

occipital pole

corpus callosum

corpus callosum section in treatment of epilepsy

visual fields

optic chiasm

eye

left hemisphere

right hemisphere

verbal tasks

spatial tasks

analytical tasks

emotional response

some spatial tasks

some verbal input

sectioned corpus callosum

left   right

corpus callosum section

Epilepsy

Epilepsy is a chronic brain disorder characterized by recurrent synchronous discharges of neuronal groups in the cortex. The discharges, which are also called **seizures**, may be localized or generalized. About 0.5–1% of the population suffer from epilepsy, and about 75% will suffer their first attack before age 18. Seizures are symptoms of brain damage, caused by factors including tissue trauma, anoxia, infection, toxic conditions, or tumor growth. Symptoms range from temporary disorders of thought to massive convulsions, depending on the extent of spread of the synchronous electrical activity. Seizures have been classified as **partial** or **generalized**, depending on the spread, and medication is selected on the basis of the classification.

Partial (focal) seizures result from localized discharges that spread from the focus to adjacent brain areas. The patient may remain conscious, and the nature of the seizure depends on the area of the brain affected. Discharges in the motor cortex may involve first the seemingly purposeful movement of extremities (fingers), with spread up the arms to the face, and down to the legs as neuronal groups are progressively recruited into the discharge. Motor seizures are also called jacksonian motor seizures, after Hughlings Jackson, who originally described the motor cortex. In **simple** partial seizures, the patient remains conscious, but if activity spreads to the other hemisphere, the patient may lose consciousness and the seizure is termed **complex** or **psychomotor**, since there may be hallucinatory experiences.

In **generalized**, or non-focal, seizures, there is a massive spread of electrical activity over both hemispheres. **Petit mal** (**absence**) seizures, which begin in childhood, involve a transient loss of consciousness without a loss of muscle tone, so those patients rarely fall down. In **grand mal** (**tonic-clonic**) seizures, the patient suddenly loses consciousness and falls down. Convulsions consist of increased muscle tone (tonic) periods alternating with jerking movements (clonic). After the convulsions, loss of consciousness may persist. **Status epilepticus** is a dangerous, uninterrupted series of seizures that requires urgent intravenous administration of drugs.

The various seizures are characterized by distinct **EEG patterns**. A focal seizure produces a characteristic EEG **spike**, whereas a generalized seizure produces a series of spikes that are picked up all over the skull simultaneously. The EEG also distinguishes between the **tonic** and **clonic phases** of the generalized discharge. In experimental induction of epilepsy in animals, the discharges are characterized by distinct patterns of intracellular activity. During absence seizures, there are characteristic **spike wave** patterns of discharge.

The synchronization of neuronal discharge during epilepsy appears to involve the inhibition of the inhibitory **GABAergic system**. Convulsants such as **picrotoxin**, which binds to and blocks the $GABA_A$ receptor, cause epileptic-type synchronous discharges. The normal inhibitory function of the GABAergic system may be overcome during seizures through the summation of discharge by several excitatory neurons firing simultaneously. This idea is supported by the fact that drugs that target the GABAergic system are powerful chemotherapeutic agents in the treatment of different types of epilepsy.

Temporal lobe epilepsy is due to lesions in CAI in the hippocampus (see also p. 334).

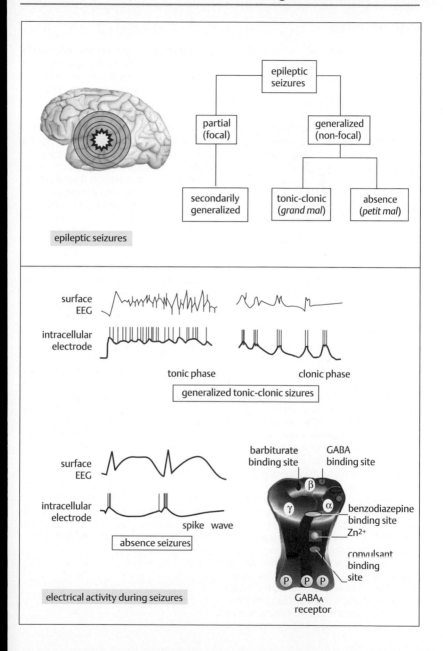

epileptic seizures

```
                              epileptic
                              seizures
                    ┌─────────────┴──────────────┐
               partial                      generalized
               (focal)                      (non-focal)
                  │                  ┌───────────┴───────────┐
            secondarily         tonic-clonic            absence
            generalized         (grand mal)            (petit mal)
```

epileptic seizures

surface EEG

intracellular electrode

tonic phase   clonic phase

generalized tonic-clonic sizures

surface EEG

intracellular electrode

spike   wave

absence seizures

barbiturate binding site   GABA binding site

β

γ   α   benzodiazepine binding site

Zn²⁺

convulsant binding site

P   P   P

electrical activity during seizures

GABA_A receptor

Drugs for Epilepsy

Epilepsy can be controlled with **anticonvulsant** drugs, and different drugs are indicated for different types of seizure. The drugs inhibit the spread of seizures by a variety of mechanisms, some of which are unknown, but in the main, they seem to act by enhancing the **GABAergic system**, or inhibiting the **glutamatergic system**, or both. They may act on postsynaptic receptors, or directly on ion channels to inhibit the influx of **Na⁺** or **Ca²⁺** ions into the cell.

Partial and **tonic-clonic** (grand mal) seizures are treated with orally active drugs such as **carbamazepine** or **phenytoin**. Phenytoin is by far the best known and most widely studied. Carbamazepine is often chosen for use in young women and for partial seizures. **Sodium valproate** is also widely used. These drugs control tonic-clonic seizures better than partial seizures, and in the latter case drugs such as **clonazepam**, **phenobarbitone**, or **primidone** may be used as well, but are markedly sedative in action. **Absence** (petit mal) **seizures** are treated with clonazepam, **ethosuximide**, or valproate. Status epilepticus requires urgent administration of drugs such as **chlormethiazole**, clonazepam, or **diazepam**.

The drugs have different and sometimes obscure **mechanisms of action**. Phenytoin inhibits seizures through the prevention of high-frequency repetitive neuronal discharges. The mechanism of action is unclear. Anticonvulsant doses have no observable effects on neuronal responses to **glutamate** or to **GABA**; neither do they affect neurotransmitter release. Phenytoin binds selectively to inactivated Na⁺ channels during neuronal discharges, and may therefore be more active during high frequency discharge, when many more Na⁺ channels are involved. Carbamazepine and valproate may act similarly to phenytoin, although valproate may act also by enhancing GABA synthesis and inhibiting GABA breakdown. **Vigabatrin**, too, raises GABA levels by inhibiting GABA transaminase (**GABA-T**). Phenobarbitone, a barbiturate, binds to its receptor site on the **GABA_A receptor**, and enhances Cl⁻ influx, an action possibly shared by clonazepam. The mechanism of ethosuximide is unknown, but may be through the blockade of T-type Ca²⁺ channels in thalamic neurons. Absence seizures involve oscillatory electrical discharges between the thalamus and the cortex.

Plasma protein binding and metabolism complicate the actions of antiepileptic drugs. Phenytoin is strongly bound to plasma proteins, and displaces other drugs, such as the anticoagulant warfarin, causing potentially dangerous drug interactions. Carbamazepine is activated by liver metabolism to an active epoxide. Carbamazepine, phenobarbitone, and phenytoin all induce liver microsomal enzymes, thereby stimulating the metabolism of drugs such as warfarin, bronchodilators such as theophylline, and the oral contraceptives. Anticonvulsants also have variable and sometimes dangerous **side effects**. Phenytoin may cause dose-related ataxia and nystagmus, gingival hyperplasia, and hirsutism. **Phenobarbitone** is sedative, and may also produce withdrawal symptoms. Valproate may cause relatively mild side effects, including nausea, weight gain, and occasional transient hair loss, although it has also caused potentially fatal hepatic toxicity. Clonazepam, like other benzodiazepines, is sedative in action, induces tolerance, and after prolonged use may also produce withdrawal symptoms.

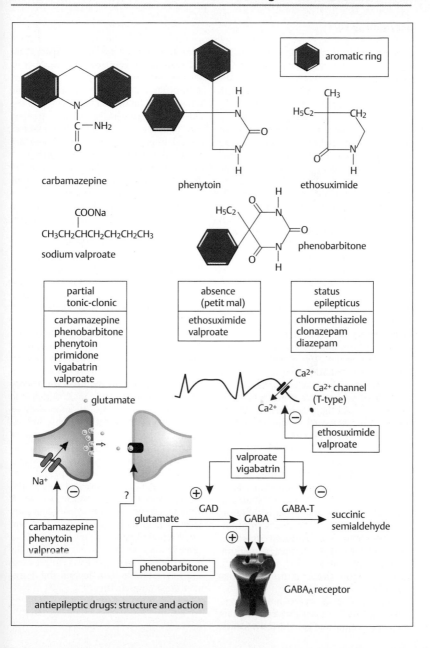

antiepileptic drugs: structure and action

Schizophrenia

Schizophrenia is a disease that usually begins in adolescence or the early twenties. Because of the early onset of symptoms, it was originally called '**dementia praecox**'. Schizophrenia occurs in 0.5–1% of the population, and is often severely incapacitating. The overall view is that of an individual in whom cognitive and emotional thought have been dissociated or split. Manic-depressive illness or the iatrogenic induction of psychosis by drugs such as phencyclidine or amphetamines have both been sometimes misdiagnosed as schizophrenia. Misdiagnoses such as these have prompted the laying down of rigorous criteria for diagnosis of schizophrenia. These are mainly descriptive. The patient has to show continuous symptoms for at least 6 months; there has to be at least one cycle of psychotic and residual episodes. During the psychotic phase, the patient must experience one delusional, or hallucinatory, or alogia symptom (see below), or a combination of these.

Symptoms of schizophrenia have been classified as **positive** or **negative**. Positive symptoms include paranoid behavior and hallucinations. Negative symptoms imply a loss of normal thought function. **Alogia**, for example, is speech lacking coherence and content. **Avolition** is an inability to execute goal-oriented behavior. **Affective flattening** is the absence of emotional content during communication. Symptoms present in episodes, sometimes long-lasting. There is usually a prodromal, pre-psychotic stage, presenting as withdrawal, odd behavior, and indifference. Intermittent **psychotic** and **residual episodes**, which include hallucination, sometimes lasting months, follow this. Residual episodes are reminiscent of the prodromal period.

The etiology of schizophrenia is unknown. It may be caused by a combination of environmental and genetic factors. Anatomical correlates are absent apart from enlarged lateral ventricles in a number of patients. The symptoms can be treated with drugs that interfere with dopamine action in the brain, and this has led to the **dopamine hypothesis**, which suggests that schizophrenia is the result of excess central dopaminergic activity. There are several dopamine receptor subtypes, and these drugs appear to act selectively on the D_2 receptor. Post-mortem analysis of brains of schizophrenic patients has revealed the presence of excessively high concentrations of dopamine receptors, and occasionally large amounts of dopamine metabolites. The hypothesis is far from dogma, however, especially since the discovery that some D_1 and $5\text{-}HT_2$ receptor antagonists are useful in the treatment of schizophrenia. (Schizophrenia is classically thought to be mediated by D_2 receptors.)

The speech disorders associated with schizophrenia have contributed to a more controversial theory, which holds that schizophrenia may be the result of **failure of hemispheric dominance**. The theory thus dismisses environmental factors, and attributes the disorder to anomalies of asymmetry. Reduced asymmetry, for example, in the planum temporale found at postmortem examination, is offered as evidence for the theory, as well as asymmetries of brain width and lateral ventricle enlargement. However, speech disorders, which might conceivably result from failure of laterality, are not usually accompanied by schizophrenia. Also, not every schizophrenic patient has failure of lateralization of the planum temporale. Nevertheless, the hypothesis is interesting, and forces one to look beyond the dominant dopaminergic theory.

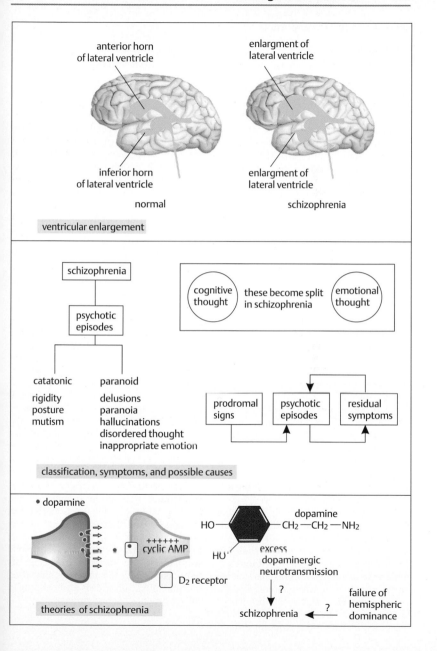

anterior horn
of lateral ventricle

enlargment of
lateral ventricle

inferior horn
of lateral ventricle

enlargment of
lateral ventricle

normal

schizophrenia

ventricular enlargement

schizophrenia

psychotic
episodes

cognitive
thought

these become split
in schizophrenia

emotional
thought

catatonic

rigidity
posture
mutism

paranoid

delusions
paranoia
hallucinations
disordered thought
inappropriate emotion

prodromal
signs

psychotic
episodes

residual
symptoms

classification, symptoms, and possible causes

• dopamine

+++++
cyclic AMP

D₂ receptor

dopamine

HO—⬡—CH₂—CH₂—NH₂

HO

excess
dopaminergic
neurotransmission

?

schizophrenia

?

failure of
hemispheric
dominance

theories of schizophrenia

Drugs Used for Schizophrenia

Schizophrenia is a psychotic condition, and is treated with **neuroleptic** drugs, also called antipsychotic, or antischizophrenic drugs, or major tranquilizers. Psychotic behavior, which perhaps reflects organic abnormalities in brain, should be distinguished from neurotic behavior, which is an inappropriate response to environmental conditions. There are three main classes of neuroleptic drugs: **phenothiazines**, **butyrophenones**, and **benzamides**. It is widely believed that blocking **dopamine receptors** in brain underlies the antipsychotic action of these drugs. This belief is supported by experiments in which it was shown that the clinical efficacy of drugs used to treat schizophrenia is directly related to their efficacy at suppressing the binding of dopamine analogs to the dopamine receptor. Indirect evidence comes from the measurement of significantly elevated postmortem dopamine levels in the left amygdala of schizophrenic patients. The ability of drugs to modulate central dopaminergic function is now a useful screening test for their possible antipsychotic activity.

Phenothiazines, which are tricyclic in structure, are further classified according to their side chains. **Chlorpromazine** (Largactil) has an aliphatic side chain, while piperazine derivatives such as **fluphenazine**, have a cyclic side chain. **Thioxanthenes**, for example **flupenthixol**, are also tricyclic, but have C substituted for N in the middle ring. Apart from this change, flupenthixol and fluphenazine are identical. The efficacy of chlorpromazine in schizophrenia was first noted in 1953. The drug was calming without significant sedation. Chlorpromazine's mechanism of action in schizophrenia is difficult to discover, since chlorpromazine blocks many different neurotransmitter receptors, including receptors for ACh, 5-HT, histamine, dopamine, and norepinephrine. **Dibenzodiazepines**, such as **clozapine**, have a 7-member middle ring (see the benzodiazepines, which are used to treat anxiety and epilepsy p. 364).

The wide-ranging actions of chlorpromazine produce several side effects. The drug causes catalepsy in animals, when they will respond to stimulation, but do not move. In patients, chlorpromazine reduces motor activity. Patients become apathetic, drowsy, and display little initiative or motivation. Patients remain conscious and retain cognitive function. The docility produced by the drug led to widespread clinical misuse when it was first introduced, since it facilitated the management of belligerent and aggressive patients. The anti-dopaminergic action of phenothiazines and other antipsychotics that block dopamine receptors in brain produces several side effects related to dopamine's central actions. The drugs may produce **Parkinson-like symptoms** (see p. 370). These are extrapyramidal motor disturbances such as tremor. **Tardive dyskinesia** may occur. The patient exhibits involuntary movements of the facial muscles, reminiscent of prolonged use of dopamine-like drugs in Parkinson's disease. Dopamine antagonists are also antiemetic, since they block the normal dopaminergic control of the vomiting reflex in the chemoreceptor trigger zone.

Haloperidol is an example of a **butyrophenone**. Haloperidol is more specific than the phenothiazines in its mechanism of action, in that it blocks mainly dopamine receptors in the central nervous system. **Benzamides**, for example **sulpiride**, were discovered during attempts to modify the antiarrhythmic drug procainamide. Sulpiride is a potent drug in the treatment of schizophrenia.

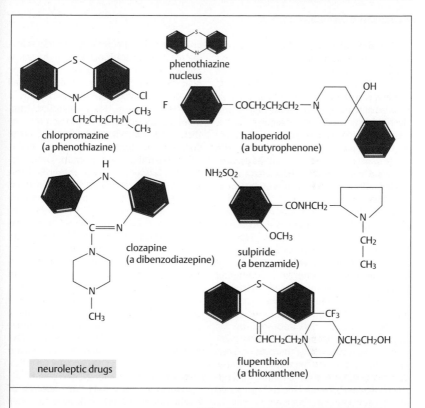

neuroleptic drugs

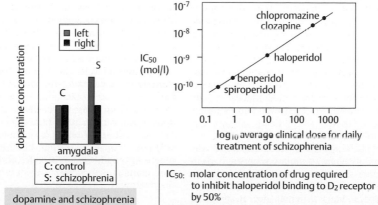

dopamine and schizophrenia

IC50: molar concentration of drug required to inhibit haloperidol binding to D_2 receptor by 50%

Parkinson's Disease

Parkinson's disease is characterized by fine tremor of the hands at rest, and the characteristic 'pill-rolling' movement of the fingers and thumb. There is muscular rigidity, which is detected as an increase in resistance to passive limb movements, and hypokinesia, which is a decrease in the frequency of voluntary movement.

Parkinson's disease is caused by the progressive degeneration of the **dopaminergic pathway** from the **substantia nigra** in the midbrain to the **corpus striatum** in the basal ganglia. These is normally a balance between dopaminergic and **cholinergic inputs to the striatum**, which controls fine movements. A loss of dopaminergic neurons unmasks an excitatory cholinergic drive, and tremor results. (**Huntington's chorea**, is a dementia resulting from a loss of GABA-mediated inhibition in the substantia nigra-striatum axis.)

The cause of the degeneration of dopaminergic cells in the substantia nigra is unknown, but a clue may have been provided by the unfortunate experiences of a group of heroin users in California in 1982. They bought illicitly prepared heroin that was contaminated with MPTP (1-methyl-4-phenyl-1, 2,3,6-tetrahydropyridine). MPTP was taken into dopaminergic cells, where it was converted by the enzyme monoamine oxidase B into a toxic metabolite, MPP^+, which destroyed the cells irreversibly, and caused parkinsonian symptoms. MPP^+ poisons cells by blocking the mitochondrial respiratory chain, which results in the generation of superoxides leading to cell death through oxidative stress.

Since this is a neurotransmitter-mediated problem, attempts have been made to mimic the dopaminergic drive with drugs. Initially, drugs, such as **benztropine** were given to block the cholinergic drive to the corpus striatum. These, however, caused unwanted side effects related to the blocking of the normal functions of the autonomic system. This approach was supplanted by the breakthrough discovery of the drug **levodopa (L-dopa)**. Dopa is a natural precursor of dopamine, and L-dopa may work by entering the synthetic pathway to flood the cell with more dopamine, or stimulate the release of existing dopamine stores from the nerve terminals. L-dopa is often prescribed together with **carbidopa**, which cannot cross the blood-brain barrier, and which blocks the conversion of L-dopa to dopamine. This minimizes unwanted dopaminergic effects outside the brain. L-dopa was a big advance. It replaced the less effective anticholinergic agents and significantly increased life expectancy in patients. Unfortunately, the drug's beneficial effects wear off progressively and are replaced after 3 to 5 years by extremely unpleasant side effects. Relief becomes what is often called an 'on-off' affair. Patients develop dyskinesias (uncontrolled, involuntary movements), especially of the limbs, mouth, and cheeks.

The disastrous long-term effects of L-dopa spurred the search for alternative approaches. An antiviral drug, **amantadine**, may alleviate symptoms through **release of dopamine**. Dopamine agonists are also extensively used. **Bromocriptine**, and a newer, longer acting analogue called **cabergoline**, activate D_2 receptors. **Transplantation of human fetal tissue** from the substantia nigra into brains of patients with Parkinson's disease is being tried. Other novel implantation treatments include **gene therapy**, which is the implantation of human cells that have been genetically engineered to produce and release nerve growth factors.

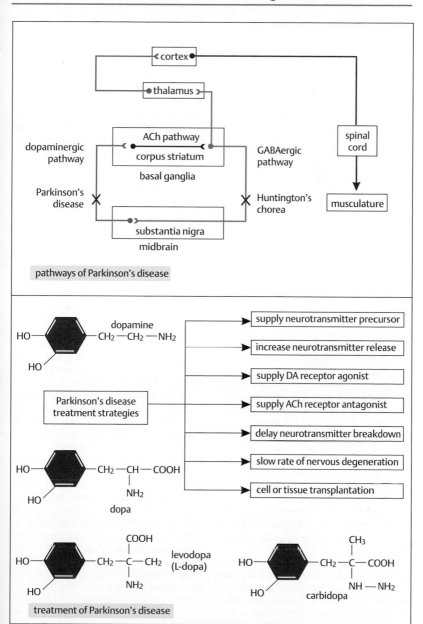

pathways of Parkinson's disease

treatment of Parkinson's disease

Affective (Mood) Disorders

Mood refers to the emotional status of the individual. It is normally confined to mild fluctuations between elation and **depression**. If, however, the mood swings become more extreme, then a pathologic condition may exist. Extremes of elation are called **manic disorders**, and extremes of depression are **depressive disorders**. **Anxiety disorders** may exist, when the individual experiences **panic** disorders or **obsessive-compulsive** disorders. This classification is a gross oversimplification, since a mood disorder may include some or even all of these states. It is nevertheless useful when considering possible neural substrates and approaches to treatment.

Depressive disorders may be unipolar or dipolar. **Bipolar depression** is a disorder in which the mood oscillates between mania and depression. There is evidence that bipolar depression is hereditary and appears when the patient is relatively young. This suggests that there may be an underlying biochemical lesion. Bipolar depression is usually accompanied by inertia and apathy. **Unipolar depression** usually occurs later in life, is not hereditary, and there are no manic episodes. Patients are not apathetic, but are frequently agitated and anxious. Some authorities classify unipolar depression as **reactive** or **endogenous**. Reactive depression is, for example, a reaction to bereavement, while endogenous depression reflects a pathological (possibly biochemical) abnormality.

Theories of depression are currently dominated by the **monoamine theory**, according to which there is an abnormally low monoaminergic drive in the brain. It arose from the fact that drugs that enhance noradrenaline (**NA**) and **5-HT** concentrations at the synapse are effective treatments for depression. Mood is lifted by drugs that inhibit the breakdown of monoamines, and which inhibit re-uptake

into the nerve terminal. Mood is depressed by drugs that deplete stores of NA and 5-HT. Electroconvulsive therapy (ECT), which increases brain responsiveness to endogenous monoamines, lifts mood. Methyldopa, a drug used to treat hypertension, inhibits NA synthesis, and depresses mood. Not all chemical manipulations of endogenous monoamines do affect mood. L-dopa, for example, which is used to treat Parkinson's disease, has no significant effect on mood.

Anxiety disorders include the so-called panic attacks, during which patients experience terror for no obvious reason, accompanied by autonomic and motor symptoms including sweating, trembling, chest pains, and flushing. Panic attacks are sometimes associated with agoraphobia, when the patient dreads leaving the home. The cause of panic attacks is unknown, although the monoaminergic system has been implicated, as well as hypersensitivity to carbon dioxide, catecholamines such as isoproterenol (isoprenaline) and lactate, all of which have been able to induce panic attacks when administered.

It has been suggested that anxiety is driven from the **locus ceruleus**, **periaqueductal gray matter**, and **raphe nuclei**, which project NA and 5-HT fibers, respectively, to limbic structures such as the **hypothalamus**, **amygdala**, and **hippocampus**. Some of these, notably the hypothalamus, project excitatory amino acid (glutamatergic) pathways to the **septum**, and there are also excitatory reciprocal **cholecystokinin** pathways between these structures and the cortex. **GABAergic** (**GABA$_A$**) pathways can inhibit these excitatory pathways at all levels from midbrain through limbic structures to the **cortex**. Panic disorders have been treated with antagonists to cholecystokinin, 5-HT$_{2C}$ and β-adrenoreceptor antagonists.

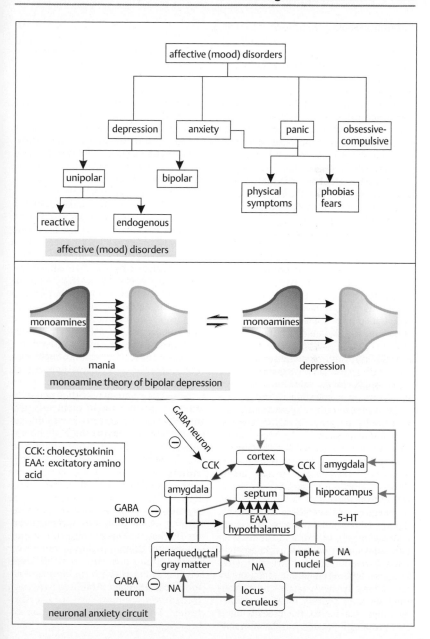

affective (mood) disorders

monoamine theory of bipolar depression

CCK: cholecystokinin
EAA: excitatory amino acid

neuronal anxiety circuit

Antidepressants

Clinical depression is treated with drugs or with electroconvulsive therapy (ECT). The main classes of drugs used are the **monoamine oxidase inhibitors** (**MAOI**), the **tricyclic antidepressants**, the **atypical drugs**, and **lithium**. The **MAOI**s were the first clinically effective drugs to be used. Two MAO enzymes have been found: MAO-A and MAO-B. MAO-A has a higher substrate affinity for NA and 5-HT, and is the enzyme targeted by MAOI antidepressants. The first was **iproniazid**. Others, e.g. **pargyline** and **tranylcypromine**, followed.

MAOI drugs rapidly raise and maintain elevated levels of NA, 5-HT, and dopamine. By inhibiting breakdown, MAOI drugs increase cytoplasmic neurotransmitter stores in the nerve terminal without affecting the vesicular stores normally released by nerve stimulation. Cytoplasmic neurotransmitter leaks into the cleft. Amines such as tyramine (found in wine and cheese) or amphetamines displace vesicular stores of neurotransmitter, and are therefore contraindicated when MAOI drugs are prescribed. Side effects of MAOI drugs include hypotension, atropine-like effects, and several drug interactions. They have been superseded largely by the tricyclic antidepressants.

Imipramine is a **tricyclic antidepressant** related to chlorpromazine. Imipramine blocks **uptake 1**, an active process whereby NA and 5-HT are taken back into the nerve terminal. This prolongs synaptic cleft concentrations. The relative importance of the two neurotransmitters in the mediation of action of the tricyclic antidepressants is unknown. It is possible that both are important since both noradrenergic and serotonergic brain nuclei are probably involved in mood. It has been proposed that 5-HT is more concerned with the mood status, while NA is more concerned with the degree of motor activation associated with a lift in mood out of depression.

Chlorination of imipramine yields **clomipramine**. Imipramine is a pro-drug, since it is demethylated in vivo to **desipramine**, the active metabolite. Clomipramine, too, is demethylated to the active substance. **Amitriptyline** and **nortriptyline** are Dibenzocycloheptadienes, produced by insertion of a dimethylene bridge into the thioxanthene ring.

Antidepressants, especially the tricyclics, are not specific for uptake 1, but also bind to cholinergic muscarinic receptors in the brain, as well as to 5-HT and histamine H_2 receptors, thereby blocking the actions of the endogenous neurotransmitters. There is also evidence that antidepressants down-regulate $5-HT_2$ and β-adrenoreceptors, which may contribute to their antidepressant action. Although tricyclics have a rapid onset of action, the antidepressant effect does not appear for some weeks, and the cause of the delay is unknown. Tricyclics interact strongly with other drugs and cause several side effects, especially hypotension and atropine-like actions. They interact with alcohol to cause respiratory depression. Atypical antidepressants such as the non-tricyclic **nomifensine** and **maprotiline** inhibit uptake of NA selectively, while **zimelidine** and **iprindole** inhibit uptake of 5-HT. **Lithium** is prescribed to prevent the manic phase in bipolar depression, and has no effect on the depressive phase. It may work by blocking the IP_3 second messenger system in the brain. **Electroconvulsive therapy (ECT)** is the electrical stimulation of the scalp of lightly anesthetized patients given a muscle relaxant. ECT reliably lifts mood, perhaps by altering brain sensitivity to NA and 5-HT.

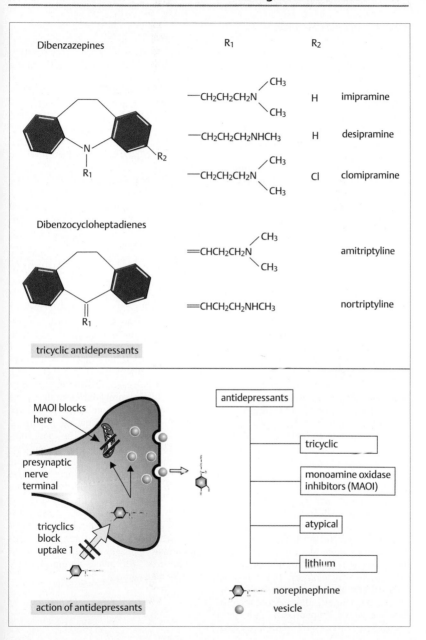

Dibenzazepines	R₁	R₂	
	$-CH_2CH_2CH_2N\begin{smallmatrix}CH_3\\CH_3\end{smallmatrix}$	H	imipramine
	$-CH_2CH_2CH_2NHCH_3$	H	desipramine
	$-CH_2CH_2CH_2N\begin{smallmatrix}CH_3\\CH_3\end{smallmatrix}$	Cl	clomipramine
Dibenzocycloheptadienes			
	$=CHCH_2CH_2N\begin{smallmatrix}CH_3\\CH_3\end{smallmatrix}$		amitriptyline
	$=CHCH_2CH_2NHCH_3$		nortriptyline

tricyclic antidepressants

MAOI blocks here

presynaptic nerve terminal

tricyclics block uptake 1

antidepressants

- tricyclic
- monoamine oxidase inhibitors (MAOI)
- atypical
- lithium

norepinephrine

vesicle

action of antidepressants

Brain Aging and Dementia

The human **brain** undergoes noticeable physical changes during **aging**. Brain **weight decreases** and **neuronal loss or shrinkage** occurs, together with **lowered protein concentrations**. Catecholamine-metabolizing enzymes fall, as do the numbers of neurons in the substantia nigra and locus ceruleus. These changes do not necessarily signal a pathological change. There is, however, a gradual **decline in memory skills** and **reduced postural reflexes** in some individuals, although some people can retain excellent memory skills into advanced old age. Sleep-waking patterns change, and older people tend to have less sleep time. In some people, however, age brings pathological changes in the brain that may result in, for example, Parkinson's disease, Huntington's chorea (see p. 370), or dementias, the most common of which is **Alzheimer's disease**.

Dementia is a blanket term that describes chronic, persistent, behavioral disorders involving **deterioration in lucidity**, **reasoning ability**, **personality**, and **personal self-care**. Alzheimer's disease is caused by the **degeneration of certain brain neuronal populations**, especially in the **cortex** and the **hippocampus**. The patient becomes forgetful, particularly when short-term memory and memory acquisition are required. Disease progression is noticed first by others, and presents as forgetfulness, mild stress, lethargy, and judgmental errors. As the disease progresses, patients will suffer psychotic episodes, with hallucinations that may cause aggression, confusion, and fear.

Examination of the living brain of an Alzheimer's patient may reveal thinning of the cortical gyri and reduced blood flow to the parietocortical areas, but this may occur in the absence of the disease. Although Alzheimer's disease occurs predominantly in older people, it can occur in younger patients as well. In the latter case,

there is a strong disease congregation within families. Evidence suggests that a combination of genetic and environmental factors may produce the disease. Late-onset disease has been linked with heritable mutations in mitochondrial DNA that encodes cytochrome-*c* oxidases I and II, and the e4 allele of the apolipoprotein E (Apo E) gene may be a risk factor for the disease.

Postmortem examination of the brain, however, reveals characteristic signs. There are large numbers of lesions called **neuritic plaques** and **neurofibrillar tangles**. The plaques are deposition of a peptide called **amyloid**, which is laid down between nerve cells (i.e. extracellularly), and which displaces the cells and may interfere with their normal function. The tangles are caused inside the nerve cells (i.e. intracellularly) by twisted strands of the so-called **tau protein**. Tau is a cytoskeletal protein that helps to maintain normal cell structure. The possible role of amyloid in Alzheimer's disease is still controversial. Brains of patients with Alzheimer's disease are also found at postmortem to be severely **deficient in several neurotransmitters**, notably ACh, 5-HT, and NA. Drugs that mimic the actions of ACh are used extensively. The most common approach is the use of anticholinesterases e.g. **rivastigmine**. The drug has been reported to improve cognitive function in some cases of mild to moderate disease. Patients may be prescribed a 'cocktail' of mood stabilizing, antidepressant drugs and antipsychotic drugs. Newer approaches include treatment with anti-inflammatory drugs such as indomethacin and antioxidants such as vitamin E to try to slow degeneration.

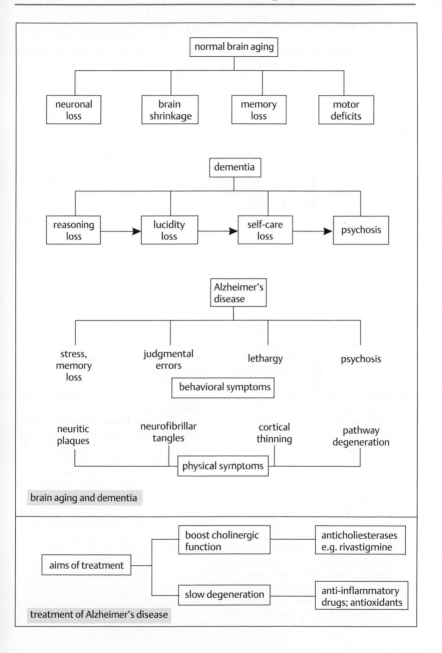

brain aging and dementia

treatment of Alzheimer's disease

β-Amyloid Precursor Protein in Alzheimer's Disease

The role of **amyloid plaques** in **Alzheimer's disease** is unknown. However, much good evidence has recently been provided that β-**amyloid**, the principal component of amyloid, and possibly some of its metabolic fragments may be involved in the etiology of Alzheimer's disease through an action on ionic permeability. This may be through an interaction with existing **ion channels** or through the *de novo* creation of ion channels or both. These interactions may mediate, at least in part, the toxic actions of amyloid in Alzheimer's disease.

β-amyloid is a 4 kDa protein of between 39 and 43 amino acids. Normally, it is a metabolic product of a membrane-spanning amino acid precursor molecule termed βAPP. Normally, βAPP is processed to both amyloidogenic and non-amyloidogenic products, some of which are membrane-associated, and some are secreted into the extracellular space. βAPP is metabolized along two main pathways by **secretase** enzymes, either to **C-100** fragments, or to so-called **P3** fragments. Some of the fragments, particularly those at the **C-terminus** of βAPP (C-100) may be important in the interactions with and generation of new ion channels. It is possible that some or all of the βAPP fragments may influence neurotransmitter release, tyrosine kinase phosphorylation, receptor activity, and transporter mechanisms.

A secreted fragment of βAPP, for example, was found to activate K⁺ channels in hippocampal tissue *in vitro*, and reduced intracellular Ca^{2+} ion concentrations through the production of cyclic guanosine monophosphate (GMP) and protein dephosphorylation. Also, β-amyloid, the peptide that is deposited in the brains of patients with Alzheimer's disease, is capable of inducing cation channels. There is a particularly toxic type of β-amyloid, β-amyloid$_{1-42}$, which aggregates rapidly. It is believed by some that β-amyloid$_{1-42}$ may react with ion channels to raise intracellular Ca^{2+} ion concentrations, which in turn injure the cell. Perhaps part of the etiology of Alzheimer's disease is the inappropriate fragmentation of βAPP into fragments that aggregate and become deposited in the tissues. The metabolite may actually inhibit the activity of cation channels. β-amyloid$_{1-40}$, for example, inhibits K⁺ channels in human fibroblasts.

There is evidence that β-amyloid and C-terminal fragments of βAPP can induce *de novo* synthesis of non-specific ion channels *in vivo*. They may do this through their incorporation into the nerve cell membrane in order to create the channel. This action is analogous to the known creation of so-called 'porin-type' channels in membranes of astrocytes, bacteria, and mitochondria. The C-terminal fragments of βAPP have a transmembrane region whose amino acid sequence is predicted to fold into a β-sheet configuration similar to that of the porins.

A familial basis of Alzheimer's disease is suggested by the discovery of mutations in the APP gene on chromosome 21, and five of these mutations have been linked with Alzheimer's disease. All mutations have in common that they lead to the production of β-amyloid$_{1-42}$, the form that is deposited as plaques in the diseased brain. Other factors apart from amyloid are possibly involved, since neurofibrillar tangles are formed in Alzheimer's diseases before the deposition of β-amyloid$_{1-42}$.

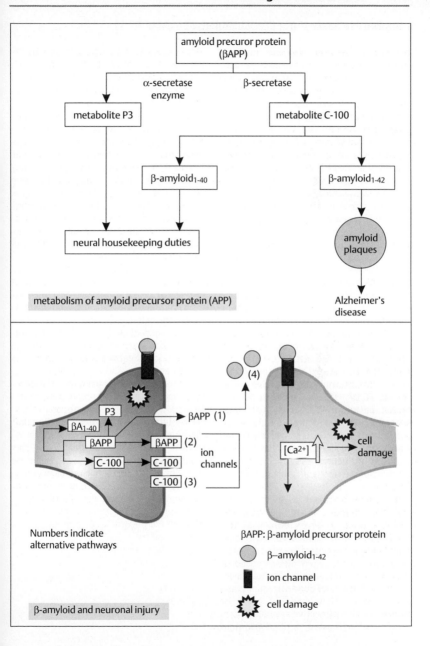

metabolism of amyloid precursor protein (APP)

β-amyloid and neuronal injury

Transmissible Spongiform Encephalopathies

Transmissible spongiform encephalopathies (**TSE**) are a group of neurodegenerative diseases that occur in man and other animals. All are transmitted experimentally and all are fatal. The term *spongiform* derives from the spongy nature of affected brain tissue described at autopsy. Clinical symptoms of TSEs in humans include progressive loss of movement coordination and dementia. Spongiform changes, amyloid deposits and gliosis are typically found during neuropathological examination.

TSEs include **scrapie**, a disease of sheep, first recorded in 1732, which can be transmitted to healthy sheep via intraocular injection with infected spinal cord. The term *scrapie* derives from the fact that infected sheep scraped off their own wool. A similar disease called **kuru** (meaning *tremor* in local language) was described in 1957 in natives of New Guinea. Tribesmen infected themselves by ingestion of infected human brains. Kuru could be transmitted across species to chimpanzees. Other human TSEs include **Creutzfeldt-Jakob Disease** (**CJD**), and a more rare variant, **Gerstmann-Sträussler-Scheinker** disease (**GSS**). **Bovine spongiform encephalopathy** (**BSE**) was discovered in November, 1986, and precipitated an international crisis when it was suspected that humans had contracted bovine BSE and CJD after eating beef from cattle that had consumed feedstuffs containing infected nervous tissue.

Pathological changes during the course of TSE progression are confined mainly to the brain. Initially, there may be hypertrophy of astrocyte end feet on blood vessels, followed by more generalized changes, notably spongiform degeneration caused by vacuoles in neurons and glial tissue. There is generalized loss of dendritic spines, and axonal degeneration.

In a search for infective agents, infected tissue was fractionated, until an infectious extract was obtained. This contained a 27-30 kDa protease-resistant protein, which was called **PrP27-30**. (PrP is abbreviated from **prion protein**.) It was found to be the protease-resistant core of an abnormal isoform of a protein normally found in the host brain. PrP27-30 accumulates in the brain during the course of scrapie. The importance of PrP protein in the etiology of scrapie was underlined by the discovery that transgenic mice without the PrP gene were resistant to infection with scrapie. PrP genes have been described in a number of species, including humans, and it is possible that the PrP gene may be a common factor in the transmission and development of the TSEs.

Despite the evidence of PrP proteins, the nature of the infectious agent involved in the transmission of TSEs remains controversial. A **virus** may transmit the disease, although no virus large enough to infect has been discovered. It has been suggested that a small nucleic acid given a coat of host protein (a **virino**) may be the infectious agent. Another hypothesis proposes that an unusual **protein** is the infectious agent. The infectious protein somehow confers its own properties on the host PrP protein. It has also been proposed that the putative infective PrP protein may associate with a host nucleic acid. This would be very interesting if correct, since it would mean that inherited characteristics could be transmitted in health and disease through proteins.

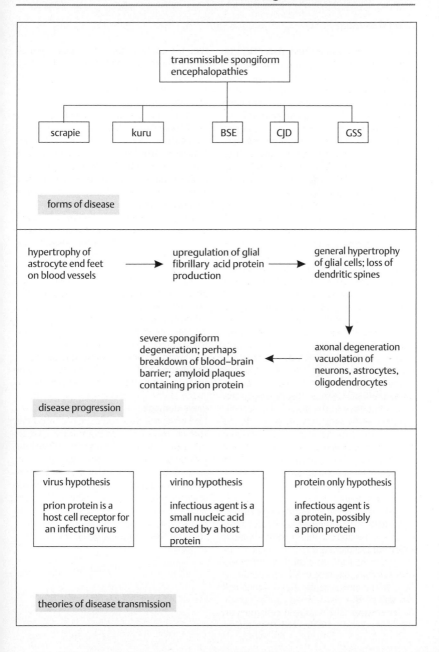

Axonal Damage

When nerves are damaged, they may recover slowly or die, depending on the nature and age of the cell, the anatomical site, and the developmental age of the animal. **Damage** may be caused through **aging**, **disease**, or through **physical**, or **chemical trauma**. We now know that the brain is susceptible to immune mechanisms, especially in the region of the meninges and perivascular microglia. More importantly, there is evidence to challenge the old dogma that adult nervous tissue cannot regenerate itself, and this promises hope for sufferers of **degenerative nervous diseases**.

When nerves, and particularly axons are damaged, the **axon** may degenerate, accompanied by characteristic morphological changes in the cell body, a process called the **axon reaction**. The cell body changes are termed **chromatolysis**. Within 24 hours after axon damage, light microscopy reveals vacuole formation, nucleolar enlargement, formation of multiple nucleoli, and displacement of the nucleus from the center of the soma of the neuron. Electron microscopy reveals breakdown of the endoplasmic reticulum and an increase in the numbers of free ribosomes. RNA synthesis increases as the cell struggles to survive by synthesizing new proteins to repair the damage. Some damaged cells, however, may not exhibit the characteristic chromatolytic response after injury, whether or not they will ultimately survive.

Axon damage may result in **retrograde cell death**, when the cell is unable to re-establish synaptic contact with healthy cells, and the damaged cell dies. The damaged cell may kill neighboring uninjured cells that are damaged through denervation. If the postsynaptically situated cell atrophies, this is termed **anterograde degeneration**. The damaged cell may, on the other hand, kill the cell that makes synaptic connection with it; this is **retrograde transneuronal degeneration**. The damaged cell may kill cells that synapse with it and with which it synapses. This is **transneuronal atrophy**.

The axon may not degenerate, but may exhibit anabolic changes that signal **regeneration**. Neurons are known to have powerful **trophic influences** on each other and on muscle. Skeletal muscle that is denervated through injury or disease will atrophy through a loss of so-called **trophic support**. Trophic support may rescue a cell whose axon is damaged, through the connections the damaged cell has with other neurons. **Trophic substances**, possibly nerve growth and other factors, are transported to the cell body of the damaged cell by retrograde axonal transport. A damaged cell may even be able to give itself trophic support through the presence of axon collaterals that feed back to the cell body. Trophic factors so far identified include nerve growth factor (NGF) and brain-derived neurotrophic factor. In the brain, NGF or brain-derived neurotrophic factor infusions have been used successfully to rescue cholinergic pathways damaged by experimental transection of septohippocampal projections. This sort of result holds promise for the treatment of degenerative diseases such as Alzheimer's disease. The mechanism of action of the trophic factors is unknown. There is evidence that they inhibit the production and release of neurotoxic proteases. There is evidence also that trophic factors may be derived not only from neurons but from supporting cells such as glia as well.

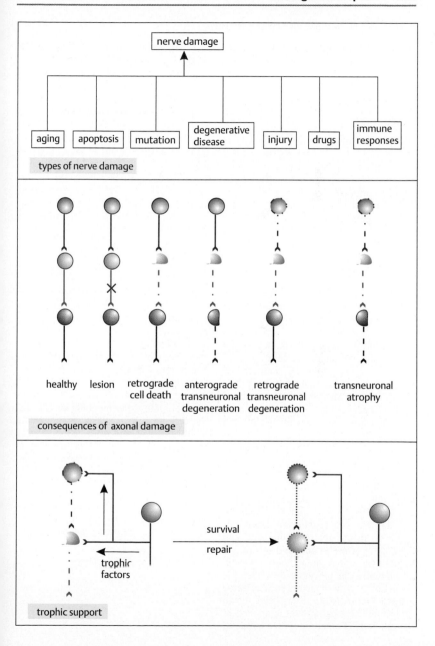

types of nerve damage

consequences of axonal damage

trophic support

Axonal Injury and Nerve Growth Factor

When an **axon** is cut, the section attached to the soma or cell body is termed the proximal segment, and the section separated from the cell is termed the distal segment. Both cut ends seal to limit leakage of axoplasm, and both cut ends swell due to accumulation of products of axoplasmic transport and flow. The synaptic terminals of the distal segment degenerate and become filled with tangled neurofilaments and ruptured mitochondria. The distal segment gradually degenerates over a period of months by a process called **wallerian degeneration**. The myelin sheath breaks away from the distal segment, which breaks up into fragments. If the damaged cell is to die, then the soma, too, shows degenerative changes called chromatolysis.

When a peripheral neuron is damaged, macrophages infiltrate and assist in the degradation of the distal segment. A similar function is performed by the microglia in the central nervous system. In both the central and peripheral nervous systems, the myelin sheath, which is composed of the processes of the glial **Schwann cell**, is also destroyed. Mention has already been made elsewhere that a degenerating neuron can cause the death of neighboring neurons. One of the first signs that neighboring cells are affected is the **shrinking away of synapses from the damaged cell**.

Damaged neurons do not always die. In the thalamus, for example, cells whose axons are cut may shrink, but they do not die. Peripheral spinal and motoneurons, for example, can **regenerate axons**. Instead of dying, the proximal cut end develops a **growth cone**, and reconnects to make functional contact with more distal elements. The process is dependent on the action of growth factors such as **nerve growth factor** (**NGF**). It has been shown experimentally that if NGF is applied to the cell body of a neuron with a damaged axon, then neighboring synapses will not shrink away from the cell but retain contact. Conversely, the application of NGF antibodies to a damaged peripheral neuron will accelerate the shrinkage of neighboring synapses away from the damaged cell. Axon regeneration may also occur if the myelin sheath of the damaged or transected axon remains intact. Infiltrating macrophages appear to stimulate Schwann cell proliferation in the vicinity of the lesion. The Schwann cells secrete axon-guiding molecules such as laminin and adhesion molecules, which somehow guide the regenerating axon to its functional target site.

Traditionally, it was thought that adult brain neurons could not be regenerated, but this dogma now seems obsolete. NGF also seems to be an active trophic substance in the central nervous system. It is especially concentrated in the hippocampus, which receives a dense cholinergic input, and application of NGF to sectioned cholinergic axons drastically reduces the degenerative damage caused. This makes NGF a potential treatment for Alzheimer's disease. Damaged CNS axons can be made to regenerate experimentally by blocking the action of the endogenous growth inhibitors N1250 and N135, coupled with the application of growth factors such as acidic fibroblast growth factor and brain-derived neurotrophic factor.

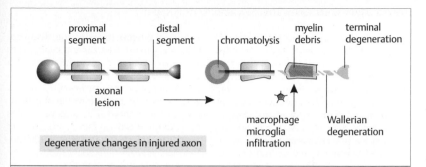

proximal segment · distal segment · chromatolysis · myelin debris · terminal degeneration

axonal lesion

macrophage microglia infiltration · Wallerian degeneration

degenerative changes in injured axon

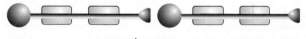

axotomy → growth cone develops · Schwann cells proliferate

regenerative changes in injured axon

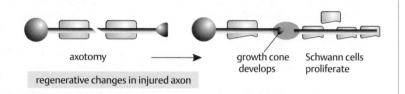

normal synapse

lesion

degeneration: presynaptic terminal shrinks away from damaged cell

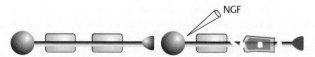

NGF

appliction of NGF to cell body rescues cell; presynaptic terminal retains contact

NGF rescues lesioned neurons

Neural Stem Cells, Gene Therapy, and Neural Repair

Approaches to the **treatment of cell damage** in the nervous system have been revolutionized by the discovery that adult nerves can **accept tissue grafts from fetal sources**. Attempts are being made to repopulate the human brain of Parkinson's patients with fetal dopaminergic grafts. A newer advance is the use of **genetically engineered cells** to repair damaged peripheral and central nervous tissue. There are two basic approaches. One is to create **cells that synthesize growth factors** such as NGF or **metabolic enzymes** that mediate neurotransmitter action. These are injected into the tissue and repopulate injured or diseased brain areas. These cells have been injected into the aging rat brain, and have been shown to partially reverse learning and memory deficits due to age-related loss of cholinergic neuronal systems. The aim, however, is to supply not only chemicals but also **genes** to the diseased tissues.

To understand modern thinking about neural cell and gene therapy, some knowledge of the principles of stem cell division and differentiation is needed. During mammalian embryogenesis, cells differentiate into the different progeny that comprise the adult organism. In some tissues, such as skin, liver, or bone marrow, cells continue to divide. This is possible because these tissues maintain subpopulations of **stem cells**, which never terminally differentiate, but can divide mitotically to produce not only more stem cells, but also **progenitor** cells that will enter a pathway that leads them to terminal differentiation as a cell type specific to the tissue. Classically, it was thought that brain did not possess stem cells, but there is now evidence that mammalian forebrain may possess stem cells capable of mitotic division into progenitor cells with multilineage potential.

This evidence includes the discovery that adult mammalian forebrain contains cells that respond to growth factors such as epidermal growth factor (EGF) and transforming growth factor-α (TGF-α) in a way similar to that of neural precursor cells of the embryo. This discovery holds out hope that growth factors may be able to activate cells in adult brains to differentiate into neurons and glial cells.

This concept is currently being explored using approaches that include the use of **immortalized progenitor** cells. Immortalized cells are those whose differentiation is suspended by using genetic engineering to induce them to remain in a process of continuous cell cycle. The immortalized cells are grown in culture and implanted into the brain. Progenitor cells have been implanted into immature and adult rat brains, and develop into neurons and glia, which become integrated with the brain area into which they are implanted. Results of experiments in rats are promising. Immortalized cells that express the enzyme tyrosine hydroxylase have been implanted into rats that have been rendered parkinsonian-like. The injection of cells significantly improved behavioral parameters to those measured in healthy control animals.

While this approach is still very much in the experimental stages, it is clearly the most hopeful on offer. It is to be hoped that diseases such as **Parkinson's disease**, **Huntington's chorea**, and **Alzheimer's disease** will eventually be treatable, and even curable, using interventions that restore cell populations lost during the course of the disease.

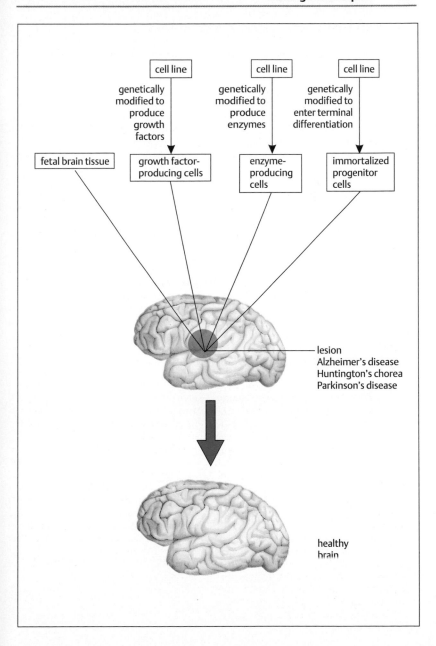

Literature

Textbooks and Reference Works

Barr, M.L. and Kiernan, J.A. *The Human Nervous System* (5th edition). Philadelphia: J.B. Lippincott Company, 1988.

Brodal, P. *The Central nervous System*, New York: Oxford University Press, 1992.

Brown, A.G. *Organization in the spinal cord. The anatomy and physiology of identified neurons*. London: Springer-Verlag, 1981.

Brown, A.G. *Nerve Cells and Nervous Systems. An Introduction to Neuroscience*. London: Springer-Verlag, 1991.

Carpenter, M.B. *Core text of Neuroanatomy* (3rd edition). Baltimore: The Williams & Wilkins Company, 1985.

Carpenter, R.H.S. *Neurophysiology* (3rd edition). London: Arnold., 1996.

Conn, P. M. (Ed). *Neuroscience in Medicine*. Philadelphia: J.B. Lippincott, 1995.

Crossman, A.R. and Neary, D. *Neuoranatomy*. Edinburgh: Churchill Livingstone, 1995.

De Groot, J. J. and Chusid, J.G. *Correlative Neuroanatomy* Connecticut: Appleton & Lange, 1988.

Eccles, J.C. and Schade, J.P. (Eds). *Organization of the Spinal Cord*. Progress in Brain Research Volume 11. Amsterdam: Elsevier Publishing Company, 1964.

Fitzgerald, M.J.T. *Neuroanatomy Basic and Clinical* (3rd edition). London: W.B. Saunders Company Ltd, 1996.

Guyton, A.C. *Basic Neuroscience Anatomy and Physiology*. Philadelphia: W.B. Saunders Company, 1987.

Haines, D.E. (Ed) *Fundamental Neuroscience*. New York: Churchill Livingstone, 1997.

Jones, E.G. (1985). *The Thalamus*. Plenum Press, 1985.

Kahle, W. *Nervous System and Sensory Organs* (4th edition). Stuttgart: Georg Thieme Verlag, 1993.

Kandel, E.R., Schwartz, I.H. & Jessell, T.H. (Eds.) *Principles of Neural Science* (3rd Edition). New York: Elsevier, 1991.

Kuffler, S.W., Nicholls, J.G. and Martin, R.WM. *From Neuron to Brain* (2nd edition). Massachusetts: Sinauer Associates Inc., 1984.

Larsen, W.J. *Human Embryology*. New York: Churchill Livingstone Ltd., 1993.

Nolte, John. *A Study Guide to Accompany the Human Brain*. (3rd edition). St. Louis: Mosby-Year Book, 1993.

Snell, R.S. Clinical Neuoranatomy for Medical Students (4th edition). Philadelphia: Lippincott-Raven, 1997.

Wilkinson, J.L. *Neuroanatomy for Medical Students* (2nd edition). Oxford: Butterworth-Heinemann Ltd, 1992.

Papers and Reviews

Neuroanatomy

Atwood, H.L. and Lnenicka, G.A. (1986). Structure and function of synapses. Emerging correlations. Trends in Neurosciences 9, 248–250.

Rexed, B. (1952). The cytoarchitectonic organization of the spinal cord in the cat. Journal of Comparative Neurology **96**, 415–495.

Embryology

Davies, A.M. and Lumsden, A. (1990). Ontogeny of the somatosensory system: Origins and early development of primary sensory neurons. Annual Reviews in Neuroscience **13**, 61–73.

Cellular Neuroscience

Dunant, Y. (1986). On the mechanism of acetylcholine release. Progress in Neurobiology **26**, 55–92.

Guy, H.R. and Conti, F. (1990). Pursuing the structure and function of voltage-gated channels. Trends in Neurosciences **13**, 201–206.

Jacobs, M. (1982). Microfilaments and cell movement. Trends in Neurosciences **5**, 369–374.

Julius, D. (1991). Molecular biology of serotonin receptors. Annual Reviews in Neuroscience.**14**, 335–360.

Kimelberg, H.J. and Norenberg, M.D. (1989). Astrocytes. Scientific American **260**, 44–55.

Levitan, J.B. (1988). Modulation of ion channels in neurons and other cells. Annual Reviews in Neuroscience **11**, 119–136.

Mason, T. (1981). Noradrenaline in the brain: progress in theories of behavioural function. Progress in Neurobiology **16**, 263–303.

Maycox, P.R. (1980). Amino acid neurotransmission: Spotlight on synaptic vesicles. Trends in Neurosciences **13**, 83–87.

Schofield, P.R. *et al.* (1990). The role of receptor subtype diversity in the CNS. Trends in Neurosciences **13**, 8–11.

Vallee, R.B. and Bloom, G.S. (1991). Mechanisms of fast and slow axonal transport. Annual Reviews in Neuroscience **14**, 59–92.

Walz, W. Role of glial cells in the regulation of the brain ionic environment. Progress in Neurobiology **33**, 309–333.

Somatosensory Processing

Hamill, O.P. and McBride D.W. (1996). A supramolecular complex underlying touch sensitivity. Trends in Neurosciences **19**, 258–261.

Hasan, Z. and Stuart, D.G. (1988). Animal solutions to problems of motor control: The role of proprioceptors. Annual Reviews of Neuroscience.**11**, 199–223.

Keegan, J.J. and Garett, F.D. (1948). The segmental distribution of cutaneous nerves in the limbs of man. Anatomical Record **102**, 409–437.

Lynn, B. and Hunt, S.P. (1984). Afferent C-fibres: physiological and biochemical correlations. Trends in Neurosciences **7**, 186–188.

Maxwell, D.J. and Rethelyi, M. (1987). Ultrastructure and synaptic connections of cutaneous afferent fibres in the spinal cord. Trends in Neurosciences **10**, 117–123.

Matthews, P.B.C. (1981). Evolving views on the internal operation and functional role of the muscle spindle. Journal of Physiology **320**, 1–30.

Rudomin, P. (1990). Presynaptic inhibition of muscle spindle and tendon organ afferents in the mammalian spinal cord. Trends in Neurosciences **13**, 499–505.

Woolsey, C.N. (1964). Cortical localization as defined by evoked potential and electrical stimulation. In: Cerebral Localization and Organization. G. Schaltenbrand, C.N. Woolsey, Eds. University of Wisconsin Press, pp. 17–32.

Motor Control

Armstrong, D.M. (1988). The supraspinal control of mammalian locomotion. Journal of Physiology **405**, 1–37.

Kennedy, P.R. (1990). Corticospinal, rubrospinal and rubro-olivary projections: A unifying hypothesis. Trends in Neurosciences **13**, 474–478.

Prochazka, A, (1989). Sensorimotor gain control: A basic strategy of motor systems? Progress in Neurobiology **33**, 281–307.

Ralston, A.D. and Ralston, H.J. (1985). III. The terminations of corticospinal tract axons in the macaque monkey. Journal of Comparative Neurology **242**, 325–337.

Brain Stem

Dean, P., Redgrave, P. and Westby, G.V.M. (1989). Event or emergency? Two systems in the mammalian superior colliculus. Trends in Neurosciences **12**, 137–147.

Foote, S.L. and Morrison, J.H. (1987). Extrathalamic modulation of cortical function. Annual Reviews of Neuroscience **10**, 67–95.

Moruzzi, G. and Magoun, H.W. (1949). Brain stem reticular formation and activation of the EEG. Electroencephalogram and Clinical Neurophysiology. **1**, 455–473.

Saper, C.B. (1987). Function of the locus coeruleus. Trends in Neurosciences **10**, 343–344.

Autonomic nervous System

Andersson, K.-E. and Sjögren, C. (1982). Aspects of the physiology and pharmacology of the bladder and urethra. Progress in Neurobiology **19**, 71–89.

Burnstock, G. (1986). The changing face of autonomic neurotransmission. Acta Physiologica Scandinavia **126**, 67–91.

Laskey, W. and Polosa, C. (1988). Characteristics of the sympathetic preganglionic neuron and its synaptic input. Progress in Neurobiology **31**, 47–84.

Simmons, M.A. (1985). The complexity and diversity of synaptic transmission in the prevertebral sympathetic ganglia. Progress in Neurobiology **24**, 43–93.

Wallin, B.G. and Fagius, J. (1986). The sympathetic nervous system in man – aspects derived from microelectrode recordings. Trends in Neurosciences **9**, 63–67.

Special Senses

Corwin, J.T. and Warchol, M.E. (1991). Auditory hair cells: structure, function, development and regeneration. Annual Reviews of Neuroscience 14, 301–333.

Dionne, V.E. (1988). How do you smell? Principle in question. Trends in Neurosciences **11**, 188–199.

Hubel, D. and Wiesel, T. (1962). Receptive fields, binocular interaction and functional architecture in the cat's visual cortex. Journal of Physiology **160**, 106–154.

Kaas, J.S. (1989). Why does the brain have so many visual areas? Journal of Cognitive Neuroscience **1**, 121–135.

Kauer, J.S. (1991). Contributions of topography and parallel processing to odor coding in the vertebrate olfactory pathway. Trends in Neurosciences **14**, 79–85.

Kinnamon, S.C. (1988). Taste transduction: a diversity of mechanisms. Trends in Neurosciences **11**, 491–496.

Martin, K.A.C. (1988). From enzymes to visual perception: A bridge too far? Trends in Neurosciences **11**, 280–287.

Nobili, R., Mammano, F. and Ashmore, J. (1998). How well do we understand the cochlea? Trends in Neurosciences **21**, 159–167.

Roper, S.D. (1989). The cell biology of vertebrate taste receptors. Annual Reviews of Neuroscience **12**, 329–354.

Shapley, R. and Perry, V.H. (1986). Cat and monkey retinal ganglion cells and their visual functional roles. Trends in Neurosciences **9**, 229–235.

Hypothalamus and Limbic System

Amaral, D.G. and Witter, M.P. The three-dimensional organization of the hippocampal formation: a review of anatomical data. Neuroscience **31**, 571–591.

Fisher, R.S. (1989). Animal models of the epilepsies. Brain Research Reviews **14**, 245–278.

Excitatory amino acids in the brain: Focus on NMDA receptors. Trends in Neurosciences 10 number **7**, 1987 (devoted issue).

Kuhar, M.J. (1986). Neuroanatomical substrates of anxiety: a brief survey. Trends in Neurosciences **9**, 307–310.

Learning and memory. Trends in Neurosciences **11** number 4, 1988 (devoted issue).

Linden, D.L. and Routtenberg, A. The role of protein kinase C in long term potentiation: a testable model. Brain Research Reviews **14**, 279–296.

McEntee, W.J. and Mair, R.G. (1990). The Korsakoff syndrome: A neurochemical perspective. Trends in Neurosciences **13**, 340–344.

Richardson, R.T. and DeLong, M.R. (1988). A reappraisal of the functions of the nucleus basalis of Meynert. Trends in Neurosciences **11**, 264–267.

Scoville, W.B. and Milner, B. (1957). Loss of recent memory after bilateral hippocampal lesions. Journal of Neurology, Neurosurgery & Psychiatry **20**, 11–21.

Zucker, R.S. (1989). Short-term synaptic plasticity. Annual Review of Neuroscience **12**, 13–31.

Higher Brain Function and Damage and Repair

Baars, B.J. (1998). Metaphors of consciousness and attention in the brain. Trends in Neurosciences **21**, 58–62.

Barlow, H. (1990). The mechanical mind. Annual Reviews of Neuroscience **13**, 15–24.

Brust, J.C. (1980). Music and language. Musical alexia and agraphia. Brain **103**, 367–392.

Brodmann, K. (1909). Vergleichende Lokalisationslehre der Grosshirnrinde. Berlin: J.A. Barth.

Caramazza, A. (1988). Some aspects of language processing revealed through the analysis of acquired aphasia: The lexical system. Annual Reviews of Neuroscience **11**, 395–421.

Connor, B.W. and Gutnick, M.J. (1990). Intrinsic firing patterns of diverse neocortical neurons. Trends in Neurosciences **13**, 99–104.

Damasio, A.R. (1990). Category-related recognition defects as a clue to the neural substrates of knowledge. Trends in Neurosciences **13**, 95–98.

Foote, S.L. and Morisson, J.H. (1987). Extrathalamic modulation of cortical function. Annual Reviews of Neuroscience **10**, 67–95.

Fraser, F.P., Suh, Y-H. and Djamgoz, M.B.A. (1997). Ionic effects of the Alzheimer's disease _-amyloid protein and its metabolic fragments. Trends in Neurosciences **20**, 67–72.

Frey, U. and Morris, R.G.M. (1998). Synaptic tagging: implications for late maintenance of hippocampal long-term potentiation. Trends in Neurosciences **21**, 181–188.

The Frontal Lobes-Uncharted provinces of the brain. Trends in Neurosciences **7**, number 11, 1984 (devoted issue).

Goldman-Rakic, P.S. (1988). Topography of cognition: Parallel and distributed networks in primate association cortex. Annual Reviews of Neuroscience **11**, 137–156.

Jones, E.G. and Powell, T.P.S. (1970). An anatomical study of converging sensory pathways within the cerebral cortex of the monkey. Brain **93**, 793–820.

Auld, D.S., Har, S. and Quirion, R. (1998). _-Amyloid peptides as direct cholinergic neuromodulators: a missing link? Trends in Neurosciences **21**, 43–44.

Mattson, M.P. (1997). Mother's legacy: mitochondrial DNA mutations and Alzheimer's disease. Trends in Neurosciences 20, 373–375.

Miller, R. (1989). Schizophrenia as a progressive disorder: Relation to EEG, CT, neuropathological and other evidence. Progress in Neurobiology **33**, 17–44.

Neve, R.L. and Robakis, N.K. (1998). Alzheimer's disease: a re-examination of the amyloid hypothesis. Trends in Neurosciences **21**, 15–19.

Pandya, D.N. and Selzer, B. (1982). Association areas of the cerebral cortex. Trends in Neurosciences **5**, 386–390.

Parnavelas, J.G. and Papadopoulos, G.C. (1989). The monoaminergic innervation of the cerebral cortex is not diffuse and nonspecific. Trends in Neurosciences **12**, 315–319.

Posner, M.I. and Petersen, F.E. (1990). The attention system of the human brain. Annual Reviews of Neuroscience **13**, 25–42.

Ross, E.D. (1984). The right hemisphere's role in language, affective behavior and emotion. Trends in Neurosciences **7**, 342–346.

Swindale, N.V. (1990). Is the cerebral cortex modular? Trends in Neurosciences **13**, 487–492.

van Ree, J.M. and Matthysse, S. (1986). Psychiatric disorders: Neurotransmitters and neuropeptides. Progress in Brain Research **65**, 1–28.

Wall, J.T. (1988). Variable organization in cortical maps of the skin as an indication of the lifelong adaptive capacities of the circuits in the mammalian brain. Trends in Neurosciences **11**, 549–558.

Weinberger, D. (1988). Schizophrenia and the frontal lobes. Trends in Neurosciences **11**, 367–370.

Weiss, S., Reynolds, B.A., Vescovi, A.L., Morshead, C., Craig, C.G. and van der Kooy, D. (1996). Is there a neural stem cell in the mammalian brain? Trends in Neurosciences **19**, 387–393.

Woods. B.T. (1983). Is the left hemisphere specialized for language at birth? Trends in Neurosciences **6**, 115–117.

Glossary of Terms

abasia
inability to walk without falling i.e. cannot maintain equilibrium due to damage to the **flocculonodular node** of the **cerebellum** (see also **astasia**)

abducens
means drawing away

abducens
6th cranial nerve; controls the lateral rectus muscle of the eye that drives the direction of the gaze away from the midline

ablation
(means carried away) removal by cutting of a part of the body or diseased tissue or organ

accessory
means an appendage (something added on)

accessory nerve
(also called spinal accessory or 11th **cranial nerve**) essential for certain movements of shoulder and head, and for swallowing and speech

accommodation
ability of a system or tissue (usually nervous) to adjust or adapt so that it no longer responds to a previous stimulus, whose duration and/or intensity needs to be increased to elicit the same response

acetylcholine
(**ACh**) neurotransmitter chemical of the CNS and peripheral nervous system

acetylcholinesterase
(**AChE**) enzyme that inactivates acetylcholine by breaking it down to acetate and choline

acromegaly
disease caused by over-secretion of growth hormone in adults

action potential
electrical impulse transmitted across an electrically excitable cell membrane (also sometimes called action current)

adenohypophysis
see **pituitary**

ADP
adenosine diphosphate

adrenal medulla
inner portion or core of the adrenal gland; secretes **epinephrine** and **norepinephrine**

adrenaline
see **epinephrine**

adrenergic
epinephrine-containing

afferent
directed towards the center e.g. afferent nerve, which conducts electrical impulses away from the periphery towards the spinal cord or brain (see also **efferent**)

agnosia
inability to understand the significance of all sensory inputs

agonist
chemical having affinity for a specific **receptor** and producing a predictable response; or means a muscle whose contraction is opposed by an **antagonist** muscle

agraphia
inability to express thoughts in writing

akinesia
total lack of spontaneous movement

allele
one of two or more alternative forms of a gene occupying corresponding positions (loci) on **homologous chromosomes**

allocortex
ancient or phylogenetically older part of cortex (see also **paleocortex; archeocortex**)

alexia
inability to understand written words or sentences

all-or-none law
if a stimulus is strong enough to trigger an electrical impulse in an excitable membrane (nerve or muscle), it will trigger a maximal impulse i.e. there is no gradation of response (it either happens or it doesn't)

alveus	layer of white matter that covers the ventricular surface of the hippocampus
Alzheimer's disease	presenile dementia thought to be due primarily to cholinergic neurodegeneration; characterized by intra-and extracellular degenerative changes, especially in the neocortex and hippocampus
amblyopia	loss of binocular vision due to incomplete development of the lateral geniculate connections within the columns in the **visual cortex** for one of the eyes
amacrine cell	retinal nerve cell
ambiguus	name given to cranial nerve nucleus (see also **nucleus ambiguus**)
Ammon's horn	alternative name of the hippocampus
amygdala	also called the amygdaloid body or nucleus, found in the cerebral hemisphere, in the temporal lobe; part of the **basal ganglia**
anencephaly	congenital (born with) absence of brain and spinal cord
angiotensin	polypeptide in blood that forms part of the renin-angiotensin system for the control of salt/water balance
anopsia	arrested development of the eye
ANS	autonomic nervous system
antagonist	chemical with affinity for a **receptor**, opposing the action of an **agonist**; or a muscle that opposes the contraction of another muscle
anterior horn of the spinal cord	anterior projection of gray matter into white matter of the spinal cord
anterograde	(also called antegrade) means moving forward e.g. anterograde degeneration of a nerve (see also **retrograde**)
antidromic	impulse propagation along an axon in the direction opposite to the normal flow
antipyretic	able to decrease body temperature (see also **pyretic**, **pyrogen**)
apex	end, tip or top of any structure
aphasia	partial or complete inability to understand language (**sensory** or **receptive aphasia**) and/or inability to express language in speech (see **dysphasia**) or writing see **dyslexia**, **alexia**)
apraxia	impaired ability to manipulate objects or perform purposeful movements without pre-existing paralysis. It is also an impaired ability to perform speech due to brain damage (**apraxia of speech**)
aquaporin	water channel in apical cell membrane of the collecting ducts in the kidneys
aqueous humor	clear fluid that fills the anterior and posterior chambers of the eye
arachnoid	any fibrous, delicate structure reminiscent of a spider's web.
arachnoid membrane	delicate membrane (also called **arachnoid mater**) that surrounds the brain and spinal cord. The part surrounding the brain is also called the **arachnoid of the brain** or **arachnoidea encephali**; that part surrounding the spinal cord is called the **arachnoid of the spinal cord** or **arachnoidea spinalis**

archeocortex	phylogenetically older cortex, consisting of three layers, found mainly in dentate gyrus and hippocampus (see also **allocortex**; **paleocortex**)
archicerebellum	phylogenetically older part of the cerebellum, also referred to as **archeocerebellum**; controls body equilibrium (see **paleocerebellum**)
arcuate nucleus	nucleus of neuronal cells in the basal **hypothalamus**, concerned with the control of reproductive function
area postrema	caudal part of the floor of the 4th ventricle; relatively permeable part of the blood-brain barrier
association areas	areas of the cerebral cortex not believed to receive direct sensory inputs or send outputs to motoneurons, but communicate with other cerebrocortical areas
associative learning	learning through the experimental procedure of pairing of two more events (see also **learning**; **non-associative learning**)
astasia	inability to stand or sit without falling due to damage to the **flocculonodular node** of the **cerebellum** (see also **abasia**)
astrocyte	large, star-shaped neuroglial cell
ataxia	impaired ability to co-ordinate motor activity, due to cerebellar or spinal cord lesion, or can be hereditary
atheroma	abnormal deposition of lipid on lining of arterial wall
athetoid	refers to **athetosis**; a disease characterized by uncontrollable writhing of distal limbs, caused by lesions in the **basal ganglia** that may cause a disturbance of normally inhibitory pallidothalamic pathways (see also ballismus)
ATP	adenosine triphosphate
atresia	absence of normal body opening, such as the external ear, anus or vagina
atrophy	shrinking or wasting of a tissue, organ or limb
auditory	associated with the special sense of hearing
auditory cortex	(primary auditory cortex) area of the **cerebral cortex** that is the final destination for auditory inputs; situated in the floor of the lateral sulcus in the superior **temporal gyrus**
autism	poorly understood mental disorder that presents in childhood, usually before age three, in which the child becomes withdrawn, uncommunicative and seems to be absorbed in fantasy; usually associated with enlarged temporal lobes and abnormal EEG patterns
autoreceptors	receptors on a nerve terminal, usually presynaptic, that, when acted on by the released neurotransmitter, limit the further release of the neurotransmitter
autonomic	property of independent function without inputs (hence the autonomic nervous system is incorrectly named)
autonomic N.S.	N.S. stands for nervous system; the A.N.S. regulates involuntary activity, and is composed of parasympathetic and sympathetic divisions
autoradiography	also called **radioautography**; detection of radioactive isotopes in tissue sections

autosome	chromosome that is not a sex chromosome
autosomal	refers to the characteristics of an autosome, or a property conferred by it
axoaxonic	synapse where the axon of one neuron contacts the axon of another neuron
axodendritic	synapse where the axon of a neuron contacts dendrites, usually of another neuron
axolemma	another name for the axon plasma membrane
axon	cylindrical process of the nerve cell, which conducts the electrical impulse generated in the cell body away to another cell
axon hillock	area of the neuron cell body (other terms for the cell body are: **perikaryon**, **soma**) where the axon arises, and where the nerve impulse is generated
axon reaction	degenerative changes in axons and cell bodies of damaged nerves
axon reflex	(not a true reflex arc) when an impulse travels along an axon, reaches a branch and then travels to a target organ such as skin, without entering another nerve cell body; an example is flushing i.e. vasodilation of skin when skin is stimulated e.g. by a nettle sting
axoplasm	cytoplasm of the axon
axoplasmic flow	pulsatile flow of cytoplasm from the soma to the axon, supplying it with necessary metabolites to maintain axon integrity
axosomatic	synapse where a nerve axon contacts a cell body
ballismus	(**ballism**) **basal ganglia** lesion causing involuntary (ballistic) jerking of upper or lower limb (see also **athetoid**)
bands of Baillarger	fiber bands in the **cerebral cortex**
baroreceptor	pressure-sensitive nerve ending in the aortic arch, atria of the heart, carotid sinus and vena cava
basal ganglia	also called basal nuclei; bilateral masses of gray matter within each **cerebral hemisphere**, composed of the **amygdaloid nucleus**, **claustrum** and **corpus striatum**
basement membrane	non-cellular tissue layer that underlies and secures overlying epithelium
basilar membrane	membrane throughout the **cochlea** that partitions it
behavior	motor expression of motivation
binocular zone	central zone of the retinal **visual field** constructed by left and right retinae (see also **monocular zone**)
biopsy	removal of small fragment of living tissue for examination
bipolar depression	mental disorder in which mood oscillates between mania and depression (see unipolar depression)
blind spot	see optic disc
bovine spongiform encephalopathy	(**BSE**); one of a group of **transmissible spongiform encephalopathies** (**TSE**)
brachial	means an arm or like an arm
brady	means slow e.g. **bradykinesia, bradykinin**
bradycardia	slow-beating heart
bradykinesia	abnormally slow voluntary movements, in, for example, **Parkinsonism**

bradykinin	endogenous peptide causing vasodilation; slow-acting, hence the name
brain	part of central nervous system contained within the bony cranium
brainstem	part of the brain consisting of the medulla oblongata, pons and mesencephalon
Broca's area	area of the inferior frontal gyrus of the frontal lobe, identified by the French anthropologist and pathologist **Pierre Paul Broca** as the motor speech area of the brain, which when damaged impaired or destroyed the power of speech, although the patient still understood speech (see **Wernicke's area**)
Brodmann's map	a cytoarchitectural map of the surface of the cerebral cortex by the German neuropsychiatrist **Korbinian Brodmann**, based on the microscopic structure and arrangement of nerve cells; still very useful and widely referred to
bromocriptine	dopamine receptor **agonist**
BSE	see **bovine spongiform encephalopathy**
calcarine	means shaped like a spur e.g. calcarine cortex, calcarine fissure
capacitor	reservoir of stored charge
catecholamine	chemical name for an aliphatic amine with an attached catechol group; examples are **epinephrine** and **norepinephrine**
cauda aquina	(means horse's tail) the lower end of the spinal cord, where lumbar, sacral and coccygeal spinal nerve roots emerge from the spinal cord
caudal	towards the distal (tail) end of the body
caudate nucleus	crescent-shaped mass of gray matter, part of the **corpus striatum**, situated lateral to the thalamus in the floor of the third ventricle
cell nuclei	(often confusing) can mean the nucleus of a single cell; in nerves, the nucleus is found in the cell body or perikaryon; also can mean a clump of nerve cell bodies e.g. the **arcuate nucleus** in the **hypothalamus**
cells of Martinotti	multipolar cells in the cerebral cortex
central canal	canal or conduit running the length of the spinal cord, lying centrally between the ventral and dorsal commissures; it opens out in the medulla oblongata into the 4th ventricle
central nervous system (CNS)	division of nervous system consisting of brain and spinal cord
central sulcus	deep groove dividing the cerebrum into cerebral hemispheres
cerebellum	part of brain behind the brainstem, located in the posterior cranial fossa; concerned with integration of motor function
cerebral	referring to the cerebrum
cerebral cortex	layer of gray matter lying on the surface of the cerebral hemisphere
cerebral dominance	specialization of a cerebral hemisphere for a specific structure or certain functions
cerebral hemisphere	one half of the cerebrum

cerebral aqueduct	(also called aqueduct of Sylvius) narrow passage for cerebrospinal fluid between the 3rd and 4th **ventricles** in the **midbrain**
cerebral peduncles	bilateral pair of pillars of nerve fiber bundles that project from the rostral **pons** to the left and right **hemispheres**
cerebroside	member of a group of glycolipids found in nervous tissue, particularly in myelin
cerebrospinal	refers to anything involving the brain and spinal cord
cerebrospinal fluid (CSF)	fluid flowing through the spinal canal, subarachnoid space, and ventricles of the brain
cerebrospinal pressure	pressure of CSF in the CNS, typically 100–150 mm of H_2O
cerebrovascular	referring to cerebral blood vessels and blood supply
cerebrum	largest and most rostral part of the brain, consisting of the two cerebral hemispheres, connected by the corpus callosum
cervical flexure	bending of the human fetal brain between the spinal cord and hindbrain
chiasm	means lines that cross (often used as **chiasma**)
chordotomy	(also called **cordotomy**) surgical operation to divide the spinoreticular and spinothalamic tracts, in order to reduce intractable pain
chorea	Greek word meaning a dance; rapid, involuntary, apparently purposeless movements e.g. **Huntington's chorea**
choreiform movements	jerky, rapid involuntary movements, usually caused by lesions of the **basal ganglia** (see also **athetoid**, **ballismus**)
choroid	thin, delicate, highly vascularized membrane e.g. **choroid plexus** in the brain ventricles, or choroid membrane covering part of the eye between the sclera and the retina
chromatolysis	degenerative changes in the damaged neuronal cell body
ciliary body	thickened portion of the vascular tunic of the eye; joins the **iris** with the anterior part of the choroid; contains the circular **ciliary muscles**
ciliary muscles	circular bands of semitransparent smooth muscle fibers that are attached to the **choroid** of the eye. When they contract they relax the suspensory ligaments attached to the crystalline lens, which allows the lens to become more convex, and thus accommodate for near vision.
cingulate	means having a girdle e.g. cingulate gyrus
cingulum	bundle of association fibers in the white matter of the cingulate gyrus
circle of Willis	vascular network at the base of the brain, formed by interconnection of anterior cerebral, anterior communicating, internal carotid, posterior cerebral and posterior communicating arteries; named after an English physician, **Thomas Willis**, born 1621 and a founder of the British Royal Society
circuit of Papez	essentially correct circuit that mediates emotion, proposed by the American anatomist **John Papez** in 1937
claustrum	thin sheet of gray matter situated lateral to the **internal capsule** and separating it from the white matter of the **insula**

CNS	central nervous system
cochlea	(means snail shell) bony conical structure resembling a snail shell in the inner ear; constructed as a spiral tunnel of graded diameter approximately 3 cm long
cochlear nerve	a principal division of the 8th cranial nerve that carries electrical impulses generated by the cochlea to the brain stem **cochlear nuclei**
colliculus	means a swelling; e.g. swelling of the **inferior** and **superior colliculi** (also called the **corpora quadrigemina**) comprising the midbrain tectum; also the **facial colliculus** on the floor of the 4th ventricle
commissure	here, means band of nerve fibers connecting the two hemispheres, or the two sides of the spinal cord
conditioned response	automatic reaction learned through training with use of an applied stimulus (see also **unconditioned response**)
conditioned stimulus	stimulus designed by the experimenter e.g. a bell ringing or a flash of light (see also **unconditioned stimulus**)
conditioning	stereotyped responses to an applied stimulus
conduction aphasia	language disorder caused by lesions in the supramarginal gyrus, when patients cannot write dictated language, although hearing is normal and patients can copy written language.
cone cells	photoreceptor cells in the retina that detect colors (see also **rods**)
congenital	means born with
conjugate movements	identical movements of the two eyes (see **disconjugate movements**)
conjunctiva	specialized epithelium that covers the sclera
connexons	pairs of cylinders composed of **connexins** that make up the **electrical gap junction**
contralateral	on the opposite side (see **ipsilateral**)
cornea	transparent, convex layer of tissue that allows light to pass into the eye
corona radiata	(corona means crown) a spreading network of fibers radiating out from the internal capsule to the cerebral cortex
corpus callosum	principal commissure of the **cerebral hemispheres**
corpus striatum	means striped body; bilateral mass of gray matter lateral to the **thalamus**, important in motor function, and divided almost completely by the **internal capsule** into the **caudate nucleus** and **lentiform nucleus**
cranial nerves	12 pairs of nerves that emerge from the cranial cavity
craniopharyngioma	congenital pituitary tumor consisting of remnants of **Rathke's pouch** after development of the **pituitary** gland
cranium	see **skull**
Creutzfeldt-Jakob disease	(**CJD**) one of a group of transmissible **spongiform encephalopathies** (**TSE**)
crus	means a leg, or structure resembling a leg
crus cerebri	ventral part of the **midbrain cerebral peduncle**, comprising descending fiber tracts from the **cerebral cortex** (also called the basis pedunculi cerebri)

CSF	cerebrospinal fluid
cuneate	means wedge-shaped e.g. cuneate fasciculus
cutaneous	referring to the skin
cytoarchitectonic	cellular arrangement within structures, tissues
decibel	(dB) unit of sound intensity
decussation	crossing of nerve fibers from left to right side and *vice versa*
dentate	(means toothed) e.g. cerebellar dentate nucleus, dentate gyrus in temporal lobe
dendrite	process branching out from the nerve cell body; receives incoming impulses from an axon or other dendrites
dendrodendritic	synapse where the dendrite of one neuron contacts another dendrite, usually of another neuron
denervation	prolonged interruption of nerve impulse to a target organ or tissue; denervation of skeletal muscle causes the muscle to atrophy
diencephalon	division of brain between midbrain and the cerebrum; consists of hypothalamus, thalamus, epithalamus, subthalamus and most of the third ventricle
depolarization	reduction of the **membrane potential** to a less negative value
diploid	having two sets of **homologous chromosomes**
disconjugate movements	eyes moving in opposite directions (see **conjugate movements**)
dominant gene	gene that can express itself whether or not its **allele** is different or similar (see **recessive gene**)
dopamine	(**DA**) is the major **catecholaminergic neurotransmitter** of the **CNS**
dorsal horn	dorsal (posterior) projection of gray matter into the white matter of the spinal cord
duct of Schlemm	(canal of Schlemm) drains the aqueous humor from the anterior chamber (see **glaucoma**)
dura mater	tough outer membrane, part of the **meninges,** surrounding the spinal cord and brain
dysgraphia	impaired ability to write
dyskinesia	impaired ability to execute voluntary movement
dyslexia	impaired ability to read
dyssynergia	(also called decomposition of movement) partial or complete loss of co-ordinated movement e.g. **ataxia**)
eardrum	see **tympanic membrane**
ectoderm	the outermost (dorsal) of the three primary embryonic cell layers; gives rise to the **nervous system**, special sense organs e.g. eyes, the epidermal tissues e.g. skin glands, nails, hair, and mucous membranes of anus and mouth (see also **endoderm, mesoderm**)
efferent	directed away from the center e.g. **efferent nerve**, which conducts electrical impulses away from the brain or spinal cord (see also **afferent**)
ejaculation	explosive emission of semen from the male urethra

electrical gap junction	junction between two cells where the electrical impulse is transmitted electrically
electrical synapse	junction between two cells across which an electrical impulse is transmitted directly without transduction to chemical neurotransmitter
electrocardiogram	the graphic output produced by an **electrocardiograph**
electrocardiograph	machine that records the passage of the electrical impulse through cardiac tissue through electrodes placed on the skin of the chest
electroencephalogram	the graphic output produced by an **electroencephalograph**
electroencephalograph	machine that records brain electrical activity through electrodes placed on the scalp
emboliform nucleus	nucleus deeply situated in the cerebellar medulla
embryo	in humans, the developmental stage between two weeks after conception and the end of the 7th or 8th week of pregnancy (see also **fetus**)
endoderm	innermost of the three primary embryonic cell layers; gives rise to (e.g.) epithelium of gut, respiratory tissue, urinary bladder, liver, pancreas, thyroid, and forms the lining of body cavities and the outer coat of most of the internal organs (see also **ectoderm**, **mesoderm**)
endolymph	potassium-rich fluid that fills the **cochlear duct** and the **semicircular canals** (see also **perilymph**)
endoneurium	connective sheath surrounding an individual nerve fiber
endorphins	**pituitary** neuropeptides that reduce pain
end plate potential	(**EPP**) depolarization of the postsynaptic membrane by the neurotransmitter (see also **miniature end plate potential**)
enkephalins	pain-alleviating pentapeptides discovered in brain, pituitary and gut; they bind to morphine-sensitive receptors
enzyme	protein that catalyzes chemical reactions i.e. reduces the energy level required to initiate and sustain the reaction, and thereby makes life possible at 37°C
entorrhinal cortex	(Brodmann area 28) part of the lateral olfactory cortex in the temporal lobe
ependyma	(means upper garment) layer of ciliated epithelium lining the spinal cord central canal and brain **ventricles**
epilepsy	group of neurological disorders involving recurrent electrical discharges from foci in the cerebral cortex, resulting in seizures of variable severity; the causes are variable, but most seem to involve trauma to the tissue as the primary cause
epinephrine	main **catecholamine** secreted by the **adrenal medulla** and by **adrenergic** nerve terminals (called **adrenaline** in UK)
epineurium	connective tissue sheath that surrounds a nerve of the peripheral nervous system
epiphysis	see **pineal body**
epithalamus	part of the **diencephalon** above the **thalamus**; includes the posterior **commissure** and **pineal** body

EPSP	see excitatory postsynaptic potential
erection	swelling of the penis and (to a lesser extent) the clitoris due to engorgement with blood
excitatory post-synaptic potential	(**EPSP**) depolarization of the postsynaptic membrane caused by the neurotransmitter i.e. membrane potential becomes less negative (see also **IPSP**)
exteroceptor	sensory nerve ending in mucous membranes, skin and sense organs that respond to stimuli originating outside the body (see also **interoceptor**, **proprioceptor**)
extinction	loss of effectiveness of a conditioned stimulus
extradural space	space outside the dura mater (membrane)
extrapyramidal	refers to structures associated with movement apart from the **motor cortex**, cerebrospinal **pyramidal** tracts, corticobulbar tracts and **motoneurons**
extrinsic	(means outside) refers to anything originating outside a tissue, organ or organism
facial	refers to the face
facial colliculus	swelling in floor of 4th ventricle at inferior end of the median eminence, caused by the **facial nerve** winding around the root of the **abducens** nerve
facial nerve	7th **cranial nerve**; sensorimotor cranial nerve innervating the eyelids, forehead, scalp and muscles of the cheeks and jaw; essential for facial expression
fasciculus	small bundle of muscle, nerve or tendon fibers
fastigial nucleus	nucleus buried deeply in the cerebellar medulla
fetus	term for unborn animal when it attains its form as seen at birth; in humans, from about the 8th week until birth (see also **embryo**)
fimbria	bundle of nerve fibers at the medial border of the **hippocampus**; the fimbria becomes continuous with the **fornix**
fissure	groove or cleft
flocculus	means like wool; phylogenetically oldest part of the **cerebellum**
foramen	aperture, opening or passage in bone or membrane, through which (e.g.) nerve or blood vessel pass
foramen magnum	aperture in occipital bone through which the spinal cord enters the bony spinal (vertebral) column
foramen of Monro	passage between the third and lateral ventricles of the brain
fornix	nerve fiber tract that leaves the **hippocampus**, curves of the **thalamus** and terminates in the hypothalamic **mamillary body**
fovea	means a depression e.g. the fovea (also called fovea centralis) of the retina where **cone cells** are concentrated
fractured somatotopy	fragmented somatotopic representation of the body in a brain area e.g. the **cerebellum**, where a part of the body may be represented in more than one area
frontal lobe	lies beneath the frontal bone of the skull; largest of the lobes of each **cerebral hemisphere**
frontal plane	perpendicular plane dividing body into front and back parts (see **horizontal plane, sagittal plane**)

fusiform	means like a spindle; tapered at both ends e.g. fusiform cells of the **cerebral cortex**
GABA	gamma-aminobutyric acid; an inhibitory **neurotransmitter**
ganglion	group or knot of cells outside the CNS; plural: **ganglia**
genu	means knee; describes bend in nervous tissue tracts e.g. genu of the **corpus callosum**
Gerstmann-Sträussler-Scheinker disease	(**GSS**) one of a group of transmissible **spongiform encephalopathies** (**TSE**)
Golgi neuron	cerebellar neuron named after **Camillo Golgi**, an Italian anatomist
glabrous	smooth e.g. glabrous (hairless) skin
glaucoma	elevated pressure in eye due to obstruction of the canal of Schlemm
globose nucleus	nucleus deeply buried in the cerebellar medulla
globus pallidus	medial, smaller part of the **lentiform nucleus**; divided into external and internal parts, and separated from the **putamen** by the lateral medullary lamina
glossopharyngeal	means tongue and throat (pharynx)
glossopharyngeal nerve	9th **cranial nerve**; essential for special sense of **taste**, and for some salivary secretion and some visceral sensation
gracile	means slender e.g. gracile fasciculus in spinal cord
gray matter	also called gray substance; inner core of spinal cord; contains mainly cell nuclei and interneurons
gray rami communicantes	unmyelinated postganglionic nerve fiber bundles of the sympathetic nervous system return to the spinal nerve through the **gray rami communicantes** (called gray because they are unmyelinated; see also **white rami communicantes**)
growth cone	growing tip of a developing or proximal end of a regenerating nerve **axon**
gustation	sense of tasting foods
gyrus	convolutions on the surface of the **brain** due to cortical infolding
habituation	a type of **non-associative learning**; attenuation of a behavioral response to repeated application of a non-noxious stimulus
hair cell	ciliated cell in the sensory epithelium of the vestibular apparatus, innervated by the vestibular nerve; transduces movement of the **endolymph** into an electrical impulse
Hebbian synapse	synaptic system in which repeated activity in one presynaptic system increases activity in another; a neuronal basis for explanation of **Pavlovian conditioning**; named after the neuroscientist **D.O. Hebb**
helicotrema	hole at the apical end of the basilar membrane through which sound waves can pass from the scala vestibuli to the scala tympani of the **cochlea**
hemiparesis	muscular weakness on one side of the body
hemiplegia	unilateral paralysis i.e. on one side of the body only
heterotropic inhibition	release of one **neurotransmitter** reciprocally inhibits the release of another
hippocampal	adjective meaning anything pertaining to the hippocampus

hippocampus	(means a sea-horse or sea-monster) curved elevation of the floor of the lateral ventricle; part of the limbic system known to be concerned with emotion and memory
homeostasis	condition of constancy or stability in the body when changes in, for example, temperature and pH, are resisted, and values are kept within narrow limits
homologous	any two chromosomes within the **diploid** complement of a somatic cell having identical loci, shape and size
homunculus	means little man; representation of the human form superimposed over neuronal structures
horizontal cells of Cajal	cells in superficial layers of the cerebral cortex; named after the Spanish neuroanatomist **Ramon y Cajal**
horizontal plane	plane parallel to the horizon that divides the body or organ into upper and lower parts (see **frontal plane**; **sagittal plane**)
hydrocephalus	abnormal accumulation of cerebrospinal fluid within the cranial vault, causing abnormal dilatation of the ventricles
5-hydroxytryptamine	(**5-HT**) indolamine **neurotransmitter** and constituent of platelets, enterochromaffin cells and mast cells (see also serotonin)
hyper-	prefix meaning above, beyond or excessive
hyperphagia	eating to excess
hyperpolarization	increasing the **membrane potential** to a more negative value
hypo-	prefix meaning beneath or below
hypoglossal	means under the tongue
hypoglossal nerve	12th cranial nerve; essential for moving the tongue and swallowing
hypothalamus	brain area within the **diencephalon**; forms part of the lateral wall and floor of the 3rd **ventricle**
hypophysis	see **pituitary**
iatrogenic	medical problems induced by medical treatment
ICP	intracranial pressure
incus	ossicle (small bone) in middle ear resembling an anvil (see also **malleus**, **stapes**)
inferior colliculi	swellings on posterior surface of midbrain, composing lower auditory centers(see also **colliculus; superior colliculi**)
infundibulum	means funnel; e.g. funnel-shaped stalk from the posterior pituitary gland
inhibitory post-synaptic potential	(**IPSP**) hyperpolarization of the postsynaptic membrane caused by the neurotransmitter i.e. membrane potential becomes more negative (see also **EPSP**)
instrumental learning	(sometimes called trial-and-error or **operant conditioning**) a form of **associative learning**; through trial and error it is learned that a maneuver will elicit a reward or noxious response
insula	(means an island) area of **cerebral cortex** obscured from view, which lies at the base of the lateral **sulcus**; concerned (e.g.) with **olfaction** (smell) and **gustation** (tasting foods)
interneuron	(usually) short neuron interposed between two other neurons; common in the CNS

interoceptor	sensory nerve ending in the viscera that responds to internal stimuli related to internal organ function, e.g. respiration, circulation, digestion and excretion (see also **exteroceptor, proprioceptor**)
intrafusal muscle fiber	striated muscle fiber in muscle spindle
interstitial	refers to the spaces between **tissues e.g. interstitial fluid, interstitial cells (of testis)**
intrinsic	(means inside) refers to anything originating inside a tissue, organ or organism; **extrinsic** (means outside) refers to anything originating outside a tissue,
ion channels	integral membrane proteins that make possible the passage of ions across a membrane down their electrochemical transmembrane gradients
ipsilateral	on the same side (see **contralateral**)
iris	contractile, circular disc, situated between the cornea and the lens, suspended in aqueous humor; the iris regulates the amount of light allowed through the cornea
kinesthesia	awareness of one's own body weight, parts and movement
kinocilium	terminal cilium at one end of the apex of the **hair cell**
Klüver-Bucy syndrome	caused by bilateral lesions of the amygdaloid nuclei during temporal lobe surgery or trauma; patients are docile, may eat to excess (**hyperphagia**) and may no longer recognize objects by sight, touch or hearing
Korsakoff syndrome	amnesia (memory loss) due to alcoholism resulting in damage to the mamillary bodies, frontal cortex and medial dorsal nucleus of the thalamus
Kuru	one of a group of **transmissible spongiform encephalopathies** (**TSE**) described in 1957 in tribesmen in New Guinea, who ritually ate human brains
lamina	thin, flat layer
lateral geniculate body	elevation of the posterior lateral **thalamus** that receives impulses from the **retina** via the **optic** nerve and relays the information to the **visual cortex**
lateral horn	lateral projection of gray matter into the white matter of the spinal cord
learning	acquisition of knowledge from the external environment (see also **associative learning, non-associative learning**)
leminscus	tract of nerve fibers in the CNS, especially the ascending fibers of the lemniscal system
lentiform nucleus	means lens-shaped; part of the corpus striatum
lesion	injury or wound to any tissue, including abnormality such as a tumor or eruption
locus ceruleus	bilateral area of heavy dark-blue pigmented neuronal cell bodies on each side of the floor of the 4th ventricle; the pigment is **melanin**, and the neurons are part of a **noradrenergic** pathway in the CNS

long-term potentiation	(**LTP**) process whereby presynaptic activity promotes the development of prolonged neuronal activity in a circuit; a proposed basis of forms of memory (see also **Hebbian synapses**)
lumbar	defines the region of the body between the thoracic region and the pelvis
lumbar puncture	insertion of a hollow needle and stylet into the subarachnoid space to remove cerebrospinal fluid (CSF) or to measure CSF pressure, or to inject (e.g.) oxygen, air or radio-opaque substances
macrosmatic	describes animals with a highly developed sense of smell (see **microsmatic**)
malleus	ossicle (small bone) in middle ear resembling a hammer (see also **incus**, **stapes**)
mamillary bodies	swellings on ventral surface of the hypothalamus
mastication	chewing
M-cells	a type of retinal ganglion cell that may discriminate illumination contrasts and movement (see also **P-cells**)
mechanoreceptors	sensory receptors that fire off after mechanical deformation
medial	means towards the midline (middle) of the body
medial geniculate body (nucleus)	elevation of the dorsal posterior **thalamus** that receives auditory inputs and relays the information to the primary **auditory cortex** n the superior temporal **gyrus**
medulla oblongata	bulbous continuation of the spinal cord just above the foramen magnum, containing vital centers for life
melanin	dark brown or black pigment that gives color to iris and choroid of the eye, and to hair and skin
melanocyte	cell that synthesizes **melanin**
melanocyte-stimulating hormone	(MSH) polypeptide secreted by the **pituitary** gland
melatonin	hormone secreted into circulation by the **pineal body**; may be involved in bodily rhythms and has been used for 'jet-lag'
meninges	the three membranes enclosing the brain and spinal cord, comprising pia mater, arachnoid mater and dura mater
mesencephalon	also called the midbrain; the second of the three brain **vesicles**
mesoderm	middle of the three primary embryonic cell layers; lies between ectoderm and endoderm, and gives rise to (e.g.) bone, blood, lymphatic tissue, muscle, vascular tissue and the peritoneal and pericardial pleurae (see also **ectoderm**, **endoderm**)
metastatic	spread of malignant tumor cells throughout the body
metencephalon	anterior part of the embryonic **rhombencephalon;** develops ventrally into the **pons**, and dorsally into the **cerebellum**
microsmatic	describes animals with a poorly developed sense of smell (see **macrosmatic**)
midbrain	see **mesencephalon**
microglia	neuroglial cell of CNS with phagocytic function
middle ear	cavity in the ear bounded by the **tympanic membrane** and the **oval window**, containing the ossicles

miniature end plate potential	(**MEPP**) small potentials on the postsynaptic membrane caused by continuous release of small quanta (amounts) of neurotransmitter
monoamine oxidase	(**MAO**) presynaptic enzyme that metabolizes **catecholamine neurotransmitters;** there are two forms of MAO: **A** and **B**
monoamine oxidase inhibitors	(**MAOI**) largely obsolescent antidepressants that inhibit the action of **MAO**
monocular zone	crescent-shaped visual field constructed by each retina alone (see also **binocular zone**)
motoneuron	efferent nerve cell whose axon transmits electrical impulses from brain or spinal cord to effector organ, usually glandular tissue or muscle
M-pathway	(M-stream) pathway of inputs from retinal **M cells** to the posterior parietal cortex
multiple sclerosis	progressive demyelination of nerve fibers of brain and spinal cord
muscarinic receptors	receptors that bind **ACh**; so-called because they were originally described using muscarine from the fungus *Amanita muscaria*
muscle spindle	specialized sensory proprioceptor organ
myasthenia gravis	muscle weakness, especially in face and throat due to defective neurotransmission at the **neuromuscular junction**
myelencephalon	posterior part of embryonic hindbrain, where the **medulla oblongata** develops
myelin	fatty sheath coating axons of some nerve fibers
myelinated	has a myelin sheath
myelomeningocele	(also called meningomyelocele) failure of embryonic neural tube to close, resulting in herniation of part of the spinal cord through a cleft in the vertebral column
myenteric plexus	group of **autonomic ganglia** and **nerve fibers** in the muscular intestinal coat
nascent	newly formed e.g. nascent **CSF**
neocortex	phylogenetically youngest part of the brain; in humans consists of all cerebral cortex tissue except for **hippocampal** and **pyriform** cortex
neostratum	see **striatum**
Nernst equation	equation that relates the concentration ratio between permeable ions on both sides of a membrane with the electric potential across the membrane
nerve	electrical cable of the nervous system, consisting of bundles of **nerve fibers** that carry electrical impulses
nerve fiber	single conducting unit of the nerve, consisting of the **axon**, and it may be **myelinated** or **unmyelinated**
nerve growth factor	(**NGF**) a polypeptide, similar in structure to insulin, that promotes neuronal differentiation, growth and maintenance
nerve plexus	intersecting or interwoven network of nerves
neural crest	band of cells, derived from ectoderm, that lies along each side of the embryonic **neural tube**; neural crest cells migrate through the embryo and give rise to some of the **ganglia**

neural fold	(also called medullary fold) one of the two longitudinal folds or lips produced by the invagination of the **neural plate**
neural groove	(also called medullary groove) longitudinal depression formed by the folding of the **neural folds**
neural plate	(also called medullary plate) thick layer of ectoderm lying along the central axis of the fetus, which gives rise to the **neural tube**
neural tube	longitudinal tube formed by fusion of **neural folds** which in turn result from the invagination of the **neural plate**; gives rise to the **brain**, **spinal cord** and all other neural tissue of the CNS
neuroglia	traditionally considered the supporting tissues of CNS; now thought to interact functionally with neurons and modulate their activity
neurohypophysis	see **pituitary**
neurolemma	layer of **Schwann cells** enclosing the **myelin sheath**
neurolepsis	a state of consciousness, characterized by indifference, reduced motor activity and acquiescence
neuroleptic	an agent (usually a drug) that produces neurolepsis in disturbed psychiatric patients
neuromuscular junction	area where nerve terminal meets muscle, and where impulse information is chemically transferred from nerve to muscle by a **neurotransmitter**
neuropores	openings at cranial and caudal ends of the fused embryonic **neural tube**
neurotransmitter	chemical released from nerve terminal into the **synaptic cleft** between the nerve, another nerve or a target organ such as muscle or gland
nicotinic receptor	(anachronistic name) receptor where ACh is an agonist; so-called because nicotine was originally used to identify them
nociceptive	refers to a painful stimulus and pain-mediating mechanisms
node of Ranvier	myelin-free regions between myelin sheaths on nerve where sodium channels are concentrated; **action potentials** jump from one node to the next (see **saltatory conduction**); named after the French histologist **Louis-Antoine Ranvier**
non-associative learning	learning through the repeated application of a stimulus (see also **learning**; **associative learning**)
noradrenaline	see **norepinephrine**
noradrenergic norepinephrine	containing (e.g. noradrenergic neuron)
norepinephrine	a **catecholamine** secreted by **noradrenergic** nerve terminals and from the **adrenal** medulla (called **noradrenaline** in UK)
notochord	fetal longitudinal strip of mesodermal tissue running along the developing embryo; forerunner of the vertebrae
nuclear bag fiber	type of **muscle spindle** fiber
nuclear chain fiber	type of **muscle spindle** fiber
nucleus	can mean a subcellular compartment of a cell, containing genetic information as DNA; in Neuroscience also means a clump of neuronal cells in the CNS, often a functional unit e.g. **arcuate nucleus**
nucleus basalis	see **substantia inominata**

nystagmus	involuntary eye movement
obex	apex of the inferior part of the 4th **ventricle**
ocular dominance	occurs in cell columns in the **visual cortex** which receive inputs from only one eye
oculomotor nerve	3rd cranial nerve; supplies medial, inferior and oblique rectus muscles of the eye
olfaction	sense of smell
oligodendrocyte	neuroglial cell whose processes coil round neuronal axons; the processes become the myelin sheath
oligodendroglia	neuroglial CNS cells that produce myelin
olive	olive-shaped swelling situated bilaterally on the **medulla oblongata;** a collection of **olivary nuclei** consisting of the accessory, inferior and superior olivary nuclei
ontogeny	period of differentiation and growth
operant behavior	see **associative learning**
operculum	(means a covering or lid) part of the **temporal cerebral hemisphere** that overlaps the **insula**
opiate	narcotic substance that contains opium or natural or synthetic derivatives of opium
opioid	natural or synthetic substance with opium-like effects, although not derived from opium
optic	pertaining to eyes or sight
optic chiasma	(also called optic chiasm) point of **decussation** (crossing over) of some of the optic nerves at the base of the brain
optic disc	area adjacent to the **fovea** on the **retina** where ganglion axons converge; also called the blind spot because it has no **photoreceptors**
optic nerve	one of a pair of **cranial nerves** that arise in the ganglion cell layer of the **retina** in the eye and which transmit optical information to the **visual cortex**
optokinetic movements	impression that you are moving backwards even when stationary when something (e.g. a train alongside you) is moving forwards
organ of Corti	organ of hearing in **scala media** of the **cochlea**; it transduces sound waves into electrical impulses
oval window	oval aperture in the wall that separates the **middle** and **inner ear**; the footplate of the **stapes** vibrates against the oval window and transfers sound waves through the window to the **cochlea**
OVLT	**organum vasculosum of the lamina terminalis**; a structure in the wall of the 3rd ventricle that may mediate water balance through **vasopressin** signals
oxytocin	hormone secreted into the circulation by the posterior **pituitary**; causes milk ejection and uterine contraction
paleocerebellum	phylogenetically older portion of the **cerebellum** concerned with locomotion and postural control (see also **archeocerebellum**)
paleocortex	three-five layers of the olfactory cortex; see also **allocortex**; **archeocortex**)

paleostratum	globus pallidus; also called pallidum; phylogenetically older than the **striatum**; a component of the **basal ganglia**
parasympathetic	a division of the **autonomic nervous system** (**ANS**)
parenchyma	part of a tissue not including the connective or supporting tissues
paresis	incomplete or partial paralysis
parietal lobe	part of the mediolateral **cerebral hemisphere** covered by the parietal bone of the skull
Parkinson's disease	progressive degenerative brain disease marked by **extrapyramidal** symptoms and muscle rigidity; caused by destruction of cells in the basal ganglia
patch clamping	technique involving the sucking of a piece of membrane against a microelectrode tip to study the behavior of individual ion channels
patella	(knee cap) triangular flat bone situated at the front of the knee joint; used for the **patellar reflex**
Pavlovian conditioning	type of stimulus-reflex learning behavioral technique developed by the Russian physiologist **Ivan Petrovich Pavlov**
P-cells	a type of retinal ganglion cell that transmits information about color and acuity (see also **M-cells**)
peduncle	stalk- or stem-like connection e.g. cerebral or cerebellar peduncles
perforant path	nerve fiber tract from the entorhinal area to the dentate gyrus of the hippocampus
periaqueductal gray	(**PAG**) area of the midbrain
perikaryon	nerve cell body; usually means the cytoplasmic compartment excluding the nucleus and any processes
perilymph	fluid that separates the membranous labyrinth of the inner ear from the osseous labyrinth (see also **endolymph**)
perineurium	connective tissue sheath encasing a bundle of peripheral nerve fibers
peripheral nervous system	nerves and ganglia outside the brain and spinal cord
phagocytic	having the function of engulfing cellular debris and micro-organisms (see **microglia**)
phenothiazines	group of antipsychotic drugs e.g. chlorpromazine
phospholipid	substance containing fatty acids, phosphoric acid and a nitrogenous base
photon	the smallest amount of electromagnetic energy, having no charge and no mass and travels at the speed of light
photopic vision	daylight vision
phylogenetic	refers to the evolution of a species from simpler forms
photoreceptor	nerve cell responsive to light stimuli (see **rods** and **cones**)
pia mater	innermost and most delicate part of the **meninges**, closely apposed to the spinal cord, and highly vascularized
pilomotor	hair erection
pinna	external ear

pineal body	(also called the pineal gland) cone-shaped organ in the brain situated between the **pulvinar**, **splenium** of the **corpus callosum** and the **superior colliculi**; secretes **melatonin** into the circulation
pituitary	(also called the **hypophysis**) gland suspended beneath the **hypothalamus**; made up of anterior pituitary gland (**adenohypophysis**) and posterior pituitary gland (**neurohypophysis**)
planum temporale	part of **Wernicke's area** in the temporal lobe that is lateralized in size, being much larger in the left hemisphere
plexus	network of intersecting blood vessels and nerves
pons	means 'bridge'; here, a prominence on the ventral surface of the brainstem between the cerebral peduncles of the midbrain and the medulla oblongata
pontine flexure	bending of the human fetal brain in the area of the future **pons**
portal system	capillary network that carries hormones from the **hypothalamus** down the **pituitary** stalk
P-pathway	(P-stream) pathway of inputs from retinal **M-cells** to the inferior temporal cortex
projection	here means the direction forward of a nerve or nerve tract to its destination or termination site
proprioceptor	sensory receptors in the inner ear, muscle, tendons and joints that respond to changes in body movement and position
prosencephalon	(also called the forebrain) part of brain including the **diencephalon** and **telencephalon**
prosody	phenomenon whereby patients with brain lesions that destroy speech processing and understanding are still able to make sounds and sing
pseudo-conditioning	see **sensitization**
ptosis	drooping eyelid due to weakness of levator muscle or paralysis of the 3rd cranial nerve
pulvinar	part of the **thalamus** situated above the **lateral** and **medial geniculate bodies**
punctate	means pointed; here refers to point-by-point innervation of skin by nerve endings e.g. temperature sensing in skin is **punctate**
Purkinje cell	large neurons that provide efferent fibers from the **cerebral cortex**
putamen	part of the **lentiform nucleus** lateral to the **globus pallidus** in the **corpus striatum**
pyramid	describes tissue mass rising to a crest
pyramidal cell	neuron with pyramid-shaped **perykaryon** in the **cerebral cortex**
pyramidal nucleus	gray matter lying between the midline and the **olivary nucleus**; projects fibers to the cerebellar **vermis**
pyretic	able to increase body temperature (see also **antipyretic**)
pyriform	(means pear-shaped) e.g. pyriform cortex; part of the **olfactory cerebral cortex**
pyrogen	any agent that causes fever i.e. temperature rise; examples are bacterial toxins

raphe nuclei	(raphe means a seam) nuclei lying in the midline of the **midbrain**, **pons** and **medulla oblongata**
RAS	see reticular activating system
Rathke's pouch	embryonic depression in the roof of the mouth during the 4th week of embryogenesis; develops into the **anterior pituitary gland**
recessive gene	member of a pair of genes that cannot express itself in the presence of a **dominant allele** (see **dominant gene**)
receptive field	area (e.g. of skin) within which a stimulus must occur in order to activate the fiber that subserves that field
receptor	structure that receives, recognizes and may transduce a specific stimulus that may be chemical, electrical or physical
red nucleus	bilateral motor nuclei in the midbrain tegmentum; called red because of rich blood supply
referred pain	pain felt distant from the site of injury
reflex	(means to bend backward; think of a reflected image) here means a reflected movement that may be chemical, electrical or physical, and in the body is an involuntary response to a stimulus
refractory period	period during which a pulse generator such as an excitable nerve membrane is unable to respond to an incoming signal
repolarization	restoration of the **membrane potential** after **depolarization**
retina	nervous tissue; 10-layered membrane continuous with the **optic nerve** in the retina; transduces incident light into electrical impulses transmitted to the brain via the optic nerve
retinopic map	orderly arrangement of photoreceptors and associated ganglion cells in the retina that makes possible the accurate transmission of the received visual layout to the brain
reticular	like a net
reticular activating system	(**RAS**) anatomically diffuse CNS system, including the brain stem, hypothalamus thalamus and cerebral cortex that make possible attention, consciousness, introspection and wakefulness
reticular formation	diffuse, poorly understood cluster of cells in the brain stem that controls circulation, consciousness, respiration and other processes
retinal slip	inability to focus the eyes on an object when turning the head
retrograde	moving backwards e.g. retrograde degeneration of a nerve (see also **anterograde**)
Rexed's layers of The spinal cord	cytoarchitectural division of the gray matter of the spinal cord into layers or laminae, by the Swedish neuroanatomist **Bror Rexed**
rhinencephalon	term not much used these days to describe the structures of the limbic and olfactory systems
rhodopsin	purple pigment that allows the **rod** cells in the **retina** of the eye to detect light
rhombencephalon	embryonic posterior primary brain vesicle, giving rise to the **metencephalon** and **myelencephalon**
rods	cells of the retina that detect light through the pigment **rhodopsin** (see also **cones**)

rostral	(means beak-shaped) towards the front of the brain or head
rubro-	prefix meaning red; here refers to the **red nucleus**, which gives rise to (e.g.) the rubrospinal tract
saccadic eye movements	fast alteration in direction of gaze; allows gaze to focus on still object in the visual field when the head moves or turns
sagittal	anteroposterior plane; an imaginary line extending through the midline from the front of the body to the back (see **frontal plane, horizontal plane**)
sacral	referring to the sacrum, defines anatomical location of nerves
sacrum	triangular dorsal bone of the pelvis, wider and shorter in women than in men
saltatory conduction	jumping of action potentials from one node of Ranvier to another
scala media	chamber of the cochlea, containing the **organs of Corti**
scala tympani	chamber of the cochlea
scala vestibuli	chamber of the cochlea
Schwann cell	cell that forms the neurolemma
schizophrenia	(means split mind) umbrella term for a large group of mental disorders characterized by inability to grasp reality and often gross distortion of it; speech may be affected and hallucination is common; cause is unknown, but may be due to temporal lobe dysfunction and disturbance of brain dopamine metabolism
sclera	strong outer layer of connective tissue that covers the eyeball
scrapie	one of a group of **transmissible spongiform encephalopathies** (**TSE**), originally described in sheep; the term derives from the behavior of infected sheep that literally scraped off their own wool
second messenger	first chemical mediator that conveys the information that a chemical has bound to its receptor on the surface of the cell
semicircular canals	fluid-filled, bony loop-like structures in the osseous labyrinth of the inner ear
sensitization	(also called pseudoconditioning) increased response to a noxious or intense stimulus
septal area	consists of the subcallosal (beneath the **corpus callosum**) area and the paraterminal **gyrus**
septal nuclei	a group of nuclei lying beneath the septal area
septum	a partition
septum pellucidum	double membrane separating the anterior (frontal) horns of the lateral **ventricles**; separates the **corpus callosum** and the **fornix**
serotonergic	5-HT-containing)
serotonin	(see **5-hydroxytryptamine**)
skull	bony cranium of the head and skeleton of the face
smooth pursuit	movements of the eyes to track a moving object
somatic	derived from 'soma', meaning the body; anything to do with the body
somatosensory	anything to do with the sensory systems of the body
somatostatin	hormone released by the hypothalamus into the pituitary **portal system**; inhibits growth hormone release from the anterior **pituitary** gland (also called growth hormone release inhibitory hormone or GHRIH)

somatotopic	representation of the body or any of its parts in the brain
somite	one of a pair of segmented **mesodermal** tissue masses lying along the length of the neural tube early in embryogenesis;
splenium of the corpus callosum	widened posterior part of the **corpus callosum**
spina bifida	incomplete fusion of the **neural tube**; a congenital defect
spinal cord	part of the central nervous system, extending from base of foramen magnum to the upper lumbar region
spinal dysraphism	see **spina bifida**
split brain	brain in which the **corpus callosum** has been sectioned
stapes	ossicle (small bone) in middle ear resembling a stirrup (see also **incus** and **malleus**)
status epilepticus	dangerous, uninterrupted series of epileptic seizures
stellate	star-shaped e.g. stellate **neuron** or **ganglion**
stereocilia	cilia at the apex of the **hair cells** of the sensory epithelium in the **semicircular canals**
stress	(biological) any condition of tension in mind, or in physical or chemical system that requires a reaction to reduce tension
stretch receptor	sensory nerve endings in e.g. **muscle spindle** specialized to fire off when stretched
stria	means a streak
striatum	also called **neostratum** because it is phylogenetically the newest part of the corpus striatum; consists mainly of putamen and caudate nucleus
striosomes	areas within the striatum that stain negatively for **acetylcholinesterase**, but stain positively for **opioid** receptors and several neuropeptides
stripe of Gennari	thick white band of afferent inputs running through the primary visual cortex, which is why it is also called the **striate cortex**; named after the Italian physician **Francesco Gennari**, who discovered it (while still a medical student)
subfornical organ	structure in the dorsal wall of the 3rd **ventricle**; mediates drinking behavior via **angiotensin** signals
substance P	a neurotransmitter
substantia	means 'substance' e.g. **substantia gelatinosa** of spinal cord gray matter; **substantia nigra** of the midbrain
substantia gelatinosa	column of small neurons in a column that runs the length of the **spinal cord** at the apex of the **dorsal horn gray matter**
substantia inominata	area under the **anterior commissure** (**subcommissural region**); often called the basal nucleus, or **nucleus basalis** of Meynert, after the Austrian neuropsychiatrist; has widespread cholinergic projections to the cerebral cortex; of special current interest since these neurons selectively degenerate in **Alzheimer's disease**
substantia nigra	dark band of cells, many being pigmented with **melanin**, lying between the **tegmentum** and **crus cerebri**; destruction of these cells causes **Parkinson's disease**

subthalamus	lies beneath the **thalamus**; correlates optic and vestibular impulses that are relayed to the **globus pallidus**
superior colliculi	swellings on posterior surface of midbrain, comprising centers for visual reflexes (see also colliculus; inferior colliculi)
sulcus	shallow furrow or groove on the surface of the **cerebral hemisphere**
sympathetic	division of the **autonomic nervous system** (**ANS**)
synapse	junction between two nerves or nerve and effector organ where the impulse may be transmitted across chemically or electrically; word coined by the English physiologist **Charles Sherrington**
synaptic cleft	extracellular space between presynaptic nerve terminal and the postsynaptic membrane, across which the **neurotransmitter** diffuses
synaptic plasticity	property of **synapses** to change their characteristics
synaptic transmission	passage of an electrical impulse across a synapse through transduction to chemical neurotransmitter presynaptically and transduction back to electrical signal postsynaptically
syndrome	collection of symptoms
Tabes dorsalis	progressive degeneration of the body, especially the dorsal columns and roots of the spinal cord with loss of deep tendon reflexes; caused by syphilis
tardive dyskinesia	repetitive, involuntary movements, especially in the elderly; an **iatrogenic** disease caused by prolonged administration with **phenothiazines**, which disturb **CNS dopamine** metabolism; can be treated with cholinergic drugs
tectum	roof of midbrain, comprising the **inferior** and **superior colliculi**
tegmentum	dorsal part of the **pons** and most of the midbrain **cerebral peduncles**
tela choroidea	vascularized connective tissue membrane continuous with the **pia mater**
telencephalon	part of embryonic brain from which the cerebral hemispheres will develop
temporal	relates a brain structure to the temporal bone of the **skull**
tendon	fibrous, glistening white band of tissue attaching muscle to bone
tentorium cerebelli	tent-shaped extension of the **dura mater** that separates the **cerebellum** from the **occipital lobe** of the **cerebral hemispheres**
thalamus	(means wedding couch) bilateral large oval bodies, part of the **diencephalon**, making up most of the walls of the lateral **ventricle**; relay station for sensory inputs to the **cerebral cortex**
thermoregulation	control of temperature
thoracic	referring to the chest
thoracic nerves	twelve pairs of spinal nerves in thoracic region of the spinal cord
tonsil	means a small, rounded structure e.g. lymphatic tissue in the oropharynx; here, the name of a lobule that overlies the inferior **vermis** of the **cerebellum**
tract	group of tissues forming a pathway

tractus solitarius	(solitary tract) tract of visceral afferent fibers running caudally from the inferior ganglia of the **glossopharangeal** and **vagal** nerves to the solitary nucleus
transcortical sensory aphasia	a form of **Wernicke's aphasia** in which repetition is spared
transcortical motor aphasia	a **conduction aphasia**; patient can understand and repeat verbal language but cannot write dictated language
transcription	formation of RNA from a DNA template
transducer	a mechanism that converts one form of energy to another
transmissible spongiform encephalopathies	(**TSE**); a group of neurodegenerative disease (see also **BSE**)
trapezoid body	transverse network of fibers in the **pons** carrying auditory inputs
trigeminal	literally means three born together; refers to the three main divisions of the trigeminal nerve
trigone	means three-cornered
trigones	swellings in the 4th ventricle representing the nuclei of the **hypoglossal** and **vagal** nerves
trochlear	means a pulley; refers to the trochlear nerve, which passes through a pulley-like fibrous ring called the trochlea, and which innervates the superior oblique muscle of the eye
trophic support	maintenance of tissue integrity through intercellular influence e.g. muscle integrity is maintained through trophic support of its innervating neuron
TSE	see **transmissible spongiform encephalopathies**
tumor	enlargement or swelling (does not necessarily imply or mean cancer)
tympanic membrane	(also called the **eardrum**) a semi-transparent membrane, about 1 cm in diameter, that transmits sound waves from the **outer** to the **middle ear**
unconditioned response	automatic response to an **unconditioned stimulus** e.g. salivation (unconditioned response) to the sight of food (unconditioned stimulus; see also **conditioned response**)
unconditioned stimulus	(also called reinforcement) a stimulus not devised by the experimenter)
uncus	(means a hook) hook-shaped anterior end of the **hippocampal gyrus** in the **temporal lobe**
unipolar depression	mental disorder when the patient is depressed but suffers no manic period (see also **bipolar depression**)
uveitis	inflammation of the uvea
uvea	collective name for the choroid, ciliary body and iris
uvula	(means a grape) part of the **vermis** of the **cerebellum**; is also the name of a small process suspended from the posterior border of the soft palate
vagus nerve	(means wandering nerve) the 10th cranial nerve; so-called because of its extensive distribution in the thorax and abdomen
vasopressin	(also called antidiuretic hormone; ADH) hormone secreted by

	the posterior **pituitary**; increases water re-absorption in the kidneys and is a potent vasoconstrictor when injected
velum	(means a sail or curtain) e.g. inferior medullary velum and superior medullary velum, which form the roof of the 4th ventricle
venous plexus	network of veins and venule
ventral horn	Anterior columns of spinal cord gray matter
ventricle	means a small cavity, here being one of the various brain cavities filled with CSF
vergence	movement of the eyes in different directions (see **disconjugate movements**)
vermis	(vermiform means resembling a worm) median lobe of the **cerebellum**
vertebra	any one of the 33 bones of the spinal (vertebral) column
vertebral canal	passage along the spinal (vertebral) column through which the spinal cord travels
vesicle	means a blister; in the nervous system means a small swelling
vestibular	(vestibule means courtyard) refers to biological chambers
vestibular apparatus	inner ear structures concerned with balance
vestibular nuclei	nuclei lying in the floor of the 4th **ventricle**; receive afferents from the **vestibular apparatus** and relay the information to the **cerebellum**
visual cortex	area of cerebral cortex which occupies lower and upper lips of the calcarine sulcus on the medial surface of each cerebral hemisphere
visual field	picture received by the retina with both eyes open
vitreous humor	gel in the posterior chamber of the eye
voltage clamp	clamping the membrane potential at a fixed value; this enables the electrical behavior of the membrane (e.g. ionic permeabilities) to be studied at chosen values of the membrane potential
wallerian degeneration	process of axon degeneration in which the distal portion of a damaged axon fragments; named after **Augustus Waller**, an English physiologist and physician
Wernicke's area	area in the posterior legion of the temporal lobe described by the German neuropsychiatrist **Carl Wernicke**, which, when damaged, impaired or destroyed the patient's ability to understand speech, although still able to speak; called **Wernicke's aphasia** (see **Broca's area**)
white matter	also called white substance; tissue surrounding gray matter in spinal cord, consisting mainly of myelinated nerve fiber bundles, with some unmyelinated fibers, embedded in neuroglia
white rami communicantes	myelinated preganglionic nerve fiber bundles of the sympathetic nervous system leave the spinal cord in a spinal nerve and enter the paravertebral ganglia through the **white rami communicantes** (called white because they are myelinated; see also **gray rami communicantes**)
zona incerta	extension of the **reticular formation** gray matter into the **subthalamus**; involved in the control of drinking behavior

Index